Molecular Diseases

3

MOLECULAR CHARACTERIZATION OF OVARIAN TUMOR

Sami A. Al- Mudhaffar

First

MOLECULAR CHARACTERIZATION OF LH IN SOME OF OVARIAN TUMOR

Sami A. Al-Mudhaffar
Lanja Ehsan Omar

Contents

Title	Page
Molecular Diseases 3	1
First Molecular Characterization of LH in Ovarian Tumors	2
Contents	3
Chapter One	8
Introduction and Literature Survey	8
ChapterTwo :- Experimental	27
Chapter Three :- Result and Discussion	49
References	88
The second Biochemical Characterization Of CA125 in ovarian tumors	100
Chapter One :- Introduction	104
Chapter Two :- Preliminary studies for the binding of ^{125}I-antiCA125 antibody to the CA125	133
Chapter Three :- Chromatographic purification of CA125 by Gel Filtration and Binding Characterization to Its Specific Antibody	173
Chapter Four :- Kinetic & Thermodynamic Studies of the Binding of CA125 with ^{125}I-antiCA125 antibody in Ovarian Tumor Homogenates	186
Chapter Five :- Spectroscopic StudiesOn Isolated (^{125}I-anti 125 antibody/CA125) Complex	215
Third :- Molecular Characterization of Prolactin in Ovarian Tumors	259

Chapter One Introduction

1- The Ovaries

The mature ovaries are paired nodular structures 2.5 – 5 * 2* 1cm, weighing from 4gm to 8gm, the weight varyies during the menstrual cycle [1,2,3]. Usually the ovary lies with its long axis vertical but it shares in any movement of the broad ligament and uterus [4]. The human ovaries are attached to the posterior surface of the broad ligament by a peritoneal fold called the mesovarium. Nerves, blood vessels and lymphatics traverse the mesovarium and penetrate the ovary at its hilum [5,6]. The blood supplied to the ovaries are derived from the ovarian and uterine blood vessels. The medullary and cortical branches supply the entire ovary, with arborizations virtually supplying every follicle. The venous drainage is by the ovarian veins, which enters the inferior vena cava just below the entry of the renal veins [7].

The ovary is comprised of three distinct regions [8,9]

- An outer cortex containing the ovarian follicles.
- A central medulla consisting of ovarian stroma.
- An inner hilum around the area of attachment of the ovary to the mesovarian.

The ovarian cortex contains the ovarian follicles in various stages of maturation (Primary, Secondary, Tertiary, Graafian and atretic) together with corpora lutea and corpora albicantia for those that have reached full maturation [10]. Figure (1-1).

The ovarian stroma consists of three specific cell types:-
Contractile cells, connective tissue cells and interstitial cells [8].

The hilum consist of specific type of interstitial cells known as the hilus cell. Normal hilus cells have been shown to synthesize and secrete testosterone in response to Luteinizing hormone (LH)[11,12].

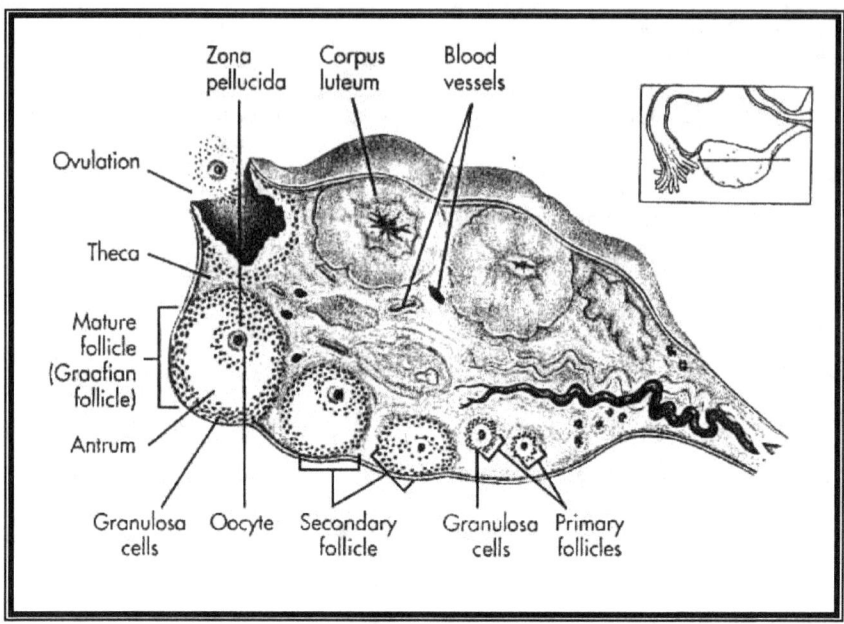

Figure (1-1): Structure of the ovary [6]

The ovary serves dual functions of storing the female germ cells or ova and producing the female sex hormones [13,14] through the regulation and release of sex hormones. The ovaries influence the development of secondary sexual characteristic, regulation of menstrual cycles, maintenance of pregnancy and advent of menopause [13].

The term menstrual cycle refers to the series of changes that occur in sexually mature, nonpregnant females and that culminate in menses [6].

Regular cyclic changes that may be regarded as periodic preparation for fertilization and pregnancy. Its most conspicuous feature is the periodic vaginal bleeding that occurs with the shedding of the uterine mucosa (menstruation) [15].

The mean cycle length is 28 days, but regular cycle lengths of 23 to 35 days may be considered normal [16].

At the start of each cycle, the primordial follicles enlarge and cavity forms around the ovum (antrum formation). One of the follicles in one ovary starts to grow rapidly on the 6th day, while the others regress [15]. At the 14th-16th day of the cycle, the follicle ruptures and the ovum is extruded in to the abdominal cavity. This process is called ovulation [15]. The precise cause of ovulation is not known, but ovulation occurs 1 to 24h after the LH peak [17]. The ovum is picked up by the fimbriated ends of the uterine tubes and transported to the uterus [15]. The follicle that ruptures at the time of ovulation filled with blood. The granulosa and theca cells of the follicles lining promptly proliferate and the clotted blood is replaced with yellowish lipid-rich luteal cells, forming the corpus luteum [15]. If successful fertilization and implantation occurs the corpus luteum function is sustained by hCG produced by the trophoblastic cells of the developing embryo [17].

The function of the corpus luteum is to support the ovum in the early days after fertilization and implantation into the endometrium, before the placenta is established [18]. If there is no pregnancy, the corpus luteum begins to degenerate about 4 days before the next menses and is replaced by fibrous tissue forming corpus albicans [15,19] within a few days of the corpus luteum beginning to degenerate, another follicular phase commences in the ovary and the whole process is repeated [19].

The cessation of menstruation in western women occurs at a median age of 50.8 year [20]. Premature menopause is defined as ovarian failure and menstrual cessation before age of 40 years, this often has a genetic or autoimmune basis . Surgical menopause due to bilateral oophorectomy is common and can cause more severe symptoms owing to the sudden rapid drop in sex hormone levels [21].

During the menopause, women lose the ability to reproduce and develop symptoms include spontaneously occurring hot flushes, sweat eruptions, irritability, palpitations, lethargy sleeplessness and depression [22,23].

During menopause, low estradiol and progesterone concentrations are found in the menopause as an expression of ovarian regression [23]. Thus, circulating levels of LH and FSH are high reflecting primary gonadal failure and the fact that few if any functional follicles remain in the ovary [24].

The lowered Estradiol concentration results in osteoporosis in roughly one third of women [23].

1.1. Ovarian Hormonal System

The ovaries produce estrogens, progesterone and androgens. Ovarian hormones are secreted in a cyclic pattern as a result of the interaction between the hypothalamic releasing hormones and the pituitary gonadotrophic hormones [13].

The hypothalamus secrete adecapeptide called gonadotrophin releasing hormone (GnRH) passed by the hypophseal portal veins to the anterior lobe of the pituitary gland. Where it causes the release of two gonadotrophic hormones. These are FSH and LH. GnRH is released in pulses, in turn the pituitary gland release FSH and LH in a pulsatile manner [25].

In addition the ovary secretes peptide hormones as well as steriods. Inhibin is produced by granulosa cells in the preovulatory period where it is thought to play a paracrine role (on the inhibting the secretion of FSH) and secrete relaxin it so named because it relaxes the myometrium [26].

Estrogen

The estrogen is secreted primarily by the ovaries via ovarian follicle and corpus luteum and during pregnancy by the placenta. Adrenal and tests are also believed to secrete small quantities of estrogens [17, 27].

Only three estrogens are present in significant quantities in the plasma of the human female: B-estradiol, estrone and estriol. The principle estrogen secreted by the ovaries is B-estradiol [28].

Estrogens stimulate the development of tissue involved in reproduction. Under estrogen stimulation vaginal epithelium proliferates and differentiate uterin endometrium proliferates, the myometrium develop intrinsic rhythmic motility and breast ducts proliferate. Estradiol also has anabolic effects on cartilage so its growth promoting. By the effect on peripheral blood vessels, estrogen typically causes vasodilation and heat dissipation [29].

Progesterone
Progesterone is a C_{21} steroid secreted by the corpus luteum the placenta and in small amounts by ovarian follicle and small amounts also enter the circulation from the tests and adrenal cortex [30].

On the uterus. Promote secretory changes in the uterine endometrium preparing the uterus for implantation fertilized ovum, also progesterone decrease the frequency and intensity of uterine contraction helping to prevent expulsion of implanted ovum [28].

On the fallopian tubes. Progesterone promotes secretory changes in the mucosal lining of the fallopian tubes thus maintaining the nutrition of the fertilized ovum [28].

On the breast tissue. Progesterone stimulate the development of lobules and alveoli. It induces differentiation of estrogen prepared ductal tissue and supports the secretory function of the breast during lactation [30, 31].

Androgen

The adult female produces androgen as well as estrogens and progesterone. About 25% of these androgens are secreted from the ovaries. 25% from the adrenal cortex and 50% from either ovarian or adrenal precurosors. In the female androgens contribute to normal hair growth at puberty [13].

1.2 Ovarian Tumors

Ovarian tumors are known. Most are benign, but malignant ovarian tumors are the leading cause of death from reproductive tract cancer [21]. Ovarian cancer represents one fourth of the malignancies of female genital tract, but is the most common cause of death among women who develop gynecologic cancer [32].

Ovarian cancer accounts 5% of all cancer death in women [33].

Epithelial tumors account for 70% of all ovarian tumors, 20% are germ cell derived 10% stromal and 5% metastatic [34].

Epithelial tumors account for 90% of all malignancies [34, 35] and epithelial tumors are divided into histologic subtypes (table (1-1)). Within each of these various histological subtype there are three types of tumors. Benign, borderline and malignant [34, 36]. Two third of epithelial cancer are malignant and one third are borderline [34].

Epithelial carcinoma of the ovary metastasizes primarily by direct extension, implantation of tumor cell on the peritoneal surface and lymphatic spread [37].

The most common form of ovarian cancer is of the serous histopathologic subtype [34].

Table (1-1) Histological types of Epithelial Ovarian Tumors [38].

I	Serous tumors.
II	Mucinous tumors.
III	Endometrioid tumors.
IV	Clear cell (mesonephroid) tumors.
V	Brenner (transitional cell) tumors.
VI	Mixed tumors
VII	Undifferentiated tumors.
VIII	Unclassified and miscellaneous tumors.

Etiology

Several factors contribute to the etiology of ovarian cancer include:

1- Genetic: cases of familial ovarian cancer may constitute (5-10)% of total cases [39, 40]. Ovarian cancer is a component of three hereditary cancer syndroms: hereditary breast and ovarian cancer syndrome, hereditary site-specific ovarian cancer and the Lynch II syndrome [34, 41-43]. All these three syndromes appear to be a result of autosomal dominant genes with incomplete penetrance [39].

The majority of hereditary ovarian cancers results from inherited mutation in two genes, BRCA1 and BRCA2 [44, 45].

2- Ovulation: reproductive risk factors associated with an increase risk of ovarian cancer include those associated with an increased number of ovulation such as early age of menarche and late menopausal [34, 46, 47]. Also women with low number of pregnancies, nulliparious women are at increased risk which suggests that continual ovulation, uninterrupted by pregnancy may predispose women to develop this malignancy [39, 48, 49]. Conversely, female who uses oral contraceptives at low risk from ovarian cancer [39, 50] and actually protects against subsequent ovarian cancer [34]. Pregnancy has consistently been shown to protect against the development of ovarian cancer [51]. Also hyperstimulation of the ovary using clomiphene citrate or gonadotrophins resulting in raised estrogen concentrations and multiple follicle production over many cycles may predispose infertilite patients to ovarian cancer [38, 52, 53].

3- Environmental factors: Carcinogen in the peritoneal cavity may lead to the malignant transformation of ovarian epithelium. It has shown that women who uses talcum powder as part of their perineal hygiene are at increased risk to develop ovarian carcinoma[54]. Other environmental factors may play a role in the etiology of ovarian cancer as the incidence of ovarian cancer appears to be higher in all industrialized countries excepts Japan [54].

4- Viral etiology of ovarian cancer has also been suggested with mumps virus a leading contender [46, 54].

Pathology

Although the serous tumors may be solid, they are usually cystic, so they are commonly known as cystadenoma or cystadeno carcinoma [55]. Appearance of serous tumors varies from smooth-walled cystic forms (simple serous cystodenoma) to superficial papillary neoplasms without cystic cavity (superficial papilloma). Unilocular cystadenomas are more frequent than multilocular forms. They can be of any size up to 25cm in diameter. Bilaterality increases with the degree of malignancy from (5-8%) in benign tumors to (40-50%) in carcinomas [56].

Papillary projections constitute a hallmark of serous tumors. They may be small or large, single or numerous. In benign forms the papillae are small less numerous than in malignant tumors, whose papillae have proliferated so much that they fill the cavity, ultimately perforating the capsule [56, 57].

Cystic cavities are filled mostly with clear fluid-hence the term serous, but they may also contain thicker mucoid-appearing material derived from the vast surface of the papillary projections that may undergo degenerative changes. It may also be flocculated or bloody depending on the degree of secondary changes in the wall [56].

Many serous tumors contain laminated structures encrustated by calcium, so called "psammoma bodies". Their number increases in tumors with a greater degree of cellular proliferation, but they cannot be used as a criterion of malignancy, as some benign tumors also may contain a large quantity of them [56].

Staging

Staging of ovarian cancer is a well defined surgical process and must be performed meticulously [58] and staging of ovarian cancer is based on the findings at the time of surgery and pathological review. Because of the clinically occult spread, surgical exploration is mandatory [54, 59].

The international Federation of Gynecology and Obstetrics (FIGO) staging for ovarian cancer Table (1-2) [38, 58].

Table (1-2) FIGO staging for ovarian cancer [38, 58].

Stage I	Growth limited to the ovaries.
Ia	Growth limited to one ovary, capsule intact; no ascites; no tumor on the external surface.
Ib	Growth limited to both ovaries; capsule intact; no ascties and no tumor on the external surface.
Ic	Tumor either stage Ia or Ib, but with tumor on surface of one or both ovaries; or with capsule ruptured; or with ascites present containing malignant cell; or with positive peritoneal washing .
Stag II	Growth involving one or both ovaries with pelvic extension
IIa	Extension and/or metastases to the uterus and/or the tubes
IIb	Extension to other pelvis tissues.
IIc	Tumor either stage IIa or IIb, but with tumor on surface of one or both ovaries; or with capsules ruptured; or with ascites present containing malignant cells; or with positive peritoneal washing.
Stage III	Tumor involving one or both ovaries with peritoneal implants outside the pelvis and/or positive retroperitoneal or inguinal nodes. Tumor is limited to the true pelvis but histologically proven malignant extension to the small bowel or omentum. Superficial live metastases equal stage III disease.
IIIa	Tumor grossly limited to the true pelvis with negative nodes but with histologically confirmed microscopic seeding of abdominal peritoneal surfaces.
IIIb	Tumor involving one or both ovaries histologically confirmed implants of abdominal peritoneal surfaces; none exceeding 2cm in diameter; nodes are negative.
IIIc	Abdominal implants greater than 2cm in diameter and/or

	positive retroperitoneal or inguinal nodes.
Stage IV	*Growth involving one or both ovaries with distant metastases; if pleural effusion is present, there must be positive cytology to allot acase to stage IV; parenchymal liver metastases are stage IV disease.*

Clinical Features

Epithelial tumors of the ovary have been described as silent killers [60,61]. Because the overwhelming majority of patients presents with disease that has spread outside of the ovary and indeed out side of the pelvis at the time of initial presentation [61,62]. The majority of patients with ovarian malignancies is a symptomatic when the disease is confined to the ovary [39] in some of these patients, however, there are nonspecific symptoms associated with the presence of the enlarging ovary. Pressure on the pelvic viscera that results in symptoms of the lower intestinal or urinary tract can occur. Some patients reported urinary frequency or dysuria and gastrointestinal symptoms, particularly constipation or obstipation [32]. The physician must maintain a high index of suspicion for ovarian cancer when diagnosing patient who experience nonspecific gastrointestinal symptoms [24]. Metastatic lesions are often asymptomatic, when symptoms develop, they tend to be nonspecific such as abdominal distension, pressure and nonspecific gastrointestinal symptoms thus advanced - stage ovarian cancer is confused frequently with other clinical diagnose of the urinary and gastrointestinal tracts [32]. Vaginal bleeding is also an uncommon symptom in postmenopausal women, although premenopausal patients may present with irregular or heavy menses [32].

Detection of an adnexal mass by pelvic examination might permit the early diagnosis of ovarian cancer [32].

Signs of advanced disease include abdominal distension and a fluid wave consistent with ascites. These signs are nonspecific and can be associated with many conditions arising in the abdominal cavity, especially malignancies of other primary sites or carcinomatosis from metastatic tumors of the gastrointestinal tract and breast [32].

Diagnosis

The diagnostic work up and preoperative evaluation of a patient suspected of having ovarian malignancy include an initial full history and physical assessment including bimanual pelvic examination [63]. An adnexal mass in a premenarchal girl or postmenopausal women is usually an indication for exploratory laparotomy. Functional ovarian cysts should not occur in these age groups and a mass often indicates neoplastic growth [39].

The diagnosis of ovarian cancer is surgical, usually by a laparotomy but occasionally at laparoscopy [32].

Ultrasonography is a safe, noninvasive procedure that can be used to define intrapelvic disease. It can also be used to differentiate ascites from a large ovarian cyst [39].

Ultrasonographic signs of malignancy include an adnexal pelvic mass with areas of complexity such as irregular borders, multiple echogenic patterns within the mass and dense multiple irregular septae [64].

Newer techniques using doppler color flow imaging may enhance the specificity of ultrasonography for demonstrating findings consistent with malignancy [65].

Computed tomography (CT) adds useful diagnostic and staging information to the results of ultrasonography, lymphangiography and surgery [39]. CT scanning is useful in preoperative evaluation of extent of disease [66]. CT can delineate liver and pulmonary nodules, large abdominal and pelvic masses and retroperitoneal nodal involvement [39]. Diagnostic laparoscopy is now being used for evaluation of unexplained pelvic pain and evaluation of small adnexal masses. The difficulty with the laparoscopic approach to the evaluation of pelvic masses is rupturing a malignant tumor [61]. Another technique for the diagnosis of ovarian cancer is peritoneal cytology, aspiration of obvious ascites for cytologic assessment is routinely performed to identify malignant cells . If no ascites is present, saline may be instilled percutaneously or through the vaginal apex to flush the abdominal cavity and pelvic . The fluid is then with drawn and sent for cytologic assessment [61].

Tumor Markers

In malignant disease there is aberrant expression of a number of genes. Many of the products of these genes, including hormones, enzymes, immunoglobulins and a variety of other proteins may be over expressed on the cell surface of the cancer cell and are often secreted by the tumor cell [67].

Epithelial ovarian cancers are associated with an elevation in Carbohydrate antigen-125. It is elevated in 80% of clinically apparent ovarian cancer , but in only 50% of stage I ovarian cancers [68] . Ovarian tumor speciments screened for CA-125 tissue expression using immunohistochemistry, CA-125 expression was noted in 50% of benign serous tumors , in 75% of serous tumor of low malignant potential and 84% of malignant serous tumors, no expression of CA-125 was noted in mucinous tumors [69,70]. The clinical use of CA-125 has been primarily employed in the management of patients with an established epithelial ovarian cancer diagnosis. There is a close correlation of progression or regression of disease [71 - 73]. The CA-125 is also utilized to follow patients in order to detect recurrent disease in 90% of cases of ovarian cancer recurrence, the CA-125 began to rise before sign and symptoms developed [34]. The CA-125 is also clinically applied to evaluation before second-look surgery in virtually all patients with an elevated CA-125 prior to second-look evaluation disease will be found if the CA-125 is elevated [74].

CA-125 is useful in the management and follow up of the patients (it reflects the response to therapy in 80% of cases) [71,75]. CA-125 antigen serum concentrations have been reported to be an excellent predictor of response not only in patients who are treated with platinum-containing therapy but also in patients with recurrence or progression of ovarian carcinoma who are treated with paclitaxel [76,77]. The protein gene (P53) has been classified as a tumor suppressor gene acting as negative regulators of cell growth [78]. Recent studies have shown that P53 gene is commonly mutated in a varity of human cancer [79-83]. The P53 mutation are common (50-80%) in ovarian cancer. The frequency of mutations increases in advanced stage tumors [84 - 88]. There was little or no permanent effect in vivo on P53 expression by chemotherapy and that the P53 gene did not appear to be activated by the mutagenic effect of chemotherapy [89,90].

Tumors associated glycoprotein (TAG-72) level is elevated in 50% of patients with ovarian carcinoma and only in 4% of patients with benign diseases [91].

Combined TAG-72 and CA-125 may provide a more sensitivity for the detection of primary ovarian cancer [92].

Carcinoembryonic antigen (CEA) levels are elevated in approximately 58% of patients with stage II epithelial ovarian tumor. The frequency of elevated CEA levels progressively increases with advancing stage and bulk tumor [39].

Treatment

1- For benign neoplasma, tumor removal or unilateral oophorectomy is usually performed.

2- For malignant (ovarian cancer) in an early stage , the standard therapy is complete surgical staging followed by abdominal hysterectomy and bilateral salpingo- oophorectomy with omentectomy and selective lymphadenectomy. With more advanced disease, aggressive removal of all visible tumor improves survival [21].

Chemotherapy

Several chemotherapeutic regimens are effective, cisplatin based combinations have been the mainstay of treatment for advanced ovarian cancer [93-96].

Twenty years ago, systemic treatment consisted of giving a single alkylating agent, usually melphalan about 40% of the women responded, the overall median survival time was one year and survival for more than five years was rare [97].

After the introduction of combinations of cisplatin and an alkylating agent, the response rate increases to 70% and the median survival to two years. Now 30% of women treated with cisplatin-based combination regimens are a live at 5 years and 10 to 20% are a live at 10 years [98].

A good strategy is to treat women with ovarian cancer until a complete clinical remission occurs (including a normal serum concentration of CA-125) and subsequently to add another 6 cycles [97].

Unfortunately, the majority of women who have complete remission will relapse later and need retreatment. A number of prognostic factors is of value in identifying women who are likely to respond to retreatment, a tumor of less than 5cm, a serous cell type, a normal hemoglobin concentration and an interval since the last chemotherapy of more than six months [99,100].

Paclitaxel has recently demonstrated efficacy against ovarian cancer [101]. Paclitaxel is a novel chemotherapeutic agent that is isolated from the western yew tree. Taxus brevifolia . paclitaxel promotes microtubule assembly by preferentially binding to polymerized tubulin [102].

Recent results from the gynecologic oncology group study III (GOG-III) inducated that the use of paclitaxel and cisplatin increase median survival from 24.4 to 37.5 months (54%) over usual care in the treatment of advanced ovarian cancer [103].

Also paclitaxel prove to be an active agent in platinum-refractory ovarian cancer [101].

Ifosfamide has shown activity in the treatment of patients who previously demonstrated clinical resistance to a platinum-cyclophosphamide combination. Recently a synergistic activity of taxol combined with ifosfamide has been reported in ovarian cell lines [104].

The usual mode of administration of chemotherapeutic regimen is intravenous but that other route of administration like intraperitoneal is also present. Recent study suggest that among patients with microscopical disease (no gross residual disease) the rate of complete pathological response differed in the intravenous and intraperitoneal (complete response rate 56% and 80% respectively) [105].

Hormonal Therapy

Recent studies have revealed that hormones, hormone agonists, hormone antagonists provide beneficial and sometime dramatic results in cancer treatment and chemoprevention. In many cases they provide similar therapeutic results and can replace the conventional cancer therapies (chemotherapy, surgical therapy and radiation therapy) thus becoming new adjuvant systemic therapy for cancer [106].

Hormonal receptors have been extensively studied in ovarian cancer, estrogen and progesterone receptors are reported in approximately 50% of tumors [107,108], and 98% of ovarian cancer contains androgen receptors [109].

Progestational agents and estrogen antagonists such as tamoxifen have been used either single or in combination with cytotoxic chemotherapy in patient with advanced disease [110]. Some patients with epithelial ovarian tumors have had response to endocrine therapy although it appears that the overall response rate is 10% [32].

The trials using flutamide which is antiandrogen drug, these trials suggest that flutamide does not have significant activity against ovarian cancer and it is not recommended in patients pretreated with more than one chemotherapy regimen [111]. Therefore, hormonal therapy for patients with advanced ovarian cancer should primarily be reserved for those who have failed chemotherapeutic regimens and who are not candidates for aggressive salvage drug regimen or investigative approaches [32].

Radiotherapy has been used in ovarian cancer as an adjuvant where optimal debulking surgery has been performed and as a consolidation therapy when added to surgically and chemotherapeutically complete treatments [58].

Glycoprotein Hormones

The glycoprotein hormone of the pituitary (LH, FSH, TSH) and of the placenta (hCG) are composed of two peptide chains, usually referred to as α and β subunits, each with carbohydrate substituent group attached. The carbohydrate moiety, which accounts for 15-31% of the molecular weight include fucose, mannose, galactose, N-acetyl glucose amine, N-acetyl galactose amine and sialic acid [112-114].

Each of these hormones consists of two subunits α and β joined by non-covalent bonding [115].

The α-subunit is almost identical for all of these hormones but the β subunit differs considerably from one hormone to another, this suggests that the β subunit carries the hormonal specificity. Isolated α subunit lack biological activity while isolated β subunit may have little intrinsic biological activity, but full activity is attached when α and β subunits are recombined. This suggests that the presence of both α and β subunit is important for specific receptor recognition and that the β-subunit is responsible for eliciting the specific biological response [116,117].

The carboxyl terminal pentapeptide of α subunit is essential for receptor binding but not for α/β association. The feature that distinguishes hormones in the glycoprotein group from hormones of other groups is their glycosylation in each glycoprotein hormone, the α subunit contains two complex asparagine-linked oligosaccharides and the β subunit has either one or two. The glycosylation may be necessary for α/β interaction. The α subunit has five s-s bridges, and the β moiety has six [115].

The glycoprotein is water soluble molecules circulate in a free form not bound to plasma proteins [118]. The half life of peptide hormones is short, varying between 8-60 minutes. A percentage of intact hormone and fragments of hormone is filtered by the kidney and excreted in urine, they are also degraded by proteases and peptidases in plasma and at the target gland after internalization other organs such as the liver and lunges, which also metabolize glycoprotein hormones [119].

Luteinizing Hormone (LH)

LH is a glycoprotein hormone consists of two polypeptide called α and β subunit. The α-subunit of LH is identical to FSH, TSH and hCG.

The sequence of β subunit of human LH and hCG are very similar differing at about 20% of all residues [116].

The amino acid sequence of the α subunit contains 92 amino acid, 5 disulfide bridge and 2-carbohydrate moieties. The β subunit is longer contain 6 disulfide bridges and 3 carbohydrate moieties [116].

The molecular weight of the LH is 28KD. Expected values for LH in serum is as shown in table (1-3) [120,121].

Table (1-3): Expected values in serum for LH in normal adults [120,121].

	LH (IU/L)
Males, 23-70 years	1.2-7.8
Females	
Follicular phase	1.7-15.0
Midcycle peak	21.9-56.6
Luteal phase	0.6-16.3
Postmenopausal	14.2-52.3

Action of LH

In the female LH induces ovulation and stimulates formation of corpus luteum after ovulation has occurred. In response to LH corpus luteum secrete progesterone and estrogens.

In males LH stimulate the interstitial cells in the testis to secrete testosterone [118,122].

Hypothalamic Control of Luteinizing Hormone

The release of (LH and FSH) is controlled by one releasing hormone GnRH. This in turn is a primarily regulated by circulating levels of gonadal hormone that reach the hypothalamus [115].

The hypothalamus secretes GnRH in a pulsatile manner lasting for several minutes that occur every 1-3 hrs. The pulsatile release of GnRH also causes pulsatile output of LH [123].

Estrogen in small amounts has a strong effect in inhibiting the production of both LH and FSH, also when progesterone is available, the inhibitory effect of estrogen is multiplied even through progesterone by itself has little effect. These feedback effects seem to operate mainly directly on the anterior pituitary gland but to a lesser extent on the hypothalamus to decrease secretion of GnRH especially by altering the frequency of the GnRh pulses [28].

Another negative feedback by a hormone called inhibin, which secreted along with the steroid sex hormones by the granulosa cells of the corpus luteum. This hormone has the same effect in the female as in the male of inhibiting the secretion of FSH by the anterior pituitary gland and LH to a lesser extent as well [28].

A decline in ovarian hormones secretion during menopause or following castration cause increased secretion of LH and FSH. Ovarian steriod and peptide hormones are also able to exert positive feedback, which is important in the regulation of the LH surge required to induce ovulation and is regulated by sharply rising levels of estrogen in the late first half of the menstrual cycle [8].

Mechanism of Action of Luteinizing Hormone (LH)

Peptide hormones are too polar to diffuse passively through lipoprotein membranes. Peptide and protein hormones are also too large to pass through membrane pores. Instead these hormones initiate their response by binding to receptors located on or in the cell membrane. This binding interaction results in the generation of an intra cellular signal or "second messenger" that in turn mediates the hormones effects on intra cellular enzymes gene expression and membrane transport. Whereas the "first messenger" of intracellular communication is the hormone the second messenger may be a small organic molecule such as cyclic adenosine monophosphate (cAMP)[17,124 – 126].

After the binding of peptide hormones to their specific plasma membrane receptors on the cell surface, the majority of hormone induced responses are believed to be mediated by the second messenger molecule, cyclic adenosine monophosphate (cAMP). The binding of peptide hormones to their receptors activates the membrane-bound enzyme adenylate cyclase and results in the synthesis of cAMP.

The cAMP synthesis from ATP as the result of adenylate cyclase activation interacts with at least two types of enzyme in the cell, it can bind protein kinase molecules to proceed with its normal action or it can be rapidly degraded to $\bar{5}$-AMP by another enzyme phosphodiesterase and thus is devoid of any activity as second messenger [127,128].

ChapterTwo

Experimental

2.1. Patients

Three groups of ovarian tumors patients were included in this study. Group I contained (8) premenopausal patients with benign epithelial ovarian tumor (serous cystadenoma), group II consisted of (4) premenopausal patients with epithelial ovarian cancer (serous cystadenocarcinoma) and group III consisted of (10) postmenopausal patients with benign epithelial ovarian tumor (serous cystadenoma).

The patients were newly diagnosed and were not underwent of any type of therapy. Patients suffered from any disease that may interfere with our study were excluded.

2.2. Sampling

Blood samples (5-7ml) were obtained from premenopausal patients before surgery by veinpuncture. Age matched sera were obtained from (10) healthy premenopausal women.

Blood samples were centrifuged at 1500xg for 10 minutes after allowing the blood to clot at room temperature. The sera were aliquoted and frozen at $-20\ ^oC$ until assaying.

Collection of Ovarian Tissue Specimens

The tumors tissues were surgically removed from ovarian tumor patients by either unilateral salpingo oophorectomy or total abdominal hysterectomy with bilateral salpingo oophorectomy. The specimens were cut off and immediately rinsed with ice-cold isotonic saline solution. They were collected individually in plastic receptacles and stored at $-20\ ^oC$ until homogenization.

Preparation of Ovarian Tumor Tissue Homogenate

The frozen tissue were thawed, weighed , pulverized finely with a scalpel in petri dish standing on ice bath, and then homogenized at 4^oC in buffer solution with a ratio of 1:5 (weight-volume) by using a manual homogenizer.

The buffer used was Sucrose-Tris (ST) buffer (0.01 M, PH 7.4). The homogenate was filtered through several layers of nylon gauze to eliminate fibers of connective tissue, then centrifuged at 1000xg for 15 minutes at 4°C. The supernatants were used throughout our study.

2.3 Determination of LH Levels in Sera of Benign and Malignant Serous Ovarian Tumor Patients and Controls

Serum levels of LH were measured on samples collected from premenopausal patients and healthy premenopausal women by immunoradiometric assay (IRMA).

The assay details in the following procedure:

1- A set of coated tubes containing 100 μl of LH standards or sera of patients and controls, 50 μl of ^{125}I-anti LH antibody was added to each tube, then mixed well by hand.

2- Two additional non-coated tubes containing 50 μl of ^{125}I-anti LH antibody only, for total activity computation, set aside until counting.

3- All tubes were incubated for 90 minutes at 25°C on a horizontal shaker.

4- The mixture was aspirate, then washed twice with 2 ml wash solution.

5- The radioactivity of all tubes were measured by gamma counter.

The assay protocol of serum LH was described in Table (2-1).

Table (2-1) IRMA assay protocol of serum LH (IU/L)

	LH						Control	Unknown Samples	
Conc (IU/L)	0	0.5	3	30	90	180	-	1	2,,etc
Coated tube number	1,2	3,4	5,6	7,8	9,10	11,12	13,14	15,16	17,18
Standards	100	100	100	100	100	100	-	-	-
Control serum or samples	-	-	-	-	-	-	100	100	100
^{125}I-anti LH antibody	50	50	50	50	50	50	50	50	50

All volumes are in microliters.

Calculations

1- The mean of the c.p.m was determined for each pair of duplicate tubes.

2- The (B/T) ratio was computed for each standard and unknown sample as follows:

$$B/T\% = \frac{\text{standard or sample mean counts (B)}}{\text{total activity mean counts (T)}} * 100$$

3- A standard curve was drawn by plotting the percent value (B/T)% for each standard on the Y-axis against their concentration on the X-axis (in log-log paper), as shown in figure (2-1).

4- Sample concentration (unknown) was calculated from the standard curve.

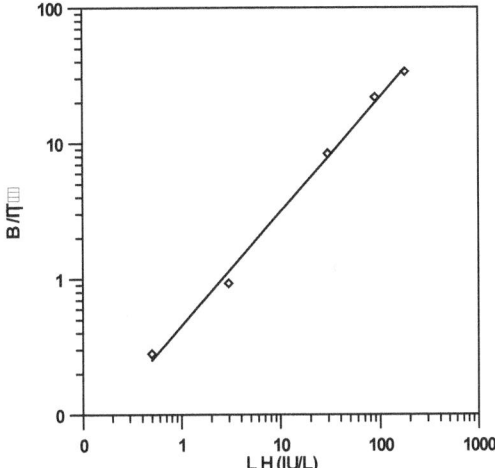

Figure (2-1): Standard curve of LH determination in human sera by IRMA

2.3 Determination of Total Protein Content in Serous Ovarian Tumor Homogenate

The total protein content of serous ovarian tissue homogenate was determined by the method of Lowry et.al, using bovine serum albumin (BSA) as the standard protein [130].

Procedure

1- One milliliter of each of bovine serum albumin (0, 20, 40, 60, 80, 100, 120, 160 and 200) μg/ml protein was pipetted in a set of duplicate tubes.

2- A set of duplicate tubes containing 100 μl of serous ovarian tissue homogenate (benign and malignant), and the volumes were made to 1 ml with D.W.

3- Five milliliters of reagent C was added to all assays tubes.

4-   The tubes were shacked and allowed to stand at room temperature for 10 min.

5-   Half milliliter of reagent D was added to all assays tubes and mixed immediately.

6-   The tubes were left at room temperature for 30 min.

7-   The absorbance of the developing color was read at 750 nm against the appropriate blank.

8-   The standard curve was obtained by plotting the absorbance against the corresponding concentration of standard protein and used to determine the unknown protein concentration of the homogenate of ovarian tumors, Figure (2-2).

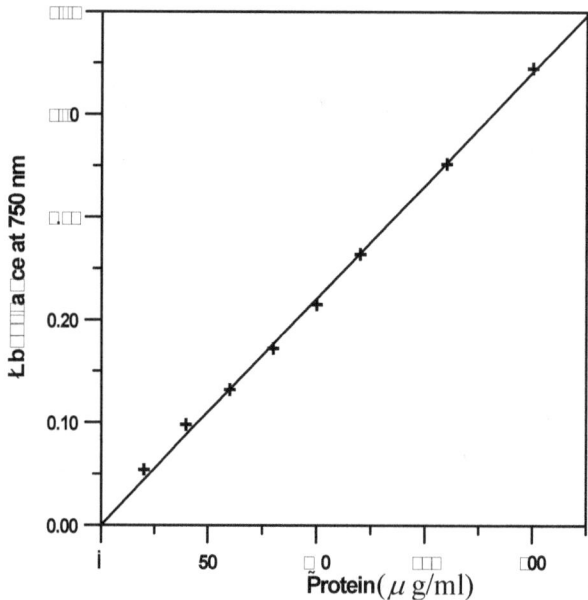

Figure (2-2): Standard curve of protein determination by Lowry's method [130].

2.4 Binding Studies of LH in Serous Ovarian Tumor Homogenate with ^{125}I-Anti LH Antibody

Preliminary Tests of LH Binding in Serous Ovarian Tumor Homogenate with ^{125}I-Anti LH Antibody

1- A volume of twenty microliter of ovarian tumor homogenate (250 μg protein) was added to 5 μl of ^{125}I-anti LH antibody, the volume of the mixture was completed to 100 μl with ST buffer (0.01M, pH7.4).

2- Two additional tubes containing 5 μl of ^{125}I-anti LH antibody only (for total activity) were set aside until counting.

3- The tubes were incubated at 25°C for 90min.

4- After incubation, the tubes were centrifuged at 1500xg for 30min at 4°C.

5- The supernatant was discarded by decanting the assay tubes, then the tubes were inverted on a filter paper for 10 min.

6- The rims of the tubes were swabbed with a cotton piece and the amount of bound radioactivity (c.p.m) were counted in a gamma counter for one minute.

Solutions

ST buffer was prepared as described in section (2.1.7).

Calculations

1- The bound fraction (B) represents the counted radioactivity in each tube, expressed in c.p.m i.e (^{125}I-anti LH antibody/LH) complex.

2-   Total activity (T) represents the counted radioactivity in the tubes containing ^{125}I-anti LH antibody only.

3-   The (B/T)% ratio for each tubes was counted as follows:

$$(B/T)\% = \frac{\text{Sample mean counts (B)}}{\text{Total activity mean counts (T)}} * 100$$

Most Appropriate Conditions of the Binding of LH in Serous Ovarian Tumor Homogenate with ^{125}I-Anti LH Antibody.

The Effect of Different Protein Concentration of Serous Ovarian Tumor Homogenate on the Binding of LH with ^{125}I-Anti LH Antibody

1-   A volume of 5 μl of ^{125}I-anti LH antibody was added to 20 μl of increasing amount (25, 50, 75, 100, 150, 200, and 250 μg protein) of ovarian tumor homogenate in a final volume of 100 μl (complete with ST buffer 0.01M, pH 7.4).

2-   Two additional tubes containing 5 μl of ^{125}I-anti LH antibody only, for total activity computation were set aside until counting.

3-   The tubes were incubated at 25°C for 90 minute.

4-   After incubation, the tubes were centrifuged at 1500xg for 30 minute at 4°C.

5-   The supernatant was discarded by decanting the assay tubes, then the tubes were inverted on a filter paper for 10min.

6-   the rims of the tubes were swabbed with a cotton piece and the amount of bound radioactivity were counted in a gamma counter for one minute.

Calculations

1- The bound fraction (B) represents the counted radioactivity in each tube, expressed in c.p.m i.e. (^{125}I-anti LH antibody/LH) complex.

2- Total activity (T) represents the counted radioactivity in the tubes containing ^{125}I-anti LH antibody only.

3- The (B/T)% ratio for each tube was counted as follows:

$$(B/T)\% = \frac{\text{Sample mean counts (B)}}{\text{Total activity mean counts (T)}} * 100$$

4- The percent of binding value (B/T)% were plotted against the increasing concentration of proteins.

The Effect of Different Concentrations of ^{125}I-Anti LH Antibody on the Binding with LH in Serous Ovarian Tumor Homogenate

1- A volume of $20\,\mu l$ ($100\,\mu g$ protein) of benign and malignant premenopausal ovarian tumors homogenate and $20\,\mu l$ ($150\,\mu g$ protein) of benign postmenopausal ovarian tumor homogenate were added to increasing volumes (1, 2, 3, 4, 5, and $6\,\mu l$) of ^{125}I-anti LH antibody then the volume were made up to $100\,\mu l$ with ST buffer (0.01M, pH 7.4).

2- A set of tubes containing the same increasing volumes of ^{125}I-anti LH antibody (1, 2, 3, 4, 5 and $6\,\mu l$) only, for total activity computation, were set a side until counting.

3- The tubes were incubated at 25°C for 90 minute.

4- After incubation, the (^{125}I-anti LH antibody/LH) complex was estimated by following the steps 4, 5 and 6 in section (2.4.2.1).

Solutions

ST buffer was prepared as described in section (2.1.7).

Calculations

1- The (B/T) percent values were determined according to section (2.4.2.1).

2- The percent of binding values (B/T)% were plotted against the concentration of ^{125}I-anti LH antibody.

The Effect of Different pH on the Binding of LH in Serous Ovarian Tumor Homogenate with ^{125}I-Anti LH Antibody

1- A volume of $20\,\mu l$ (100 and $150\,\mu g$) of the homogenate proteins were added to $5\,\mu l$ ($18.733\,\mu g$ protein) of ^{125}I-anti LH antibody, the mixtures volumes were made up to $100\,\mu l$ with ST buffer (0.01M) of different pH (6.8, 7, 7.4, 7.8, 8, 8.2, 8.6 and 9).

2- Two additional tubes containing $5\,\mu l$ ($18.733\,\mu g$ protein) of the ^{125}I-anti LH antibody only, for total activity computation, were set aside until counting.

3- The tubes were incubated at 25°C for 90 minute.

4- After incubation, the (^{125}I-anti LH antibody/LH) complex was estimated by following the steps 4, 5 and 6 in section (2.4.2.1).

Calculations

1- The values of (B/T)% were determined according to section (2.4.2.1).

2- The percent of binding value (B/T)% were plotted against their corresponding pH values.

The Effect of Temperature on the Binding of LH in Serous Ovarian Tumor Homogenate with ^{125}I-Anti LH Antibody

1-　　A volume of $20\,\mu l$ (100 and 150 μg) of the protein in homogenate were added to $5\,\mu l$ (18.733 μg protein) of ^{125}I-anti LH antibody. The volume of the mixture were completed to $100\,\mu l$ with ST buffer pH 7.4 (premenopausal benign and malignant tumors) and (postmenopausal benign tumor).

2-　　Two additional tubes containing $5\,\mu l$ (18.733 μg protein) of ^{125}I-anti LH antibody only for total activity computation, were set aside until counting.

3-　　The tubes were incubated at 25°C for 90min.

4-　　After incubation, the (^{125}I-anti LH antibody/LH) complex was estimated by following the steps 4, 5 and 6 in section (2.4.2.1).

5-　　The experiment was repeated at different temperatures (4, 10, 37, 45 and 55°C).

Calculations

1-　　The (B/T) percent values were determined according to section (2.4.2.1).

2-　　The values of (B/T)% were plotted against the different temperatures of incubation.

The Choice of the Most Appropriate Incubation Time for the Binding of LH in Serous Ovarian Tumor Homogenate with ^{125}I-Anti LH Antibody

1-　　A volume of 20 μl (100 and 150 μg) of the protein in the homogenate were added to $5\,\mu l$ (18.733 μg protein) of ^{125}I-anti LH antibody. The volume of mixture was completed to 100 µl with ST buffer (0.01M, pH 7.4).

2- Two additional tubes containing 5 µl (18.733 µg protein) of ^{125}I-anti LH antibody only, for total activity computation, were set aside until counting.

3- The tubes were incubated at 45°C (premenopausal benign tumor homogenate), 37°C (premenopausal malignant tumor homogenate) and 25°C (postmenopausal benign tumor homogenate) at different time intervals (30, 60, 90, 120, 150 and 180 minutes).

4- At the end of incubation period, the (^{125}I-anti LH antibody/LH) complex was estimated by following the steps 4,5 and 6 in section (2.4.2.1).

Calculations

1- The values of (B/T)% were determined according to section (2.4.2.1).

2- The values of (B/T)% were plotted against the different times of incubation.

The Effect of Different Halides on the Binding of LH in Premenopausal Serous Ovarian Tumor Homogenate with ^{125}I-Anti LH Antibody

1- A volume of 20 µl (100 µg protein) of premenopausal benign and malignant ovarian tumors homogenates were added to 5 µl (18.733 µg protein) of ^{125}I-anti LH antibody in a final volume of 100 µl (completed with ST buffer 0.01M, pH 7.4 containing 0.1M of each of the following halides: NaF, NaCl, NaBr and NaI). A sample without the addition of any halides was used as a control.

2-   Two additional tubes containing 5 μl (18.733 μg protein) of ^{125}I-anti LH antibody only, for total activity computation, were set aside until counting.

3-   The tubes were incubated for 120 minutes at 45°C (premenopausal benign ovarian tumor homogenate) and 120 minutes at 37°C (premenopausal malignant ovarian tumor homogenate).

4-   After incubation, the (^{125}I-anti LH antibody/LH) complex was estimated by following the steps 4, 5 and 6 in section (2.4.2.1).

Calculations

1-   The values of (B/T)% were determined according to section (2.4.2.1).

2-   The values of (B/T)% were plotted against halides concentrations.

The Effect of Mono and Divalent Cations on the Binding of LH in Premenopausal Serous Ovarian Tumor Homogenate with ^{125}I-Anti LH Antibody

1-   A volume of 20 μl (100 μg protein) of premenopausal benign and malignant ovarian tumors homogenate were added to 5 μl (18.733 μg protein) of ^{125}I-anti LH antibody in a final volume of 100 μl (completed with ST buffer 0.01M, pH 7.4 containing 25mM of each of the following salts: ($MgCl_2$, $CaCl_2$, $MnCl_2$, $ZnCl_2$ and $CuSO_4.5H_2O$) and 0.1M of each of the following salts LiCl, KCl, and NH_4Cl). A sample without the addition of any salts was used as a control.

2- Two additional tubes containing $5\,\mu l$ (18.733 μg protein) of ^{125}I-anti LH antibody only, for total activity computation were set aside until counting.

3- The tubes were incubated for 120 minutes at 45°C (premenopausal benign ovarian tumor homogenate) and 120 minutes at 37°C (premenopausal malignant ovarian tumor homogenate).

4- After incubation, the (^{125}I-anti LH antibody/LH) complex was estimated by following the steps 4, 5 and 6 in section (2.4.2.1).

Calculations

1- The values of (B/T)% were calculated according to section (2.4.2.1).

2- The values of (B/T)% were plotted against salts concentrations.

The Kinetic And The Thermodynamic Studies

The Time-Course of the Binding of LH in Pre-and Post menopausal Patient with Serous Ovarian Tumor To ^{125}I-Anti LH Antibody

1- A volume of $20\,\mu l$ (100 and 150 μg protein) of ovarian tumor homogenate were added to $5\,\mu l$ (18.733 μg protein) of ^{125}I-anti LH antibody, and the volume was completed to $100\,\mu l$ with ST buffer (0.01M, pH 7.4).

2- Two additional tubes containing $5\,\mu l$ (18.733 μg protein) of ^{125}I-anti LH antibody only, for total activity computation, were set aside until counting.

3-   The assay tubes were incubated at 4°C for different time intervals (10, 20, 30, 60, 90, 120, 150, and 180 minutes).

4-   After incubation, the steps 4 to 6 in section (2.4.2.1) were repeated.

5-   To determine the time-course of LH binding with ^{125}I-anti LH antibody at different temperatures, the above experiment was performed at four temperatures (10, 25, 37 and 45°C).

Calculation

1-   The values of (B/T)% were evaluated as mentioned in section (2.4.2.1) at each time and temperature used.

2-   The values of (B/T)% were plotted against the different times of incubation at each temperature.

Determination of Affinity Constant (K_a) and the Maximal Binding Capacity (B_{max}) of LH in Pre – and Postmenopausal Patients with Serous Ovarian Tumor Associated with ^{125}I-Anti LH Antibody

1-   A volume of 20 μl (100 μg protein) of premenopausal benign ovarian tumor homogenate was incubated with increasing volumes (1, 2, 3, 4, and 5 μl) of ^{125}I-anti LH antibody (3.746-18.733 μg protein). The final volumes were made up to 100 μl with ST buffer (0.01M, pH 7.4).

2-   Two additional tubes containing increasing volumes (1, 2, 3, 4 and 5 μl) of ^{125}I-anti LH antibody only, for total activity computation, were set aside until counting.

3-   The tubes were incubated for 120 minute at 45°C.

4-   After incubation, the steps 4, 5 and 6 of the experiment (2.4.2.1) were repeated.

5-   The previous steps were performed at different temperature (4, 10, 25 and 37°C), the time of incubation needed to get the equilibrium state were 90min at (4 and 10°C) and 120min at (25 and 37°C).

6-   The steps 1, 2 and 4 of this experiment were repeated by using premenopausal malignant ovarian tumor homogenate (100 μg protein), the time of the incubation needed to get the equilibrium state were 90min at (4 and 10°C), 60min at (25°C) and 120min at (37 and 45°C).

7-   The steps 1, 2 and 4 of this experiment were repeated by using postmenopausal benign ovarian tumor homogenate (150 μg protein), the time of the incubation needed to get the equilibrium state were 60min at (4 and 25°C), and 90min at (37 and 45°C).

Calculations

1-   The values B/F ratio were determined where:-
   B: is the bound radioactivity (mean of counts c.p.m), which represents the (^{125}I-anti LH antibody/LH) complex.
   F: is the free radioactivity (mean of the counts c.p.m), which represented the non-bound ^{125}I-anti LH antibody.
   T: is the total radioactivity mean of the counts.
   F = Total counts (T) − Bound radioactivity (B)

2-   The concentration of the (^{125}I-anti LH antibody/LH) complex in (mg/ml) that formed after time (t) was calculated from the following equation:-

$$B(mg/ml) = \frac{B(c.p.m)}{T(c.p.m)} * \text{concentration of } ^{125}\text{I-anti LH antibody in the incubation medium (mg/ml)}$$

3- The affinity constant and the maximal binding capacity were determined according to Scatchard equation [131]: -

$$\frac{B}{F} = \frac{1}{Kd}(B_{max} - B)$$

$$Ka = \frac{1}{Kd}$$

where:

Ka = Affinity constant

Kd = Dissociation constant

B_{max} = Maximal binding capacity

4- The values of the ratio B/F were plotted against the values of B in (mg/ml), gives a linear relationship. The values of the affinity constant of the binding (Ka) at each temperature can be calculated from the slop of the straight line, while the value of the total concentration of LH (B_{max}) in serous ovarian tumor tissue was calculated from the intercept with the x-axis.

The Kinetic Studies of the Binding of LH in Pre – and Postmenopausal Patient with Serous Ovarian Tumor to ^{125}I-Anti LH Antibody

The experiments was performed as described in section (2.4.3.1) in different temperatures (4, 10, 25, 37 and 45°C)

Calculations

1- The same mathematical equation mentioned in section (2.4.2.1) was used to calculate (B/T)% values in each temperature and time used.

2- Foreward reaction rate constant (k_{+1}) and also called complex formation rate constant was calculated from the following equation

$$\ln[\frac{(^{125}I-A-LH\,Ab/LH)_e}{(^{125}I-A-LH\,Ab/LH)_e - (^{125}I-A-LH\,Ab/LH)_t}]$$
$$= k_{+1}t[\frac{(^{125}I-A-LH\,Ab)_T\,(LH)_T}{(^{125}I-A-LH\,Ab/LH)_e}]$$

Where

$(LH)_T$: Total concentration of LH

$(^{125}I\text{-A-LHAb/LH})_e$: Concentration of (^{125}I-anti LH antibody/LH) complex at eqilibrium

$(^{125}I\text{-A-LHAb/LH})_t$: Concentration of (^{125}I-anti LH antibody/LH) complex at time t

$(^{125}I\text{-A-LHAb})_T$: Total concentration of ^{125}I-anti LH antibody

3- Backward reaction rate constant (K_{-1}), and also called complex dissociation rate constant was calculated from the following equation:-

Where :- $$Ka = \frac{K_{+1}}{K_{-1}}$$

Ka : Affinity constant .

Thermodynamic Studies of the Binding of LH in Pre – and Post menopausal Patients with Serous Ovarian Tumor to ^{125}I-Anti LH Antibody

According to the steps of the two experiments explained in section (2.4.3.2) and section (2.4.3.3) the thermodynamic parameters were calculated .

Calculations

1- The thermodynamic parameters of standard state (ΔH°, ΔG°, ΔS°) were obtained from Van't Hoff plot, the values of the natural logarithm of equilibrium constant (affinity constant Ka) obtained at different temperature were plotted against the reciprocal values of absolute temperatures in kelvin (1/T) was calculated according to the following equation :-

$$\ln Ka = \frac{\Delta S^\circ}{R} - \frac{\Delta H^\circ}{RT}$$

Where :-

ΔH° : The enthalpy change of the standard state.

ΔS° : The entropy change of the standard state.

R: The gas constant (8.31441 J.K^{-1} mol^{-1})

ΔH° value obtaied from the linear relationship of the plot. The change in Gibbs free energy of the standard state (ΔG°) was obtained from the following equation :-

$$\Delta G^\circ = -RT\ln Ka$$

While the standard state entropy change was obtained from

$$\Delta S^\circ = \frac{\Delta H^\circ - \Delta G^\circ}{T}$$

2- The thermodynamic parameters of the transition state were obtained from Arrhenius plot of $\ln k_{+1}$ values against 1/T values, that gives a linear relationship according to the following equation

$$\ln K_{+1} = \ln A - \left(\frac{Ea}{RT}\right)$$

Where :-

A : Arrhenius constant.

Ea: Apparent energy of activation.

T : Absolute temperature in kelvin.

The value of Ea of the binding reaction can be determined from the slop of the straight line.

The enthalpy of transition state (ΔH^*) was obtained from :-

$$\Delta H^* = Ea - RT$$

The free energy change of the transition state (ΔG^*) was calculated by using the following equation :-

$$\Delta G^* = -RT\ln K_{+1} + RT\ln\left(\frac{KT}{h}\right)$$

Where :-

K: Boltzmann constant = 1.38×10^{-23} J.deg^{-1}

H: Plank's constant = 0.662×10^{-33} J.S^{-1}

The change in entropy of the trasition state (ΔS^*) was calculated from the following equation :-

$$\Delta S^* = \frac{\Delta H^* - \Delta G^*}{T}$$

2.5 Separation of (^{125}I-Anti LH Antibody/LH) Complex by Gel Filtration Technique

Gel filtration chromotography technique was used for the separation of (^{125}I-anti LHAntibody/LH) complex from unbound ^{125}I-anti LH antibody

Preparation of The Gel

The gel (sephadex G-150) was allowed to swell in excess of Tris buffer 0.2M, PH 7.4 (20ml of buffer per gram of gel) and left to stand for three days at room temperature without stirring to equilibrate with the buffer. The buffer was decanted and the gel was resuspended in excess volume of eluent buffer three times before bed packing.

Bed Packing

The de-gassed slurry was carefully mixed before pouring into the vertical column which contains 5 ml of eluent buffer using a glass rod attached to the inner surface of the column. After the gel has settled, the column outlet was opened. Packing was continued until the gel reached a stable bed height 30 cm. The column was equilibrate with Tris buffer for 24 hr with dimensions of (1*30 cm) and a bed volume of 24 ml.

Void Volume Determination

The elution volume of blue dextran 2000 is equal to the column void volume (v_o) and it was determined as follows:

A fresh solution of blue dextran (2 mg/ml) was prepared in the eluent buffer. 0.7 ml of blue dextran solution was carried out with the same buffer, using a flow rate of 6 ml/hr. Fractions of 1 ml were collected and their absorbence were measured at 600 nm.

Sample Addition

A volume of 0.7 ml of the (^{125}I-anti LH antibody/LH) complex were prepared and then applied to the column equilibrate with Tris buffer. The fractions were eluted with same flow rate (6ml/hr). The radioactivity was measured by gamma counter and the absorbance for the eluted fractions were measured at 280nm.

2.6 Spectroscopic Studies of (^{125}I-Anti LH Antibody/LH) Complex and the Unbound ^{125}I-Anti LH Antibody

Factors Affecting the Absorption Properties of (^{125}I-Anti LH Antibody/LH) Complex and the Unbound ^{125}I-Anti LH Antibody in Premenopausal Patients with Malignant Serous Ovarian Tumor.

pH Effect

1- A volume of 100 μl (300 μg protein) of pooled fractions under peak 1 which represents the (^{125}I-anti LH antibody/LH) complex was completed to 0.5ml with different buffers at different pH values (3.8,7.4,12.0) then each of which was placed in 0.5cm cuvette in the sample beam and the buffer at the adjusted pH in the reference beam the absorption spectrum was measured in the area of (200-350) nm the above was repeated by using 100 μl of pooled fraction under peak 2 which represent the unboud ^{125}I-anti LH antibody.

Effect of Solvent Polarity on U.V Spectrum of (^{125}I-Anti LH Antibody /LH) Complex and Unboud ^{125}I-Anti LH Antibody in Premenopausal Patient with Malignant Serous Ovarian Tumor

a-Effect of 20% of Ethanol, Glycerol, Chloroform and Polyethylene Glycol(PEG)

1- A volume of 100 μl (300 μg protein) of pooled fractions under peak 1 which represent the (^{125}I-anti LH antibody/LH) complex was completed to 0.5ml with Tris buffer pH(7.4) in the presence of 20% ethanol.

2- The mixture was placed in the sample beam using 0.5cm cuvette against 20% ethanol prepared in the same buffer in the reference beam. The absorption spectrum was measured in the area of (200-350nm).

3- The steps 1,2 and were repeated to measure the absorption spectrum for unbound ^{125}I-anti LH antibody.

4- The experiment was repeated in the presence of 20% glycerol, chloroform and PEG prepared in the same buffer.

b-Effect of Urea and KCl on the U.V Spectrum of (^{125}I-Anti LH Antibody/LH) Complex and Unbound ^{125}I-Anti LH Antibody in Premenopausal Patients with Malignant Serous Ovarian Tumor.

1- One hundred microliters (300 μg protein) of pooled fraction under peak 1which represents the (^{125} I-anti LH antibody/LH) complex was completed to 0.5ml using Tris buffer containing (8 MUrea,0.03M KCl). Then each of which was placed in a 0.5cm cuvette in the sample beam against the solvent (in the same buffer) in the reference beam . The absorption spectrum was measured in the area of (200-350nm) .

2- The experiment was repeated by using 100 μl of pooled fraction under peak 2 which represent the unbound ^{125}I-anti LH antibody

Effect of Sodium Chloride (NaCl) Concentrations on the Thermal Stability of (^{125}I-Anti LH Antibody/LH) Complex by U.V Spectral Studies

1- one hundred microliter (300 μg protien) of pooled fraction under peak 1 which represents the (^{125}I-anti LH antibody/LH) complex in premenopausal patients with malignant serous ovarian tumor was completed to 0.5 ml with a mixtures (80% H_2O + 20% ethylene glycol) containing two different NaCl concentrations (0.01M and 0.1M).

2- The mixtures were incubated for 15min at different temperatures (20,30,40,50,60,70,80,90 and 100°C). The solution was placed in 0.5cm cuvette in the sample beam and the mixture of (80% H_2O + 20% ethylene glycol) containing 0.01M , 0.1M NaCl) in the reference beam .

3- The absorbance of each sample were measured at 292nm and 295nm . The absorbance at each wavelength were plotted versus the corresponding temperatures .

Chapter Three
Result and Discussion

1. Tissue Collection and Processing

Three groups of patients were included in this study. Group one consisted of (8) premenopausal patients (luteal phase) with benign epithelial ovarian tumor (serous cystadenoma), group two contained (4) premenopausal patients (luteal phase) with epithelial ovarian cancer (serous cystadenocarcinoma) and group three contained (10) postmenopausal patients with benign epithelial ovarian tumor (serous cystadenoma) as confirmed by histopathological examination. The age ranged of premenopausal patients with benign epithelial ovarian tumor was (30-35) while the age ranged of premenopausal patients with epithelial ovarian cancer was (29-36).

The age ranged of postmenopausal patients with benign epithelial ovarian tumors was (51-57).

The weights of resected tissue samples ranged between (0.5-2.5) grams. Tissue homogenization was carried out in 0.25 M sucrose. Sucrose is a hypotonic solution that enhances the rupture of plasma cell membranes, and preserves other cell organelles [132]. Homogenization was carried out in a cold medium in order to avoid protein denaturation and to decrease the proteolytic enzymes activity [133].

The tissue homogenate was filtered through several layers of nylon gauze to remove connective tissue fragments and debris, while centrifugation at 1000 xg removed the unruptured cells leaving other cytoplasmic constituents in the supernatant [134] which was used as a source of LH in our study.

2 Determination of Luteinizing Hormone Level in Sera of Benign and Malignant Serous Ovarian Tumor Patients and Controls

Serum LH levels were measured in benign and malignant serous ovarian tumors patients matched with a group of control subject. Group I contained (8) premenopausal patients (luteal phase) with benign epithelial ovarian tumor (serous cystadenoma), Group II comprised of (4) premenopausal patients (luteal phase) with epithelial ovarian cancer (serous cystadenocarcinoma). Table (3-1) show the results that obtained from this study. The level of serum LH in premenopausal patients with benign tumor was found to be (4.3 ± 0.236 IU/L), whereas that of premenopausal patients with malignant tumor was found to be (2.8 ± 0.964 IU/L). But in controls, the level was found to be (4.8 ± 0.182 IU/L).

Student's T. test analysis revealed that there is no significant decrease of serum LH level ($p>0.05$), in benign and malignant premenopausal serous ovarian tumor patients.

Previous study found that women with epithelial ovarian tumors had lower serum levels of FSH and LH than those of normal [135]. Another study reported that there were no significant differences found in serum LH levels in postmenopausal women with benign or malignant epithelial ovarian tumors while significant lower FSH level were demonstrated in women with malignant tumors [136].

Table (3-1) Serum LH levels in benign and malignant serous ovarian tumor patients and controls. Details are described in section (2.2)

Group	No. of cases	Age (year)	Serum LH (IU/L)
Premenopausal of benign serous ovarian tumor	8	30-35	4.3 ± 0.236
Premenopausal of serous ovarian cancer	4	29-36	2.8 ± 0.964
Control	10	28-38	4.8 ± 0.182

3 Binding Studies of LH in Serous Ovarian Tumor Homogenate with ^{125}I-Anti LH Antibody

Preliminary Tests of LH Binding in Serous Ovarian Tumor Homogenate with ^{125}I-Anti LH Antibody

Benign and malignant ovarian tumors homogenate were used as the source of LH in this study. The homogenate was incubated with ^{125}I-anti LH antibody for 90min at 25°C. The (^{125}I-anti LH antibody/LH) complex formed was separated from the unbound particulates by centrifugation at 1500 xg for 30min. This centrifugal speed was sufficient to precipitate complex. After centrifugation the tubes were decanted in order to get rid of unbound antibody antigen present in the supernatant fraction. While the ^{125}I-anti LH antibody/LH complex remained as a pellet in the bottom of the tube. The tumor was considered to have LH if it contained any amount of percent of binding values (B/T)%. The preliminary condition used in this experiment resulted in (15%) binding in the premenopausal patients with benign serous ovarian tumor, (17.8%) in the premenopausal patients with serous ovarian cancer and 13% binding in postmenopausal patients with benign serous ovarian tumor.

The data obtained, in this study revealed that the tumors of serous ovarian cancer patients had higher incidence of LH than those of benign groups, and the benign tumor of premenopausal patients included higher incidence of LH than those of postmenopausal patients.

Most Appropriate Conditions of the Binding of LH in Serous Ovarian Tumor Homogenate with ^{125}I-Anti LH Antibody

The Effect of Different Protein Concentration of Serous Ovarian Tumor Homogenate on the Binding of LH with ^{125}I-Anti LH Antibody

In order to determine whether the different protein concentration of ovarian tumor homogenate effects the binding, increasing amount of homogenate (increasing amounts of LH) were incubated with ^{125}I-anti LH antibody according to the details in sections (2.4.2.1) Figure (3-1) shows that the binding of LH in ovarian tumor with ^{125}I-anti LH antibody was easily detected at the lowest particulate concentration tested (equivalent to 25 μg/ml protein) and increasing with increasing amount of homogenate added to the incubation mediums, until a point of maximum binding, then a resultant decrease in the binding percent (B/T%).

These results indicate that binding of LH is principally depended on the different amount of LH protein in the reaction mixture [137].

One hundred microgram of benign and malignant ovarian tumor homogenate protein for premenopausal patients and 150 μg of benign ovarian tumor homogenate protein for postmenopausal patient were used in all the subsequent experiments since it gives maximum value of binding (B/T%).

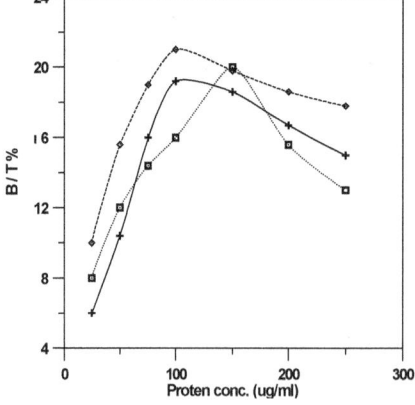

Figure (3-1): Influence of LH concentration on the binding with ^{125}I-anti LH antibody in:

+ Benign premenopausal ovarian tissue homogenate
4 Premenopausal ovarian cancer tissue homogenate
A Benign postmenopausal ovarian tissue homogenate

Details are explained in section (2.4.2.1)

The Effect of Different Concentration of ^{125}I-Anti LH Antibody on the Binding with LH in Serous Ovarian Tumor Homogenate

One of the factors that effect the binding of (^{125}I-anti LH antibody/LH) complex (Ab-Ag reaction) is the concentration of the antibody.

Fixed amount of benign and malignant tumor homogenate for premenopausal patients (100 μg/ml protein) and (150 μg/ml protein) of benign tumor homogenate for postmenopausal patient was incubated with increasing concentration ^{125}I-anti LH antibody for 90min at 25°C.

Figure (3-2) is representative of ^{125}I-anti LH antibody binding curve with LH in benign and malignant serous ovarian tumor homogenate and the results revealed that the percent of binding increased by the amount of ^{125}I-anti LH antibody added. As shown in the same figure that the binding of ^{125}I-anti LH antibody with LH is a saturable process but complete saturation however is theoretically never reached unless the amount of LH used reached infinity [138] and the LH protein used

in the incubation mixture under the conditions of the experiment were saturated with ^{125}I-anti LH antibody when the amount of the latter in the incubation mixture were equivalent to 5 μl (18.733 μg/ml protein).

Figure (3-2) Effect of different concentration of ^{125}I-anti LH antibody on the binding with LH in:
- + Benign premenopausal ovarian tissue homogenate
- ♦ Premenopausal ovarian cancer tissue homogenate
- ▲ Benign postmenopausal ovarian tissue homogenate

Details are decribed in section (2.4.2.2)

The Effect of Different pH on the Binding of LH in Serous Ovarian Tumor Homogenate with ^{125}I-Anti LH Antibody

The analysis of the influence of pH on the binding of LH in serous ovarian tumor homogenate with ^{125}I-anti LH antibody is stated in Figure (3-3). The optimum pH was found to be 7.4 for benign and malignant serous ovarian tumor in premenopausal patients and in postmenopausal patient with benign serous ovarian tumor.

The same figure shows decreasing in the binding percent at the pH higher or lower than the optimum pH. These results indicate that the shift in the pH of the environment involved in the binding, this effect includes the induction of protonation-deprotonation process occuring within the ionizable groups of the amino acids present in the binding domain of these macromolecules [139].

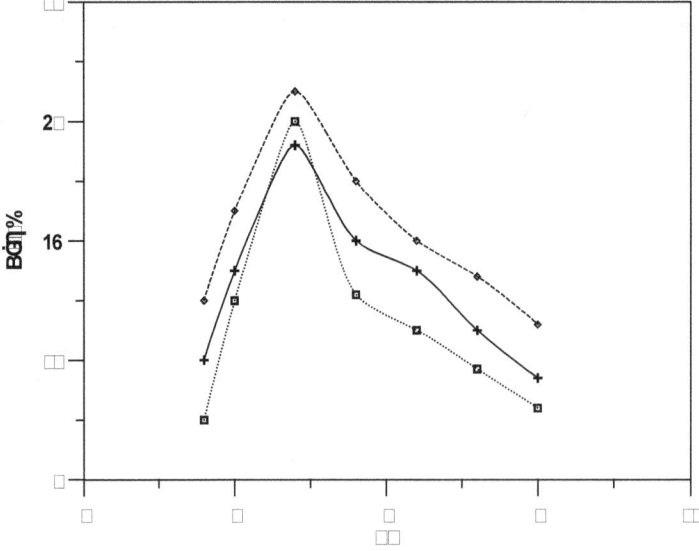

Figure (3-3) Effect of different pH on the binding of ^{125}I-anti LH antibody with LH in:
+   Benign premenopausal ovarian tissue homogenate
4   Premenopausal ovarian cancer tissue homogenate
A   Benign postmenopausal ovarian tissue homogenate

Details are explained in section (2.4.2.3).

A previous work about the ovary were done by Radioimmunoassay reported that pH 7.0 is the optimum pH for the binding in rat ovary [140]. While another work reported that the highest binding was seen at pH (7-7.5) in luteal homogenate from human ovarian corpora lutea [141].

According to the results obtained in this experiment, the pH of the buffer used in all subsequent experiment was adjusted at (7.4) as optimum pH for the three different groups used in this study.

The Effect of Temperature on the Binding of LH in Serous Ovarian Tumor Homogenate with ^{125}I-Anti LH Antibody

The temperature dependency of the association of ^{125}I-anti LH antibody with LH in benign and malignant tumor homogenate were investigated. Fig (3-4) shows the results of this analysis. It seems that binding was maximal at 45°C for benign premenopausal ovarian tumors, 37°C for malignant premenopausal ovarian tumors and 25°C for benign postmenopausal ovarian tumor.

It seems that a point of maximum binding and the binding was decreased at temperature increase after maximal value of binding. The loss of binding activity may be due to degradation of the LH or may be due to the irreversible dissociation of the (^{125}I-anti LH antibody/LH) complex.

Previous studies were done by RIA reported that the binding was temperature dependent and the optimum temperature is 25°C in granulosa cells isolated from rat ovary [142].

While other reported that 37°C is the optimum temperature in pseudo pregnant rat ovarian extract [143].

As a result of the temperature sensitivity of these complexes, we decided to study the time course of the association at different temperatures.

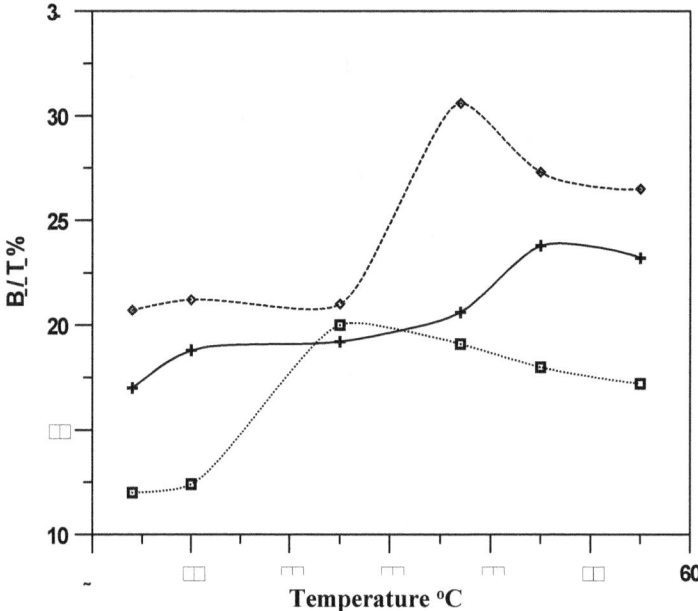

Figure (3-4): Effect of the temperature on the binding of ^{125}I-anti LH antibody with LH in:
+ Benign premenopausal ovarian tissue homogenate
♦ Premenopausal ovarian cancer tissue homogenate
▲ Benign postmenopausal ovarian tissue homogenate
Details are described in section (2.4.2.4)

The Choice of the Most Appropriate Incubation Time for the Binding of LH in Serous Ovarian Tumor Homogenate with ^{125}I-Anti LH Antibody

To choose the most appropriate incubation time at 45°C, 37°C and 25°C the experiment was carried out at different time intervals (30-180 minute).

Figure (3-5) shows that the optimal binding of ^{125}I-anti LH antibody with LH in premenopausal patients with benign tumor was occurred within 120min at 45°C, in premenopausal patients with malignant tumor was occurred within 120min at 37°C and in postmenopausal patients with benign tumor, the maximum binding was occurred within 60min at 25°C.

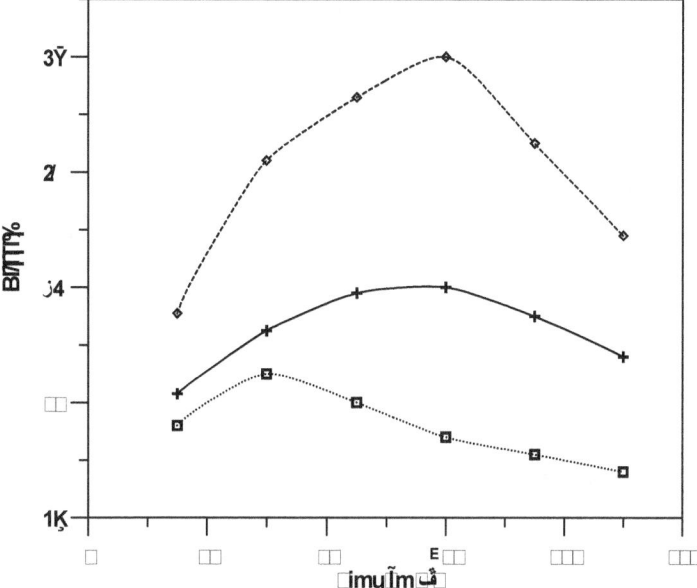

Figure (3-5): Time course of ^{125}I-anti LH antibody binding with LH in:
  + Premenopausal patient with benign tumor
  4 Premenopausal patients with malignant tumor
  A Postmenopausal patients with benign tumor
Details are described in section (2.4.2.5).

Previous studies reported that maximal binding in ovarian homogenate from pseudo pregnant rat was at 25°C for 4hr by RIA [144] and in another study they reported that the total binding was approached a plateau at 30min at 37°C in human corpora lutea homogenate was done by RIA [145].

According to our results, the binding studies of the subsequent investigations were carried out at 45°C for 120min incubation for the premenopausal patients with benign tumor, at 37°C for 120min. incubation for the premenopausal patient with malignant tumor, and at 25°C for 60min. incubation for the postmenopausal patient with benign tumor.

The Effect of Different Halides on the Binding of LH in Premenopausal Serous Ovarian Tumor Homogenate with ^{125}I-Anti LH Antibody

Different sodium halides at 0.1M concentration were investigated to study their action on the binding of ^{125}I-anti LH antibody with LH in serous ovarian tumor homogenate as shown in Figure (3-6). It seems that the sodium halides decrease the (^{125}I-anti LH antibody/LH) complex binding according to the following order:

NaI > NaBr > NaCl > NaF

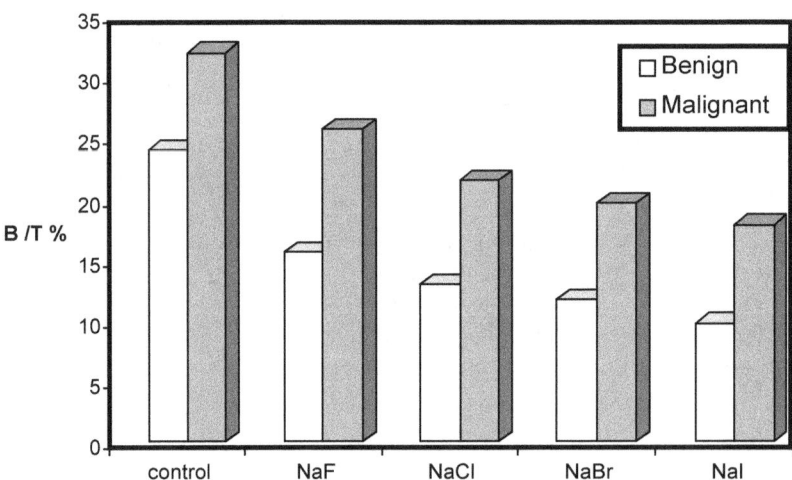

Figure(3-6) Effect of different halides on the binding of ^{125}I-anti LH antibody with LH in benign and malignant premenopausal ovarian tumors
Details are described in section (2.4.2.6)

The order corresponds to the decreasing ionic radius and increasing radius of hydration. Presumably, the lesser degree of hydration permits greater interaction of the salt with an ionic group located in the antibody or antigen combining site [146].

The Effect of Mono and Divalent Cations on the Binding of LH in Premenopausal Serous Ovarian Tumor Homogenate with ^{125}I-Anti LH Antibody

The importance of the ionic environment for the binding of ^{125}I-anti LH antibody with LH in ovarian tumor homogenate is illustrated in Figure (3-7). Monovalent cations appeared to inhibit the binding or dissociation the (^{125}I-anti LH antibody/LH) complex.

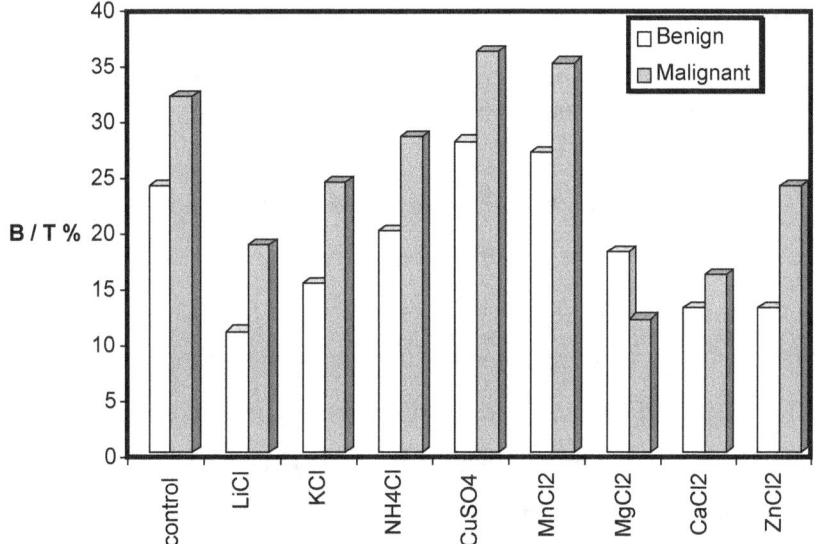

Figure(3-7) Effect of monovalent and diavalent cations on the binding of ^{125}I-anti LH antibody with LH in benign and malignant premenopausal ovarian tumors. Details are described in section (2.4.2.7)

Some of divalent cations appeared to enhance the binding reaction, while other inhibit the reaction.

Several cations have been used to study their action on the binding, these cations are Mg^{+2}, Ca^{+2}, Mn^{+2}, Zn^{+2} and Cu^{+2} in a (25mM) concentration. The presence of Mg^{+2}, Ca^{+2} and Zn^{+2} seemed to inhibit the binding, due to increasing the (^{125}I-anti LH antibody/LH) complex solubility in the presence of this cation. The interactions of these ion with the ionic groups of (^{125}I-anti LH antibody/LH) complex diminishes the complex interactions and therefore, increasing solubility of the complex [147]. The presence of Mn^{+2} and Cu^{+2} seemed to increase the binding. This is presumably due to their effect to activate the catalytic component in the antigen or in the antibody [148].

4. The Kinetic and The Thermodynamic Studies

The Kinetic of the Interaction of ^{125}I-Anti LH Antibody with LH in Pre and Postmenopausal Patients with Benign and Malignant Serous Ovarian Tumor

Figure (3-8) shows the time course of the formation of (^{125}I-anti LH antibody/LH) complex at five different temperature (4, 10, 25, 37, 45°C) in two groups of pre and postmenopausal patient with benign serous ovarian tumors and one group of premenopausal patients with serous ovarian cancer.

The results of the time-course pattern at different temperatures revealed that the binding of ^{125}I-anti LH antibody with LH in serous ovarian tumors is a temperature and time dependent process with a maximum binding occurs at 45°C with 120min for premenopausal patients with benign tumor, at 37°C with 120min for premenopausal patients with malignant tumor and 25°C for 60min for postmenopausal patients with benign ovarian tumor.

Determination of Affinity Constant (Ka) and the Maximal Binding Capacity (B_{max}) of LH in Pre- and Postmenopausal Patients with Serous Ovarian Tumor Associated with ^{125}I-Anti LH Antibody

The concentration of LH in pre- and postmenopausal patients with benign and malignant ovarian tumor homogenate (B_{max}) and the affinity constant (Ka) of the binding with ^{125}I-anti LH antibody has been measured.

The experiment was carried out at the optimal conditions, which were obtained in previous experiments.

Scatchard plot analysis gave a straight line as shown in Figure (3-9A, B, C) The results obtained indicate the presence of only one species of LH site, or more but with the same affinity and number of binding site.

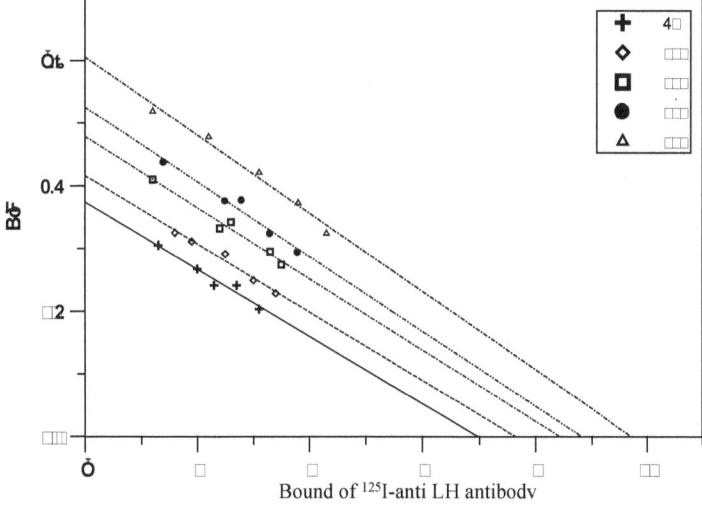

Fig (3-9A): Scatchard plot of ^{125}I-anti LH antibody binding with LH in:
   A: Benign premenopausal ovarian tissue homogenate
   Details are explained in section (2.4.3.2)

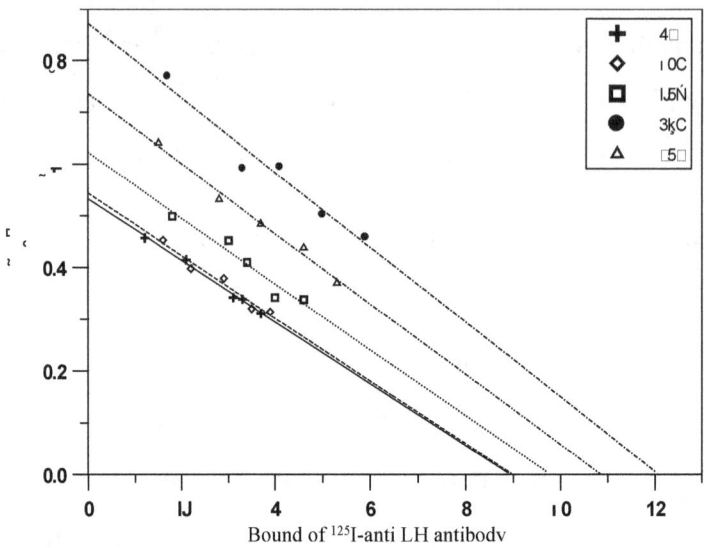

Figure (3-9B): Scatchard plot of ^{125}I-anti LH antibody binding with LH in:
B: Premenopausal ovarian cancer tissue homogenate
Details are explained in section (2.4.3.2)

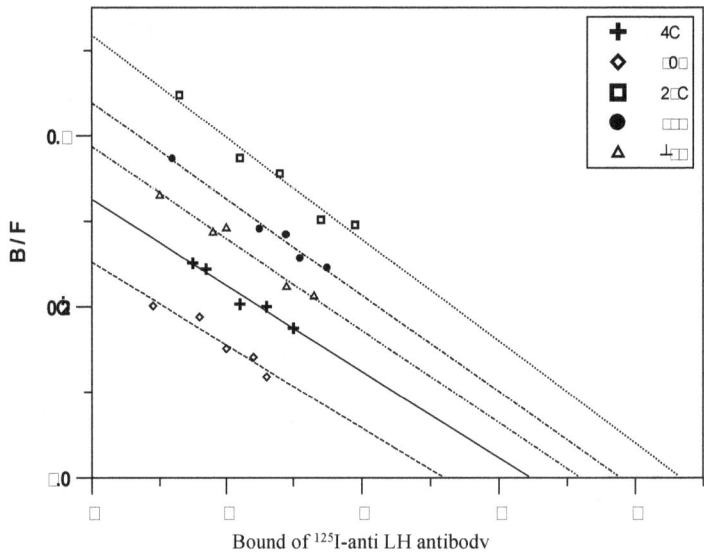

Figure (3-9C): Scatchard plot of ^{125}I-anti LH antibody binding with LH in:
C: Benign postmenopausal ovarian tissue homogenate
Details are explained in section (2.4.3.2)

The results are summarized in table (3-2) Luteinizing hormone binding capacity of premenopausal patients with benign ovarian tumors in the optimal conditions were (0.0097 mg.ml^{-1}) and of premenopausal ovarian cancer patients were (0.01208 mg.ml^{-1}) while of postmenopausal patients with benign ovarian tumors were (0.00867 mg.ml^{-1}).

Table (3-2): Concentration and affinity constant of LH in three groups of serous ovarian tumor patients. Details are decribed in section (2.4.3.2)

Group	No of cases	Binding capacity Bmax*10^{-3} (mg.ml^{-1})	Age (Year)	Ka*10^3 mg^{-1}.ml
Premenopausal patients of benign ovarian tumor	8	9.7	30-35	0.0623
Premenopausal patients of ovarian cancer	4	12.08	29-36	0.0721
Postmenopausal patient of benign ovarian tumor	10	8.67	51-57	0.0596

Determination of Kinetic Parameters of ^{125}I-Anti LH Antibody Binding with LH in Pre and Postmenopausal Patients with Serous Ovarian Tumor

The time course of ^{125}I-anti LH antibody binding with LH in pre- and postmenopausal serous ovarian tumor (benign and malignant) was carried out to describe kinetic parameters of the binding. The simplest proposed model representing the binding of ^{125}I-anti LH antibody with LH could be expressed by the following equation:

$$^{125}\text{I} - \text{anti LH antibody} + \text{LH} \underset{K_{-1}}{\overset{K_{+1}}{\rightleftharpoons}} {}^{125}\text{I} - \text{anti LH antibody/LH}$$

Where:-

K_{+1}: is the rate of the association of ^{125}I-anti LH antibody with LH.

K_{-1}: is the rate of the reverse reaction of the dissociation of the complex formed under the same condition.

At equilibrium

$$Ka = \frac{[^{125}I - \text{anti LH antibody/LH}]}{[^{125}I - \text{anti LH antibody}][LH]} \ldots\ldots\ldots (1)$$

$$Kd = \frac{[^{125}I - \text{anti LH antibody}][LH]}{[^{125}I - \text{anti LH antibody/LH}]} \ldots\ldots\ldots (2)$$

Thus

$$Ka = \frac{1}{Kd} = \frac{K_{+1}}{K_{-1}} \ldots\ldots\ldots\ldots\ldots\ldots\ldots\ldots\ldots (3)$$

Where:-

Ka: is the equilibrium constant of the association (affinity constant).

Kd: is the equilibrium constant of the dissociation (^{125}I-anti LH antibody/LH) complex.

The values of Ka and maximal binding capacity (B_{max}) were calculated from Scatchard plots at five different temperature as shown in figure (3-9A, B, C) and table (3-3). Time-course data obtained from figure (3-8A, B, C) could be used to determine the reaction order of ^{125}I-anti LH antibody binding to LH by using the following equation [149]:

$$Ln(^{125}I\text{-anti LH Ab/LH})_e \left[\frac{(^{125}I\text{-A-LH Ab})_T - (^{125}I\text{-A-LH Ab/LH})_t (^{125}I\text{-A-LH Ab/LH})_e /(LH)_T}{(^{125}I\text{-A-LH Ab})_T (^{125}I\text{-A-LH Ab/LH})_e - (^{125}I\text{-A-LH Ab/LH})_t} \right]$$

$$= K_{+1} t \left[\frac{(^{125}I\text{-A-LH Ab})_T (LH)_T - (^{125}I\text{-A-LH Ab/LH})_e}{(^{125}I\text{-A-LH Ab/LH})_e} \right] \ldots\ldots\ldots\ldots (4)$$

Table (3-3): The kinetic parameters of ^{125}I-anti LH antibody binding with LH in benign and malignant ovarian tumors. All details are described in section (2.4.3.2).

Group	Temp °C	$B_{max} \times 10^{-3}$ (mg.ml^{-1})	$K_a \times 10^{3}$ (mg^{-1}.ml)	$K_d \times 10^{-3}$ (mg.ml^{-1})
Premenopausal patients with benign ovarian tumors	4	6.97	0.05358	18.66
	10	7.63	0.05445	18.36
	25	8.42	0.05675	17.62
	37	8.80	0.05962	16.77
	45	9.70	0.06233	16.04
Premenopausal patients with malignant ovarian tumors	4	8.93	0.05959	16.78
	10	8.98	0.06054	16.51
	25	9.78	0.06355	15.73
	37	12.08	0.07219	13.85
	45	10.84	0.06783	14.74
Postmenopausal patients with benign ovarian tumors	4	6.45	0.05045	19.82
	10	5.19	0.04847	20.63
	25	8.67	0.05967	16.75
	37	7.77	0.05641	17.72
	45	7.19	0.05386	18.56

This equation could be simplified to equation 5, in order to fit the data of the first order kinetics: -

$$\text{Ln} \frac{(^{125}\text{I - A - LH Ab/LH})_e}{(^{125}\text{I - A - LH Ab/LH})_e - (^{125}\text{I - A - LH Ab/LH})_t} = K_{+1} t \left[\frac{(^{125}\text{I - A - LH Ab})_T (\text{LH})_T}{(^{125}\text{I - A - LH Ab/LH})_e} \right] \quad \ldots (5)$$

Where: -

K_{+1}: is the kinetic association constant.

$(\text{LH})_T$: is the total concentration of LH in benign and malignant serous ovarian tumor homogenate.

$(^{125}\text{I-A-LH Ab})_T$: is the total concentration of ^{125}I-anti LH antibody.

$(^{125}\text{I-A-LH Ab/LH})_e$: is the concentration of (^{125}I-anti LH antibody/LH) complex formed at equilibrium.

$(^{125}\text{I-A-LH Ab/LH})_t$: is the concentration of (^{125}I-anti LH antibody/LH) complex formed after time (t).

Since in some cases in this work, the percent of binding was small and most of the ^{125}I-anti LH antibody remained free and only a small fraction of

^{125}I-anti LH antibody was bound even at equilibrium (pseudo-first order conditions), the following equation could be used in order to fit the data of pseudo first order kinetics [150]:

$$\mathrm{Ln}\frac{(^{125}\mathrm{I\text{-}A\text{-}LH\text{-}Ab/LH})_e}{(^{125}\mathrm{I\text{-}A\text{-}LH\text{-}Ab/LH})_e - (^{125}\mathrm{I\text{-}A\text{-}LH\text{-}Ab/LH})_t} = t.K_{obs} \quad \ldots\ldots\ldots\ldots(6)$$

from equation 6, figures (3-10A, B, C) shows that the plotting of $\mathrm{Ln}\dfrac{(^{125}\mathrm{I\text{-}A\text{-}LH\text{-}Ab/LH})_e}{(^{125}\mathrm{I\text{-}A\text{-}LH\text{-}Ab/LH})_e - (^{125}\mathrm{I\text{-}A\text{-}LH\text{-}Ab/LH})_t}$ against time (t) gives a straight line with a slop equal to the observed value of first rate constant (K_{obs}) in min^{-1}. The association rate constant (K_{+1}) was calculated from the following equation [151]: -

$$K_{obs} = K_{+1} \frac{(^{125}\mathrm{I\text{-}A\text{-}LH\text{-}Ab})_T \, (LH)_T}{(^{125}\mathrm{I\text{-}A\text{-}LH\text{-}Ab}/LH)_e} \quad \ldots\ldots\ldots\ldots\ldots(7)$$

The half-life time of association (t½) ass, which represents the time needed for the formation of half amount of the complex at equilibrium, was determined from the concentration of the complex at equilibrium. The half life time of dissociation (t½)diss was determined from:

$$(t1/2)diss = \frac{\ln 2}{K_{-1}} = \frac{0.693}{K_{-1}} \quad \ldots\ldots\ldots\ldots\ldots(8)$$

The values of K_{obs}, K_{+1}, K_{-1}, (t ½)ass and (t ½)diss at five different temperatures are summarized in Table (3-4).

The results revealed that the association rate constant K_{+1} at 45°C was higher than of (4,10,25,37°C) for benign premenopausal tumors and K_{+1} at 37°C was higher than that of (4, 10, 25, 45°C) for malignant premenopausal tumors while, the K_{+1} value at 25°C was higher than that of (4, 10, 37, 45°C) for benign postmenopausal tumors and also it was found that K_{+1} values at 4, 10, 25, 37, 45°C for the two groups of benign tumors were higher than that of malignant tumors at each temperature as shown in Table (3-4).

Table (3-4): The effect of different temperatures on the kinetic parameters of ^{125}I-anti LH antibody binding with LH in benign and malignant ovarian tumors. All details are described in section (2.4.3.3)

Group	Temp °C	K_{osb} (min^{-1})	K_{+1} (mg^{-1}.ml.min^{-1})	K_{-1} *10^{-3}(min^{-1})	(t ½)ass (min)	(t ½)diss *10^{-1} (min)
Premenopausal patients with benign ovarian tumors	4	0.0402	98.27	1.834	15	3.77
	10	0.0419	103.33	1.897	21	3.65
	25	0.04413	102.67	1.809	22	3.8
	37	0.0470	111.55	1.870	11	3.7
	45	0.0527	130.31	2.090	10	3.3
Premenopausal patients with malignant ovarian tumors	4	0.0239	55.36	0.929	27	7.4
	10	0.0258	61.077	1.008	26	9.92
	25	0.0300	78.028	1.227	23	5.6
	37	0.0356	94.40	1.300	22	5.33
	45	0.0333	88.525	1.305	23	5.31
Postmenopausal patients with benign ovarian tumors	4	0.0539	134.69	2.669	11	2.59
	25	0.0819	198.37	3.324	10	2.08
	37	0.06864	167.9	2.976	10.5	2.32
	45	0.0737	184.68	3.428	10	2.02

The slow rate dissociation in malignant group may insure the hypothesis that ovarian cancer may lead to a prolongation of the half-life of LH [152]. This prolongation in the half-life can lead to regulate events leading to ovarian cancer cell proliferation and thereby, ovarian cancer under LH control can synthesize and secrete their own growth factors that can autostimulate the ovarian cancer cell [153].

The high rate dissociation in benign groups can be viewed as an indirect support to the concept that LH is involved in the proliferation of human benign ovarian tumors [149]. Thus, the results revealed that LH had a role in the growth of ovarian tumor cell in malignant group more than that in the benign groups.

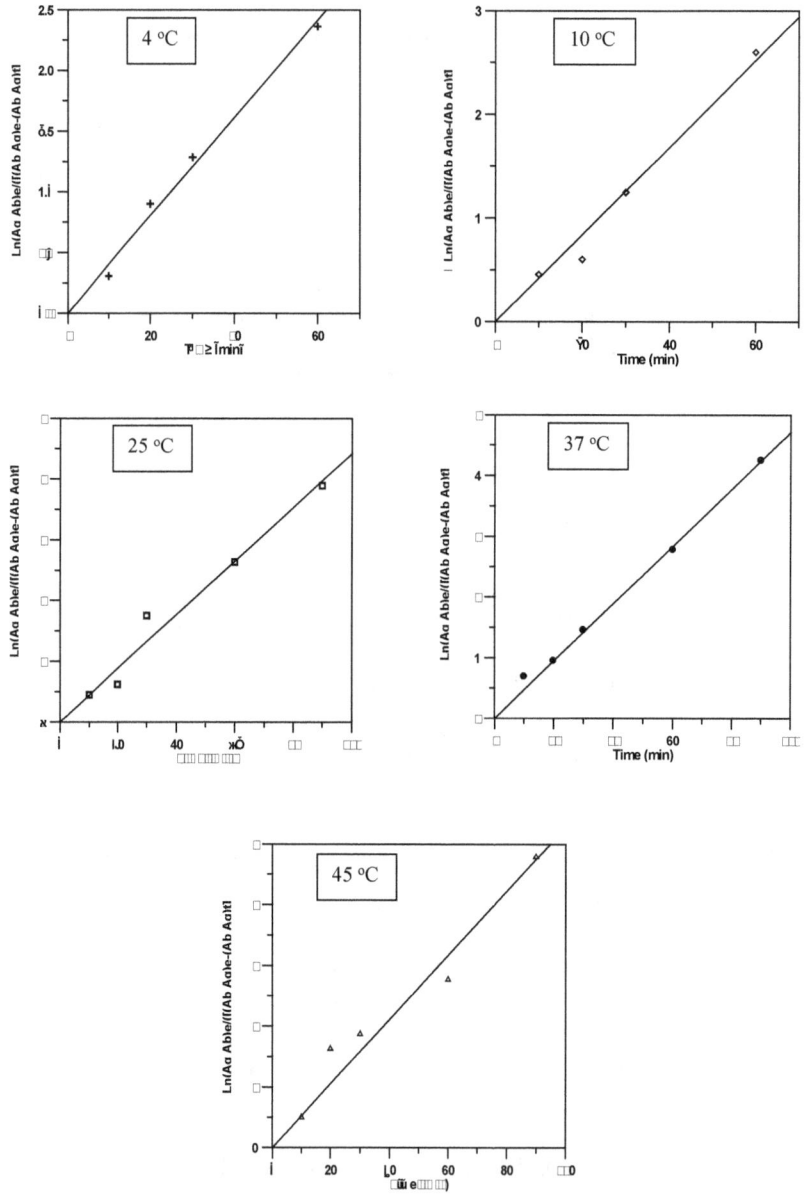

Figure (3-10A): Kinetic of ^{125}I-anti LH antibody binding with LH in
    A: Benign premenopausal ovarian tissue homogenate
    Ab: is the ^{125}I-anti LH antibody,
    Ag: is the LH

Details are explained in section (2.4.3.3)

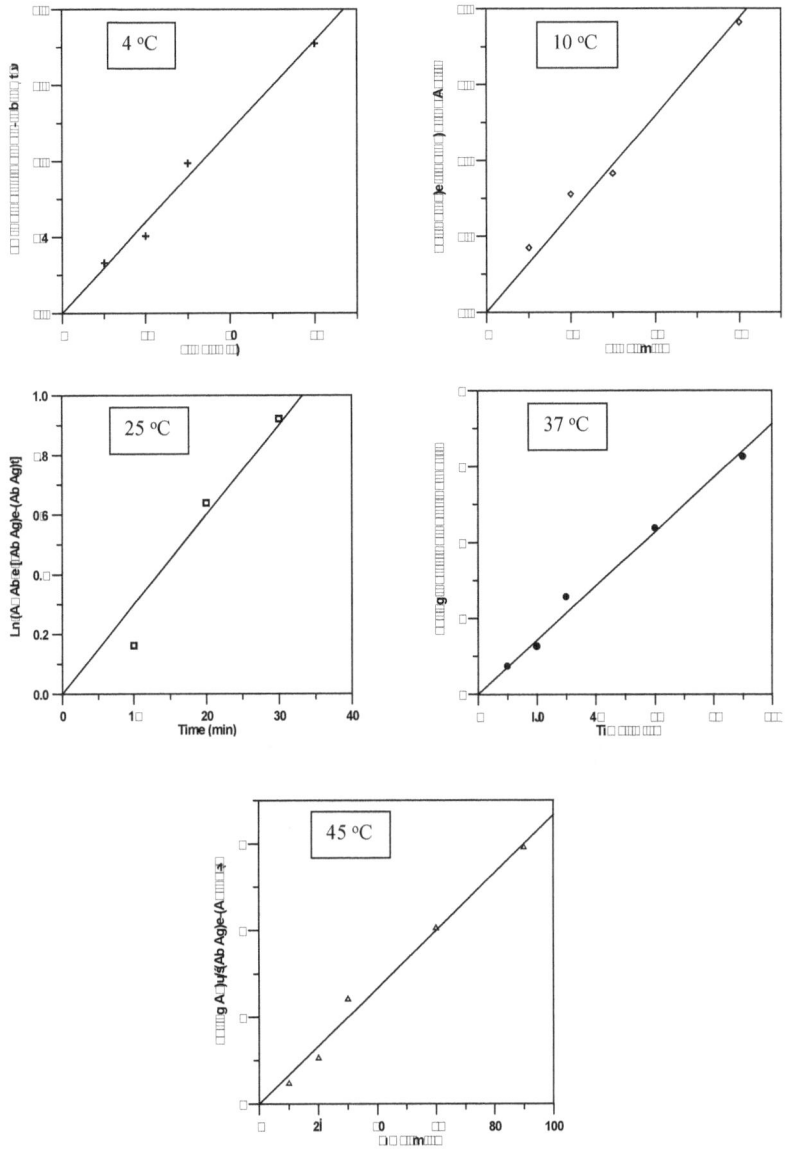

Figure (3-10B): Kinetic of ^{125}I-anti LH antibody binding with LH in
B: Premenopausal ovarian cancer tissue homogenate
Ab: is the ^{125}I-anti LH antibody,
Ag: is the LH
Details are explained in section (2.4.3.

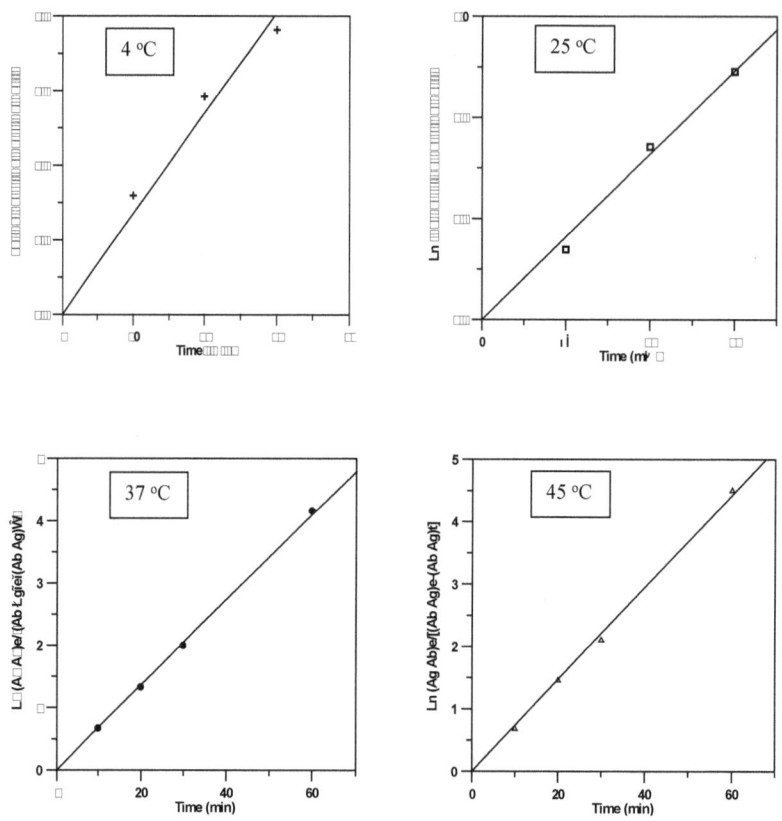

Figure (3-10C): Kinetic of ^{125}I-anti LH antibody binding with LH in
C: Benign postmenopausal ovarian tissue homogenate
Ab: is the ^{125}I-anti LH antibody,
Ag: is the LH
Details are explained in section (2.4.3.3)

The Thermodynamic of the Binding of ^{125}I-Anti LH Antibody with LH in Pre and Postmenopausal Patients with Serous Ovarian Tumor Thermodynamic Parameters of Standard State

Figure (3-11A, B and C) represents the dependence of the equilibrium binding constant (affinity constant) for the binding of ^{125}I-anti LH antibody with LH in Pre- and Postmenopausal ovarian tumor homogenate on the temperature (Van't Hoff plot). Table (3-5) shows the values of thermodynamic parameters of standard state of LH in benign and malignant ovarian tumor. The results indicate that the ΔH° in general had small values and their positive sign ascertain that the reaction was nearly endothermic.

The negative values of ΔG° reflects the stability of the complex hence, the high affinity of the reactants. So our system is characterized by the sole contribution of ΔS° to the stability of the complex formed, while ΔH° has little or no effect [154]. The positive values of ΔS° suggest that the reaction spontaneity be entropically driven.

Entropy was the driven force for the occurrence of the binding. This indicates that the hydrophobic interactions played an important role is stabilizing the complex [155].

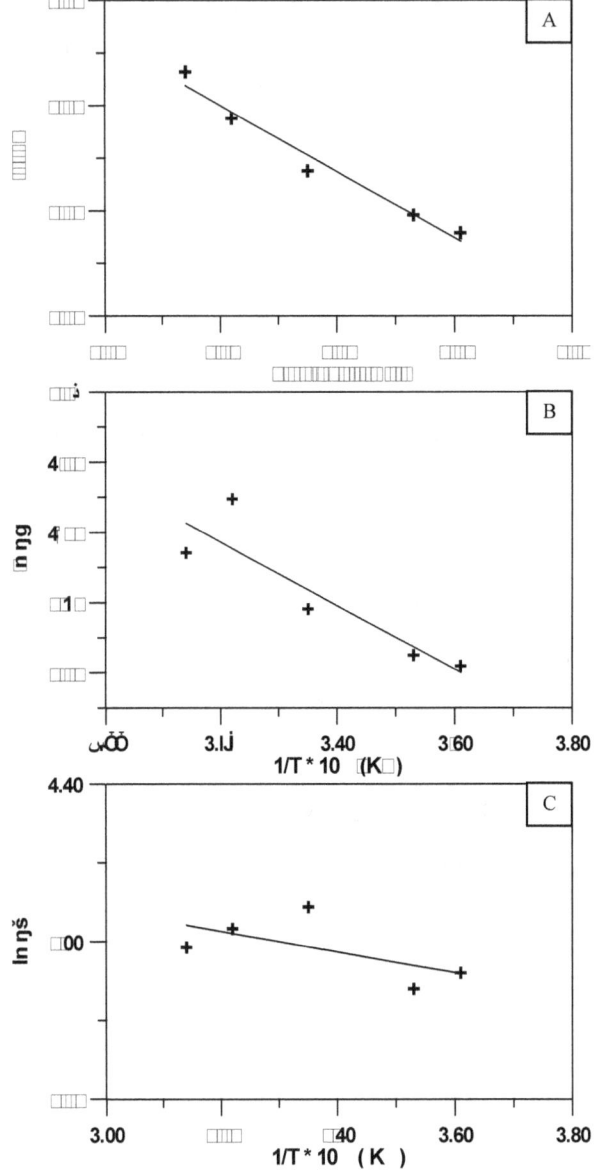

Figure (3-11): Van't Hoff plot for the ^{125}I-anti LH antibody with LH in
A: Benign premenopausal ovarian tissue homogenate
B: Premenopausal ovarian cancer tissue homogenate
C: Benign postmenopausal ovarian tissue homogenate
Details are explained in section (2.4.3.4)

Table (3-5): Thermodynamic parameters at standard state of ^{125}I-anti LH anti body binding with LH in benign and malignant ovarian tumors. All details are explained in section (2.4.3.4).

Group	Temp °C	ΔH° (KJ.mole^{-1})	ΔG° (KJ.mole^{-1})	ΔS° (J.mole^{-1}.K^{-1})
Premenopausal patients with benign ovarian tumors	4	2.609	-9.165	42.50
	10	2.609	-9.402	42.44
	25	2.609	-10.001	42.31
	37	2.609	-10.533	42.393
	45	2.609	-10.921	42.54
Premenopausal patients with malignant ovarian tumors	4	3.007	-9.412	44.83
	10	3.007	-9.651	44.727
	25	3.007	-10.286	44.607
	37	3.007	-11.025	45.264
	45	3.007	-11.146	44.506
Postmenopausal patients with benign ovarian tumors	4	2.181	-9.025	40.454
	10	2.181	-9.126	39.954
	25	2.181	-10.125	41.295
	37	2.181	-10.391	40.554
	45	2.181	-10.535	39.987

The small positive value of ΔH° may indicate a favorable interaction between ^{125}I-anti-LH antibody with LH.

These include the non-covalent interaction which are fundamentally electrostatic in nature such as charge-charge, charge-dipole, dipole-dipole, charge-induced dipole, dipole-induced dipole interactions and hydrogen bonds . The sum of these types of interactions can yield some stabilization to the folded structure of the complex. So the negative values of ΔG° showed that the overall reaction energetically favorable in the direction of complex formation.

Thermodynamic Parameters of Transition State

The transition state theory proposes that the association of two substances to form the final product proceeds through the formation of an activated complex (transition state). Consequently, the interaction of ^{125}I-anti LH antibody with LH can be represented as follows: -

$$^{125}I - A - LH\ Ab + LH \rightarrow \underset{\substack{\text{an activated complex}\\\text{(transition state)}}}{(^{125}I - A - LH\ Ab/LH)} \rightarrow \underset{\text{(product)}}{^{125}I - A\ LH\ Ab/LH}$$

The thermodynamic parameters of the transition state ($\Delta H^*, \Delta G^*, \Delta S^*$ and Ea) could be determined from Arrhenius equation and the kinetic constant.

Figure (3-12 A, B and C) shows the Arrhenius plot of $\ln K_{+1}$ against $1/T$ values. Table (3-6) shows the values of thermodynamic parameters of transition state (Ea, ΔH^*, ΔG^*, ΔS^*).

The value of Ea determined from Arrhenius plot represents the apparent energy of activation of the binding reaction and the required energy to overcome the energy barrier of the transition state for the formation of (^{125}I-anti LH antibody/LH) complex. The high positive values of $\Delta G°$ indicate that the formation of the activated complex is a non-spontaneous process and required a lot of energy (equal to Ea) to overcome the transition state energy barrier and giving the final product, whereas the high negative ΔS^* revealed that the activated complex had a more order structure than the reactance.

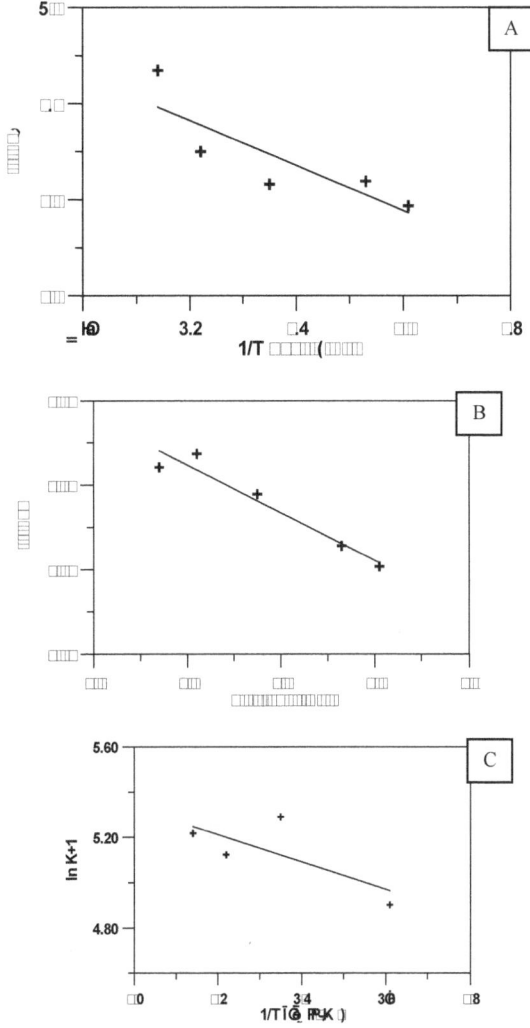

Figure (3-12) : Arrhenius plot for the ^{125}I-anti LH antibody with LH in
A: Benign premenopausal ovarian tissue homogenate

B: Premenopausal ovarian cancer tissue homogenate
C: Benign postmenopausal ovarian tissue homogenate
Details are explained in section (2.4.3.4)

Table (3-6): Thermodynamic parameters at transition state of ^{125}I-anti LH antibody binding with LH in benign and malignant ovarian tumors. All details are explained in section (2.4.3.4).

Group	Temp °C	Ea (KJ.mole^{-1})	ΔH* (KJ.mole^{-1})	ΔG* (KJ.mole^{-1})	ΔS* (J.mole^{-1}.K^{-1})
Premenopausal patients with benign ovarian tumors	4	3.898	1.595	57.105	-200.397
	10	3.898	1.545	58.273	-200.452
	25	3.898	1.420	61.506	-201.630
	37	3.898	1.321	63.870	-201.770
	45	3.898	1.254	65.176	-201.012
Premenopausal patients with malignant ovarian tumors	4	9.367	7.064	58.42	-185.397
	10	9.367	7.015	59.510	-185.494
	25	9.367	6.890	62.186	-185.556
	37	9.367	6.790	64.300	-185.514
	45	9.367	6.724	66.198	-187.025
Postmenopausal patients with benign ovarian tumors	4	5.012	2.709	56.379	-193.754
	25	5.012	2.535	59.875	-192.416
	37	5.012	2.43	62.816	-194.793
	45	5.012	2.36	64.254	-194.635

The positive values of ΔG* is mainly attributed to the decrease in entropy of the transition state (ΔS* < 0). In addition, the positive values of ΔH* shows that the heat content of the activated complex is more than of isolated species [156].

The values of the thermodynamic parameters of the binding reaction, gave an overall idea about the nature of forces that regulate the formation of complex. The thermodynamic model describing the formation of the complex was suggested by using the thermodynamic parameters of both the standard and the transition state. The model is illustrated in Figure (3-13). This model proposes that the formation of the (^{125}I-anti LH antibody/LH) complex undergo three thermodynamic state. The thermodynamic state A represents the initial energy level of ^{125}I-anti LH antibody and LH. In the thermodynamic state B, the two species bind to form the activated complex (^{125}I-anti LH antibody/LH). The last thermodynamic state C, represents the fully interacting (^{125}I-anti LH antibody/LH) complex.

In step one of the reaction, the binding of ^{125}I-anti LH antibody with LH was associated with positive ΔG^* value. This indicates that the initial step of the reaction requires input of energy for the system. The negative entropy charge ΔS^* for this step of the reaction reflects the change of (^{125}I-anti LH antibody/LH) transition complex to amore order structure. The positive ΔH^* value shows that the heat content of the activated complex is more than that of the isolated species. In step two, the activated complex participates in further interactions, giving the fully interacting complex (^{125}I-anti LH antibody/LH). It is proposed that the formation of a protein-ligand complex, occurs in these two steps. The first stabilization of the complex by hydrophobic interactions and the second is the stabilization by short range interactions, such as electrostatic interaction, hydrogen bonding and vander waal's interactions [157].

Hydrophobic interactions contribute to the complex stability via high positive entropy change ($\Delta S^* > 0$), while electrostatic interactions, hydrogen bonding and vander waal's interactions contribute to the stability of the complex via negative entropy change ($\Delta S^* < 0$) [157, 158].

The thermodynamic data from this study indicate that the binding of ^{125}I-anti LH antibody with LH are entropically driven and in agreement with the concept that hydrophobic interaction play an important role in (^{125}I-anti LH antibody/LH) interactions.

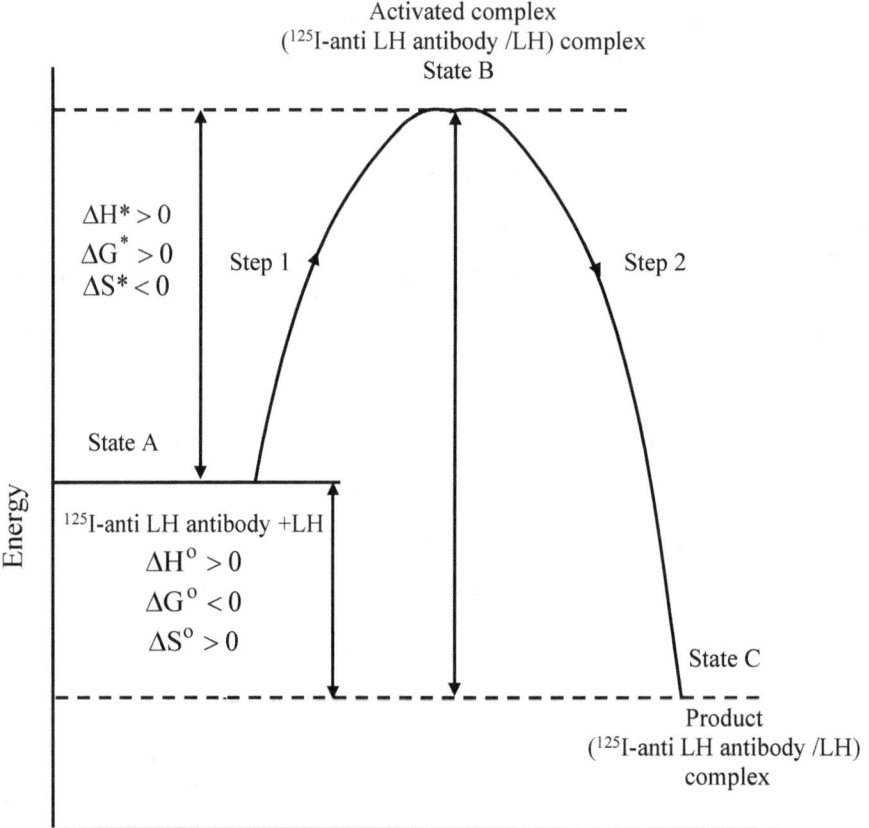

Figure (3-13): General energy diagram and thermodynamic model applied to the complex formation between ^{125}I-anti LH antibody and LH in ovarian tumor.

5. Separation of (^{125}I-Anti LH Antibody/LH) Complex by Gel Filtration Technique

Figure (3-13 A, B and C) shows the results of gel filtration technique used to separate (^{125}I-anti LH antibody/LH) complex from unbound ^{125}I-anti LH antibody for benign and malignant serous ovarian tumors.

All trials of this experiments revealed two peaks profile. The first peak represents (^{125}I-anti LH antibody/LH) complex, the second peak represents the unbound (free) ^{125}I-anti LH antibody.

The separation by gel filtration depends upon the difference of molecular weight of the compounds and because that the molecular weight of the complex is greater than that of unbound (free) ^{125}I-anti LH antibody, so the results indicate that the first peak was assigned for the complex and the second was assigned for unbound ^{125}I-anti LH antibody. Figure (3-14 A, B, C, D) shows the U.V spectrum of (^{125}I-anti LH antibody/LH) complex of benign premenopausal, malignant premenopausal and benign postmenopausal serous ovarian tumors and unbound (free) ^{125}I-anti LH antibody.

The same figure indicate that the λmax for the complex were 216.6, 216.8, and 214.6 respectively while the λmax_1 and λmax_2 for the unbound ^{125}I-anti LH antibody were 211, and 288 nm.

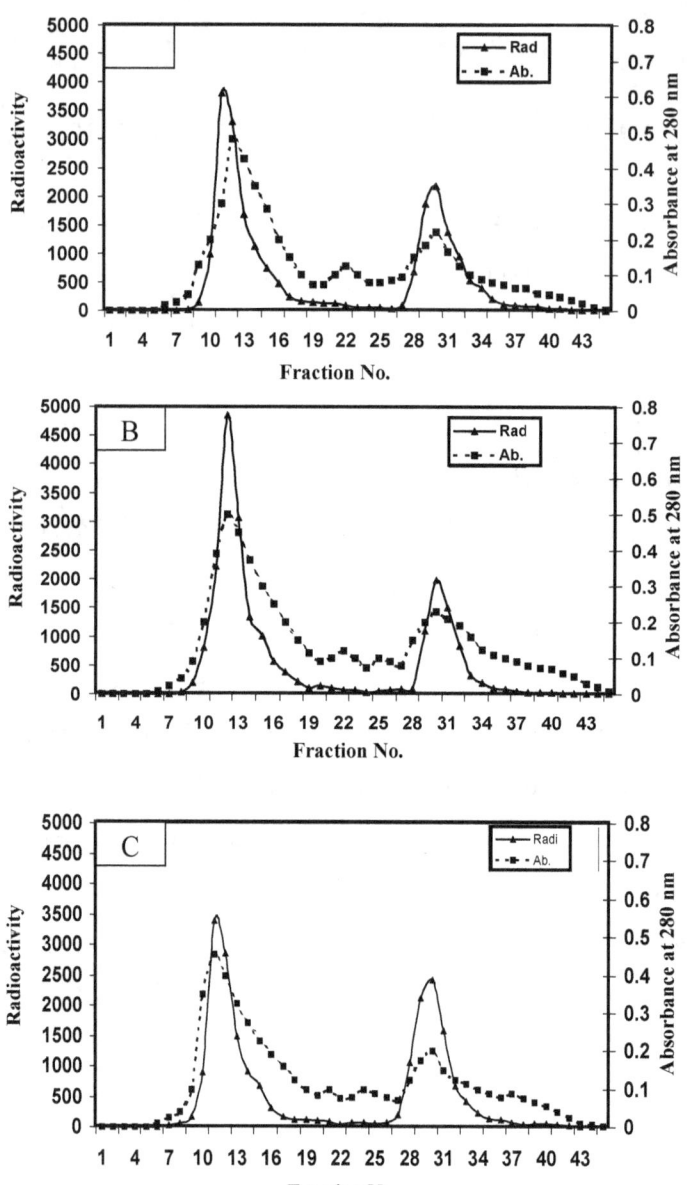

Figure (3-14): The elution profile of ^{125}I-anti LH antibody binding with LH in:
A-   Benign premenopausal ovarian tissue homogenate.
B-   Premenopausal ovarian cancer tissue homogenate.
C-   Benign postmenopausal ovarian tissue homogenate
Details are explained in section (2.5).

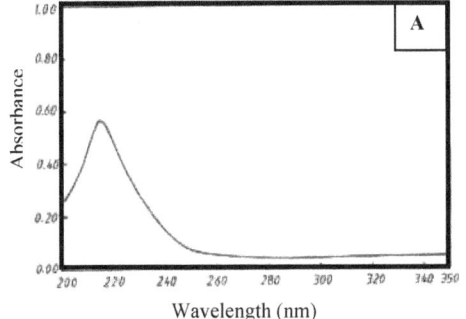
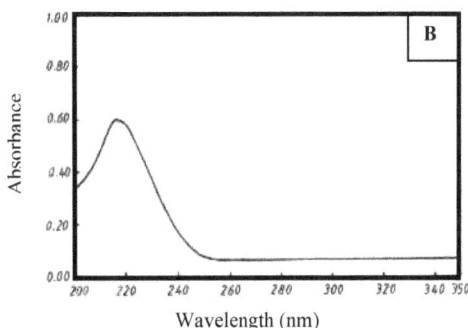
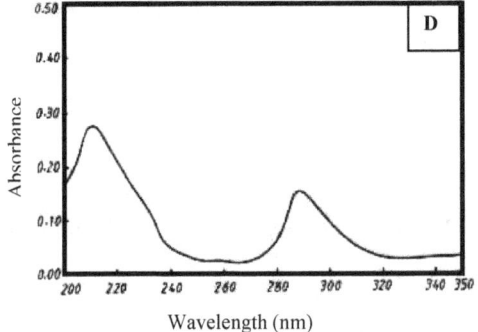
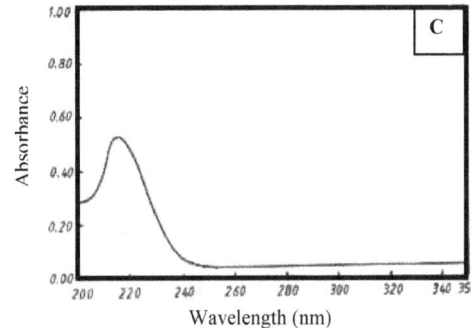

Figure (3-15): The U.V spectrum of:

A: (^{125}I-anti LH antibody/LH) complex of benign premenopausal
B: (^{125}I-anti LH antibody/LH) complex of malignant premenopausal
C: (^{125}I-anti LH antibody/LH) complex of benign postmenopausal
D: unbound (free) ^{125}I-anti LH antibody
Those fractions separated by gel filtration at pH 7.4
Details are explained in section (2.5).

3.6 Spectroscopic Studies of (^{125}I-Anti LH Antibody/LH) Complex and Unbound ^{125}I-Anti LH Antibody

The U.V Spectrum of (^{125}I-Anti LH Antibody/LH) Complex and Unbound ^{125}I-Anti LH Antibody

The U.V spectrum of (^{125}I-anti LH antibody/LH) complex.

Figure (3-14B) shows the U.V spectrum of (^{125}I-anti LH antibody/LH) complex in malignant premenopausal serous ovarian tumors homogenate at pH 7.4. The spectrum shows that there is one maximum wavelength at 216.8 nm which is assigned to the peptide bonds of the complex molecule [159].

The U.V spectrum of unbound ^{125}I-anti LH antibody.

Figure (3-14D) illustrates the U.V spectrum of unbound ^{125}I-anti LH antibody at pH 7.4. The spectrum shows that the λmax of unbound ^{125}I-anti LH antibody is consisted of two maximum wavelength, λmax_1 at 211 nm, and λmax_2, at 288 nm. The absorption at 211 nm is assigned to the peptide bonds of ^{125}I-anti LH antibody molecule [159], while the absorption at 288 nm is assigned to tryptophane.

Factors Affecting the Absorption Properties of (^{125}I-Anti LH Antibody) Complex and Unbound ^{125}I-Anti LH Antibody in Malignant Premenopausal Serous Ovarian Tumor

The absorption spectrum of a chromophore is primarily determined by the chemical structure of the molecule. However, a large number of environmental factors produce detectable change in λmax and ε. Environmental factors such as pH and polarity of the solvent [160].

pH Effect

The pH of the solvent determines the ionization state of the ionizable chromophore in the protein molecule [160].

Table (3-7) shows the λmax values of (^{125}I-anti LH antibody/LH) complex and unbound ^{125}I-anti LH antibody at different pH (4, 7.4, and 12).

When the pH value of (^{125}I-anti LH antibody/LH) complex medium was increased from 4 to 12 the λmax was increased from 214.0 nm to 226.2 nm.

When the pH values of unbound ^{125}I-anti LH antibody were increased from 7.4 to 12 the $λmax_1$ was increased from 211.0 to 217.2. While $λmax_2$ remained constant. At pH 4 the $λmax_1$ was 206.6 nm while the $λmax_2$ was 281.6 nm.

Table (3-7): The pH effect on the λmax of U.V spectrum of (^{125}I-anti LH antibody/LH) complex and unbound ^{125}I-anti LH antibody. Details are described in section (2.6.1.1)

PH	^{125}I-anti LH antibody/LH) complex λmax (nm)	Unbound ^{125}I-anti LH antibody λmax nm
4	214.0	206.6, 281.6
7.4	216.8	211.0, 288.0
12	226.2	217.2, 288.0

The spectral shifts of protein produced by pH cannot be simply attributed to the inductive effects of vicinal charges, such spectral changes must therefore be attributed mainly to rearrangement of secondary and tertiary structure, although the possibility of field effect due to an usually close conjunction of charges to aromatic groups is not excluded [161].

The Effect of Solvent Polarity

The importance of this study comes from studying of the internal configuration of proteins [162].

a- The Effect of 20% of Ethanol, Glycerol, Chloroform and Polyethylene Glycol (PEG) on (^{125}I-Anti LH Antibody/LH) Complex and Unbound ^{125}I-Anti LH Antibody U.V Spectrum.

The λmax value of (^{125}I-anti LH antibody/LH) complex and unbound ^{125}I-anti LH antibody in 20% of different organic solvent at pH 7.4 are shown in Table (3-8). It seems that the presence of 20% polyethylene glycol has an effect on the position of the λmax of (^{125}I-anti LH antibody/LH) complex, which is for the peptide bonds in the complex molecule. So there is a red shift in this λmax and a blue shift in λmax$_2$ for the unbound ^{125}I-anti LH antibody to 285.5 nm which is assigned to tryptophan. While there is a red shift in λmax$_1$ of the peptid bonds.

When the (20%) Glycerol was used a red shift in λmax of the peptide bond of the λmax for the complex and a new λmax at (279.8 nm) appeared. The new peak is related to tyrosine residue. While there was a red shift in λmax$_1$ of the unbound ^{125}I-anti LH antibody which is assigned to the peptide bond and λmax$_2$ was disappeared.

The presence of (20%) Chloroform shows a red shift in λmax of the complex and a new λmax were obtained 262.4 nm which is assigned to phenylalanine [161] and a red shift in λmax$_1$ of the unbound ^{125}I-anti LH antibody which is assigned to peptide bond and λmax$_2$ was disappeared. The presence of (20%) Ethanol has a red shift in λmax for the (^{125}I-anti LH antibody/LH) complex, which is assigned for the peptide bonds in the complex molecule and a red shift also in λmax$_1$ for the unbound ^{125}I-anti LH antibody and no effect on the λmax$_2$.

If there was no effect on the maximum absorbance, this indicates no interaction or any change that happened between the solvent and the molecules. But if one band was observed, may be attributed to the amino acids buried in the internal region of the protein and surrounded by non-polar amino acids [160]. A blue shift in wavelength in some solvent may be attributed to n → π* transitions and also may be attributed to hydrogen bonding of the solvent to the amino acid [162]. The polar chromophores show ared shift if their hydrogen bonding to solvent molecules increases in the excited state, but a blue shift if their hydrogen bonding to solvent molecules decreases in the excited state [163, 164]. Solvent may produce a blue shift by hydrogen bonding to the oxygen atom in the amino acids and withdrawing electrons from benzene chromophore [165].

Table (8-3): The effect of solvents on λmax of (^{125}I-anti LH antibody/LH) complex and free (unbound) ^{125}I-anti LH antibody in premenopausal patients with malignant ovarian tumor. Details are explained in section (2.6.1.2a).

Solvent 20%	(^{125}I-anti LH antibody/LH) complex λmax (nm)	Unbound ^{125}I-anti LH antibody
Polyethylene glycol	220.8	215.2 285.5
Glycerol	219.2 , 279.8	221.2 ____
Chloroform	221.4 262.4	223.8 ____
Ethanol	224.8	211.4 288.0

b- The Effect of Urea and KCl on the U.V Spectrum of (^{125}I-Anti LH Antibody/LH) Complex and Unbound ^{125}I-Anti LH Antibody in Malignant Premenopausal Serous Ovarian Tumor

As shown in Table (3-9) in the presence of Urea (8M) no peaks were assigned for both ^{125}I-anti LH antibody and complex. The absence of any λmax, the proteins were denaturated due to change in the secondary and tertiary structures of the protein.

Adding KCl(0.03M) caused a blue shift for (^{125}I-anti LH antibody/LH) complex to λmax 210.8 nm and a blue shift for the unbound ^{125}I-anti LH antibody to $λmax_1$ 207.1 nm and $λmax_2$ 287.0 nm this effect may be due to the change in the ionic strength of the medium.

Table (3-9): The Effect of Urea and KCl on the λmax of U.V spectrum of (^{125}I-anti LH antibody/LH) complex and unbound ^{125}I-anti LH antibody.
Details are described in section (2.6.1.2b)

Solvent	(^{125}I-anti LH antibody/LH) comlpex λmax nm	Unbound ^{125}I-anti LH antibody λmax nm	
Urea (8M)	-	-	-
KCl 0.03	210.8	207.1	287.0

Effect of Sodium Chloride (NaCl) Concentration on the Thermal Stability of (^{125}I-Anti LH Antibody/LH) Complex by U.V Spectral Studies

Figure (3-15) shows the thermal stability of (^{125}I-anti LH antibody/LH) complex in the presence of two different concentrations of NaCl. From these figure, the internal tryptophan is completely exposed to the solvent at 70°C in 0.01N NaCl and 80°C in 0.1N NaCl for (^{125}I-anti LH antibody/LH) complex. The same temperatures are sufficient for all internal tyrosine. Which are exposed to the solvent. From these result, we concluded that these proteins are more stable at higher NaCl concentrations since higher temperature is need for unfloding in 0.1N NaCl.

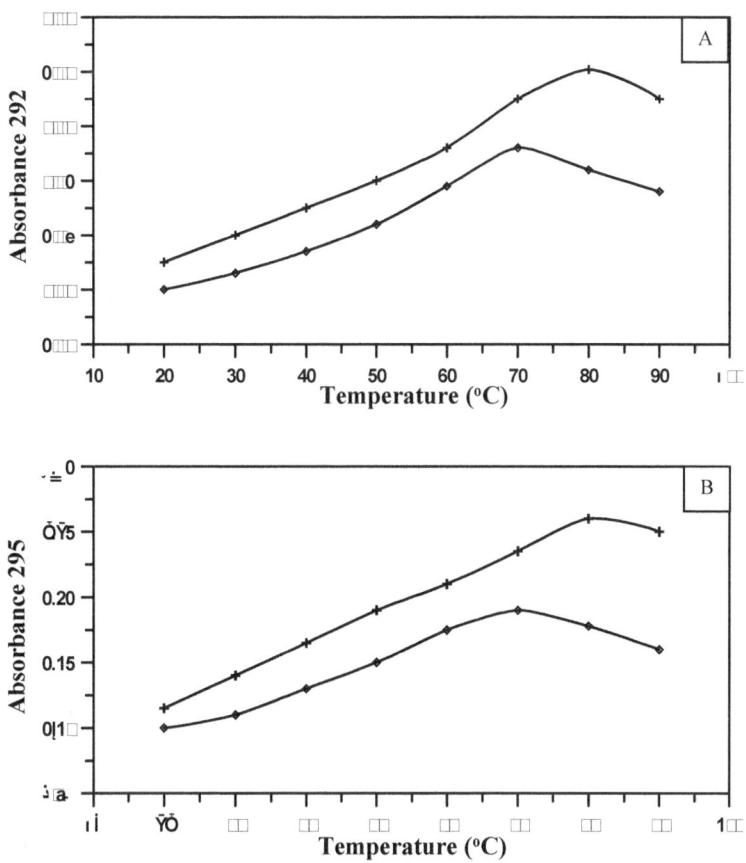

Figure(3-16): Effect of sodium chloride concentration 0.1N (+) and 0.01N (4) on the thermal stability of (^{125}I-anti LH antibody/LH) complex at 292nm (A) and 295nm (B). Details are explained in section (2.6.1.3).

References

1- Greenspan F. S., and Gardner D. G.; **Basic and Clinical Endocrinology**; 6th. ed.; The McGraw-Hill Company; 2001; P: 453.

2- Junqueira L. C., Carneiro J., and Kelley R. O.; **Basic Histology**; 8th. ed.; Lange Medical Book; 1995; P: 423.

3- Kacsoh B.; **Endocrine Physiology**; The McGraw-Hill Company; 2000; P: 503.

4- Snell R. S.; **Clinical Anatomy for Medical Students**; 5th. ed.; Little Brown and Company; 1995; P: 320.

5- Williams R. H.; **Text Book of Endocrinology**; 5th. ed.; W. B. Saunders Company; 1974; P: 368.

6- Seeley R. R., Stephens T. D., and Tate P.; **Essentials of Anatomy and Physiology**; 2nd. ed.; Mosby-Year Book; 1996; PP: 526, 532, 935,942.

7- Kannan C. R.; **Essential Endocrinology**; Plenum Medical Book Company; 1986; P: 325.

8- Carr B. R., and Blackwell R. E.; **Text Book of Reproductive Medicine**; 2nd. ed.; Appleton and Lange; 1998; PP:213-214, 225.

9- Berne R. M., and Levy M. N.; **Physiology**; 3rd. ed.; Mosby-Year Book; 1993; P: 1001.

10- Clement P. B.; **Am. J. Surg. Pathol.**; 1987; 11:277.

11- Upadhyay S., Zamboni L., and Ectopi C.; **Proc. Natal. Acad. Sci. U.S.A.**; 1982; 79:6584.

12- Dawson A. B., and McCabe M.; **J. Morphol.**; 1951; 88:543.

13- Porth C. M.; **Pathophysiology**; 4th. ed.; J. B. Lippincott Company; 1994; PP: 749-752.

14- Jubiz W.; **Endocrinology: A Logical Approach for Clinicians**; 2nd. Ed.; The McGraw-Hill Company; 1987; P: 436.

15- Pernoll M. L., and Benson R. C.; **Current Obstetic and Gynecologic Diagnosis and Treatment**; 6th. ed.; Appleton and Lang Company; 1987; PP: 111,112.

16- Pennington G. W., and Naik S.; **Hormone Analysis: Methodology and Clinical Interpretation**; volume II; CRC Press, Inc.; 1981; P: 30.

17- Burtis C. A., and Ashwood E. R.; **Tietz Text Book of Clinical Chemistry**; 3rd. ed.; W. B. Saunders Company; 1999; PP: 1615, 1608, 1678.

18- Jeffcoate W.; **Lecture Notes on Endocrinology**; 5th. ed.; Blackwell Scientific Publication; 1993; P: 206.

19- Tindall V. R.; **Jeffcoate's Principles of Gynaecology**; 5th. ed.; Butterworth and Co.; 1987; P: 57.

20- Edwards C. R., Bouchier I. A., Haslett C., and Chilvers E. R.; **Davidson's Principles and Practice of Medicine**; 17th. ed.; Pearson Professional Limited; 1995; P: 723.

21- Tierney L. M., McPhee S. J., and Papadakis M. A.; **Current Medical Diagnosis and Treatment**; 40th. ed.; The McGraw-Hill Company; 2001; PP: 746, 762.

22- Brux J. D., and Gautray J. P.; **Clinical Pathology of The Endocrine Ovary**; Philadelphia; 1984; PP: 115-118.

23- Hubl W.; **Hormone Diagnosis for Fertility Disorders: Institute for Clinical Chemistry**; Dresden-Friedrichstadt Hospital; 1992; PP: 60-62.

24- Daly W. J., Easton J. D., Hutton J. J., Kohler P. O., O'Rourke R. A., Sande M. A., Stein J. H., Trier J. S., and Zvaifler N. J.; **Internal Medicine**; 2nd. ed.; Little, Brown and Company; 1987; PP: 1969, 1122.

25- Clayton S. G., Lewis T. L., and Pinker G. D.; **Gynecology by Ten Teacher**; 14th. ed.; Edward Arnold Ltd.; 1985; P: 28.

26- Johnson L. R.; **Essential Medical Physiology**; 2nd. ed.; Lippincott-Raven Publishers; 1998; P: 650.

27- Adash E. Y., Yen S. S., and Jaffe R. B.; **Reproductive Endocrinology**; W. B. Saunders Company; 1992; PP: 181-237.

28- Guyton A. C., and Hall J. E.; **Text Book of Medical Physiology**; 9th. ed.; W. B. Saunders Company; 1996; PP: 1022, 1024, 1027.

29- Hay W. W., Hayward A. R., Levin M. J., and Sondheimer J. M.; **Current: Pediatric Diagnosis and Treatment**; 14th. ed.; Appleton and Lang Company; 1999; P: 602.

30- Ganong W. F.; **Review of Medical Physiology**; 17th. ed.; Appleton and Lange Company; 1995; PP: 408, 409.

31- Shupnik M. A.; **Gene Engineering in Endocrinology**; Human Press Inc.; 2000; P: 239.

32- Holland J. F., Bast R. C., Morton D. L., Frei E., Kufe D. W., and Weichselbaum R. R.; **Cancer Medicine**; 4th. ed.; Williams and Wilkins Awaverly Company; 1997; PP: 2289-2292, 2309.

33- Landis S. H.; **Cancer**; 1999; 49: 8.

34- Bland K. I., Daly J. M., and KaraKousis P.; **Surgical Oncology: Contemporary Principles and Practice**; The McGraw-Hill Company; 2001; PP: 919, 911.

35- Homer J.; **Lancet**; 2000; 355: 1028.

36- Haaften C. V., Russell P., Boyer C. M., Kerns B. M., Wiener J. R., Jensen D. N., Bast R. C., and Hacker N. F.; **Cancer**; 1996; 77: 2092.

37- Jain S., and Tsai C. S.; **J. Reprod. Med.**; 2001; 46: 267.

38- Peckham M., Pinedo H., and Veronesi U.; **Oxford Text Book of Oncology**; volume II; Oxford University Press; 1995; P: 1293.

39- Gunderson L. L., and Tepper J. E.; **Clinical Radiation Oncology**; Churchill Livingstone; 2000; PP: 940-943.

40- Fraumeni J. J., Grundy G. W., Creagan E. T., and Everson B. B.; **Cancer**; 1975; 36: 364-369.

41- Lynch H. T., Harris R. E., and Gurgis H. A.; **Cancer**; 1978; 41:1543.

42- Lynch H. T., and Lynch P. M.; **Am J. Surg.**; 1979; 138:439.

43- Lynch H. T., Watson P., and Bewtra T. A.; **Cancer**; 1991; 61:1460.

44- Frank T. S.; **Cancer Control**; 1999; 6:327.

45- Stratton J. F., Gayther S. A., and Russel P.; **N. Engl. J. Med.**; 1997; 336:1125.

46- Cramer D. W., Welch W. R., Cassells S., and Scully R. E.; **AM. J. Obstet. Gynecol.**; 1983; 147: 1-6.

47- Casagrande J. T.; **Lancet**; 1979; 2: 170.

48- Fathalla M. F.; **Lancet**; 1983; 71: 717.

49- Nieto J. J., Rolfe K. J., Maclean A. B., and Hardiman P.; **Lancet**; 1999; 354: 649.

50- Klapper J., Schlesselman J. J., Silberzweig S., Vergona R., Morgan M., and Wheeler J. E.; **Am. J. Epidemiol.**; 2000; 152: 233.

51- Booth M., Beral V., and Smith P.; **Br. J. Cancer**; 1989; 60: 592.

52- Rossing M. A.; **N. Engl. J. Med.**; 1994; 331: 771.

53- Fishel S., and Jackson P.; **Br. Med. J.**; 1989; 229: 309.

54- Clarke-pearson D. L., and Dawood M. Y.; **Green's Gynecology: Essentials of Clinical Practice**; 4th. ed.; Little Brown and Company; 1990; PP: 531-535.

55- Cotran R. C., Kumor V., and Collins T.; **Robbins Pathologic Basis of Disease**; 6th. ed.; W. B. Saunders Company; 1999; PP: 1068-1069.

56- Bychkoy V., Isaacs J. H.; **Pathology in the Practice of Gynecology**; Mosby-Year Book; 1995; PP: 272, 274.

57- Rosai J.; **Ackerman's Surgical Pathology**; 8th. ed.; Mosby-Year Book; 1996; PP: 1461-1492.

58- Edmonds K.; **Dewhursts TextBook of Obstetrics and Gynaecology for Postgraduates**; 6th. ed.; Blackwell Science Ltd.; 1999; PP: 592-593, 600.

59- Domjanov I., and Linder J.; **Anderson's Pathology**; 10th. ed.; Mosby-Year Book; 1996; P: 2278.

60- Bradbury J.; **Lancet**; 2000; 356: 1826.

61- Devita V. T., Hellman S., and Steven A.; **Cancer: Principles and Practice of Oncology**; 5th. ed.; Lippincott-Raven Publishers; 1997; PP: 1505,1506.

62- Yancik R.; **Cancer**; 1993; 47: 1995.

63- Clifford Chao K. S., Perez C. A., and Brady L. W.; **Radiation Oncology Management Decisions**; Lippincott-Raven Publishers; 1999; PP: 516.

64- Campbell S., Goessen L., Goswany R., and Whitechead M. L.; **Lancet**; 1982; 1: 425.

65- Bourne T., Campbell S., Steer C., Whitechead M. L., and Collins E. P.; **Br. Med. J.**; 1989; 299: 1367.

66- Kovacs L., Toldy E., Wenczl M.; **Clinical Chemistry**; 2001; 47: 124.

67- Wyngaarden J. B., Smith L. H., and Bennett J. C.; **Cecil: Text Book of Medicine**; 19th. ed.; W. B. Saunders Company; 1992; PP: 1034,1035.

68- Jacobs I., and Bast R. C.; **Human Reprod.**; 1989; 4: 1.

69- Raghavan D., Brecher M. L., Johnson D. H., Meropol N. J., Moots P. L., and Thigpen J. T.; **Text Book of Uncommon Cancer**; 2nd. ed.; John Wiley and Sons Ltd.; 1999; P: 656.

70- Kudlacek S., Schieder K., and Kolbl H.; **Gynecol. Oncol.**; 1998; 35: 323.

71- Altras M. M., Golberg G. I., and Levin W.; **Gynecol. Oncol.**; 1988; 30: 26.

72- Zygmunt A.; **Eur. J. Gynecol. Oncol.**; 1999; 20: 298.

73- Podczaski E.; **Gynecol Oncol.**; 1989; 33: 139.

74- Berek J. S.; **Obstet. Gynecol.**; 1986; 67: 685.

75- Alvarez R. D., Basts L. R., and Shingleton H. M.; **Gynecol. Oncol.**; 1987; 26: 284.

76- Rustin G. J., Nelstrop A. E., Bentzen S. M., Bond S. J., and McClean P.; **J. Clin. Oncol.**; 2000; 18: 1733.

77- Davelaar E. M., Bonfrer J. M., Verstraeten R. A., Bokkel Huinink W. W., and Kenemans P.; **Cancer**; 1996; 78: 118.

78- Harimann L. C., Podratz K. C., Keeney G. L., Kamel N. A., Edmonson J. H., Grill J. P., Su J. Q., Katzmann J. A., and Rocle P. C.; **J. Clin. Oncol.**; 1994; 12: 64.

79- Nigro J. M., Baker S. J., and Preisinger C. A.; **Nature**; 1989; 342: 705-708.

80- Harris C. C., Hollstein M.; **N. Engl. J. Med.**; 1993; 329: 1318.

81- Levine A.J., Perry M. E., and Chang A.; **Br. J. Cancer**; 1994; 69: 409-416.

82- Hollstein M., Sidransky D., and Vogelstein B.; **Science**; 1991; 253: 49-53.

83- Newcomb E. W., Sosnow Meg., Demopoulos R. I., Zeleniuch-Jacquotte A., Sorich J., and Speyer J. L.; **Am. J. Pathol.**; 1999; 154: 119.

84- Milner B. J., Allan L. A., and Eccles D. M.; **Cancer Res.**; 1993; 53: 2128.

85- Kupryjanczyk J., Thor A. D., and Beauchamp R.; **Proc. Natal. Acad. Sci. U.S.A.**; 1993; 90: 4961.

86- Seidman J. D.; **Gynecol. Oncol.**; 1995; 59: 283.

87- Vincet T., De Viat J., Hellman S. and Steven A.; **Important Advances In Oncology**; Lippincott-Raven; 1996; PP: 37-39.

88- Skomedal H., Kristensen G. B., Abeler V. M., Borresen A. L., Trope C., and Holm R.; **Am. J. Pathol.**; 1997; 181: 158.

89- White C. D., and Roberts J. A.; **J. Reprod. Med.**; 1999; 44: 840.

90- Marks J. R., Davidol A. M., and Kerns B. J.; **Cancer Res.**; 1991; 51: 2979.

91- Soper J. T., Hunter V. J., Daly L., Tanner M., Creasman W., and Bast R. C.; **Obstet. Gynecol.**; 1990; 75: 249.

92- Zuspan F. P., Gabbe S. G., Garite T. J., Kim M. H., and Manetta A.; **Am. J. Obstet. Gynecol.**; 1994; 171: 1183.

93- Casciato D. A., and Lowitz B. B.; **Manual of Clinical Oncology**; 4th. ed.; Lippincott Williams and Wilking; 2000; P: 259.

94- Covens A., Boucher S., Roche K., Macdonald M., Pettitt D., Jolain B., Souetre E., and Rivierc M.; **Cancer**; 1996; 77: 2086.

95- Tokuhashi Y., Kikkawa F., Tamakoshi K., Suganuma N., Kuzuya K., Arii Y., Kawai M., Hattori S., Kobayshi I., Furuhashi Y., Nakashima N., and Tomoda Y.; **Oncology**; 1997; 54: 281.

96- McGuire W. P., Hoskins W. J., Brady M. F., Partridge E. E., Look K. Y., Clarker D. L., and Davidson M.; **N. Engl. J. Med.**; 1996; 334: 2.

97- Neijt J. P.; **N. Engl. J. Med.**; 1996; 334: 50.

98- Neijt J. P., Ten Bokkel Huinink W. W., and Van der Burg M. E.; **Eur. J. Cancer**; 1991; 27: 1367.

99- Eisenhauer E. A., Ten Bokkel Huinink W. W., and Swenerton K. D.; **J. Clin. Oncol.**; 1994; 12: 2654.

100- Markman M., Rothman R., and Hakes T.; **J. Clin. Oncol.**; 1991; 9: 389.

101- Seewaldt V. L., Greer B. E., Cain J. M., Figge D. C., Tamimi H. K., Brown W. S., and Miller S. A.; **Am. J. Obstet. Gynecol.**; 1994; 170: 1666.

102- Schiff B. P., Fant J., and Horwitz S. B.; **Nature**; 1979; 22: 665.

103- Ozols R. F.; **Ann. Med.**; 1995; 27: 127.

104- Miglietta L., Moroso D. A., and Bruzzone M.; **Oncology**; 1997; 54: 102.

105- Alberts D. S., and Hanningan E. V.; **N. Engl. J. Med.**; 1996; 335: 1950.

106- Lupulescu A. P.; **Cancer**; 1996; 78: 2264.

107- Janne O., Kauppila A., Syrjala P., and Vihka R.; **Int. J. Cancer**; 1980; 25: 175.

108- Ford L. L., Berek J. S., Lagasse L. D., Hacker N. F., Heins Y., Esmailian F., Leuchter R. S., and De Lang R. J.; **Gynecol. Oncol.**; 1983; 15: 299.

109- Kuhneil R., De Graaf J., Rao B. R., and Stolk J. G.; **J. Steroid Biochem.**; 1987; 26: 393.

110- Thigpen J. T., Vance R. B., Balducci L., and Khansur T.; **Semin. Oncol.**; 1984; 11: 314.

111- Vassilomanolakis M., Koumakis G., Barbounis V., Hajichristou H., Tsousis S., and Efremidis A.; **Oncology**; 1997; 54: 202.

112- Pierce J. C., and Parsons T. F.; **Annal. Rev. Biochem.**; 1981; 50: 465.

113- Schulster D., and Levitzki A.; **Cellular Receptors for Hormones and Neurotransmitters**; John Wiley and Sons; 1980; PP: 149-159.

114- Frieden E. H.; **Chemical Endocrinology**; Academic Press; 1976; PP: 136-144.

115- Murray R. K., Granner D. K., Mayes P. A., and Rodwell V. W.; **Harper's Biochemistry**; 25th. ed.; Appleton and Lange; 2000; PP: 550, 555.

116- Wallis M., Howell S. L., and Taylor K. W.; **The Biochemistry of the Polypeptide Hormones**; John Wiley and Sons; 1985; PP: 150-153.

117- Talmadge K., Vamvako Poulos N. C., and Filddes J. C.; **Nature**; 1984; 307: 37.

118- Tortora G. J., and Grabowski S. R.; **Principles of Anatomy and Physiology**; 9th. ed.; John Wiley and Sons; 2000; PP: 570-577.

119- Shome B., and Pierce J. G.; **J. Clin. Endocrinol. Metab.**; 1974; 39: 199.

120- Tietz N.; **Clinical Guide To Laboratory Tests**; 3rd. ed.; W. B. Saunders Company; 1995.

121- Vankrieken L., Vander Horst F. A., Castracane V. D., Durham A. P., and El Shami A. S.; **Clinical Chemistry**; 1999; 45 (Supple 92A): 322.

122- Berlitz F. A., and Haussen M. L.; **Clinical Chemistry**; 2001; 47 (Supple 3A): 5.

123- Marshall W. J.; **Illustrated Text Book of Clinical Chemistry**; 2nd. ed.; Gower Medical Publishing; 1992; PP: 107-108.

124- Smith E. L., Hill R. L., Lehman I. R., Lefkowitz R. J., Handler P., and White A.; **Principles of Biochemistry: Mammalian Biochemistry**; 7th. ed.; McGraw-Hill Book Company; 1985; PP: 376-378.

125- Tilton R. C., Balows A., Hohnadel D. C., and Reiss R. F.; **Clinical Laboratory Medicine**; Mosby-Year Book; 1992; P: 284.

126- Orten J. M., and Neuhaus O. W.; **Human Biochemistry**; 10th. ed.; Mosby-Year Book; 1982; P: 601.

127- Rajan R.; **Postgraduate Reproductive Enodcrinology**; 3rd. ed.; Jaypee Brothers Medical Publishers; 1993; P: 28.

128- Kaplan L. A., and Pesce A. J.; **Clinical Chemistry, Theory Analysis and Correlation**; 2nd. ed.; The C. V. Mosby Company; 1989; P: 611.

129- Abu Al-Teman N. A. K.; **M. Sc. Thesis**; College of Science; University of Baghdad; 2001; P: 36.

130- Lowry O. H., Rosebrough N. J., Farr A. L., and Ronall R. J.; **J. Biol. Chem.**; 1951; 193: 265-275.

131- Scatchard G., **Ann. N. Y. Acad. Sci.**; 1949; 51: 660.

132- Chamberlain J., Jargarinec N., and Ofner P.; **Biochem. J.**; 1966; 99: 610.

133- Thompson S. A., Johnson M. P., and Brook S. C.; **The Prostate**; 1982; 3: 45.

134- Rao C. V., and Mitra S.; **Biochimica Biophysica Acta**; 1979; 584: 454.

135- Jeppson R. L.; **Acta Obstet. Gynecol. Scand.**; 1986; 65: 207.

136- Blaakaer J., Djursing H., Hording U., Bennett P., Toftager L. K., Bock J. E., and Lebech P. E.; **Acta Endocrinal.**; Copenh; 1992; 127:127.

137- Brinkinshaw M., and Falconer I. R.; **J. Endocrinal**; 1977; 55:323.

138- Shiu P.R., and Friesen H. G.; **Biochem. J.**; 1974; 149:310.

139- Haro L. S., and Talaments F. G.; **Mol. Cell Endocrinol.**; 1985; 43:199.

140- Zaltsman Y. A., and Salomon Y.; **Endocrinology**; 1980; 106:1166.

141- Raganiemi H. J., Ronnberg L., Kauppila A., and Ylostalo P.; **J. Clin. Endocrinol. Metab.**; 1981; 108:307.

142- Rao M. C., Richards J. S., Midgley A. R., Rand leo J., and Reichert E.; **Endocrinology**; 1977; 101:512.

143- Samaan N. A., Yang K., and Ward D. N.; **Endocrinology**; 1976; 98:233.

144- Lee C. Y., and Ryan R. J.; **Biochemistry**; 1973; 12:4609.

145- Lee C. Y., Coulam C. B., Jiang N. S., and Ryan R. J.; **J. Clin. Endocrinol. Metab.**; 1973; 36:148.

146- Burtis C. A., Ashwood E. R.; **Tietz Text Book of Clinical Chemistry**; 2nd. ed.; W. B. Saunders Company; 1994; P: 148.

147- Al-Gurnawi Z. A. A.; **M. Sc. Thesis**; College of Science; University of Baghdad; 1999; P: 67.

148- Joshi L. R., Boland S. R., Hewlett E. L., and Katz M. S.; **Arch. Biochem. Biophys.**; 1988; 261:137.

149- Weiland G. A., and Molinoff P. B.; **Life Science**; 1981; 29:314.

150- Stricklands S., Palmer G. and Massay V.; **J. Biol. Chem.**; 1975; 250:4048.

151- Brown E. M., Aurbach G. D., Hauser D., and Troxler F.; **J. Biol. Chem.**; 1976; 251:1232.

152- Nagasaw H.; **Prolactin in Lesion, in Breast, Uterus and Prostate**; CRC Press; 1989; P: 108.

153- Goldberg G. L., and Runowicz C. D.; **Am. J. Obstet. Gynecol.**; 1992; 166: 853.

154- Nemethy G., and Scherage H. A.; **J. Phys. Chem.**; 1962; 66:1773.

155- Waelbroeck M., Van Obberghen E., and DeMeyts P.; **J. Biol Chem.**; 1979; 254:7736.

156- Ross P. D., and Subramanian S.; **Biochem.**; 1981; 20:3096.

157- Blumenthal D. K., and Stull J. T.; **Biochem.**; 1982; 21:2386.

158- Laporte D. C., Wierman B. M., and Strom D. R.; **Biochem.**; 1980; 19:3814.

159- Delvin T. M.; **Text Book of Biochemistry with Clinical Correlation**; 2nd. ed.; John Wiley and Sons; 1986; P: 66.

160- Freifeldar D.; **Physical Biochemistry**; 2nd. ed.; 1982; PP: 494, 500-503.

161- Yanari S., and Bovery F. A.; **J. Biol. Chem.**; 1960; 235:2818.

162- Leach S. J., and Scheraga H. A.; **J. Biol. Chem.**; 1960; 235: 2827.

163- Leach S. J.; **Physical Principles and Techniques of Protein Chemistry**; Part A. Academic Press; 1969; P: 101.

164- Bayliss N. S., and McRae E. G.; **J. Phys. Chem.**; 1954; 58:1002.

165- Scheraga H. A.; **Protein Structure**; Academic Press; 1961, P: 2170.

The second

Biochemical Characterization
Of CA125 in ovarian tumors

Prof. Dr. Sami A. AL-Mudhaffar
Dr. Majid Karbon

Chapter One

Introduction & Literature Survey

1.1 Historical background of tumor marker

Bence jones protein which is exhibits unusual solubility in water was the first tumor marker identified in 1848, it appears in large amounts in the urine of patients with multiple myeloma. More than 100 years after its discovery the Bence-Jones protein was identified as a monoclonal light chain of immunoglobulin [1].

Between 1928-1963, many substances including (hormones, enzymes, isoenzymes and proteins) were discovered and used as tumor markers useful in the diagnosis of individual tumors, but the general application of tumor marker for monitoring cancer in patients did not start until the discovery of α-fetoprotein (AFP)[2] in 1963 and carcinoembryonic antigen (CEA) in 1965[3]. The production of such markers during fetal development as well as in tumors, led to the term oncodevelopmental markers.

Monoclonal antibodies were developed in 1975[4]. to detect oncofetal antigens and antigens derived from tumor cell lines such as CA125, CA 15-3, and CA 19-9.

More recent advances in molecular techniques with the use of molecular probes and monoclonal antibodies to detect chromosome or protein alteration, including the study of oncogenes, suppressor genes, and genes involved in DNA repair, have led to the rapid understanding and use of tumor markers at molecular level [5]. Unlike earlier tumor markers, these new markers can be linked to specific biological processes related to the regulation of cell growth and tumor development including malignant transformation, proliferation, apoptotic cell death and metastasis.

1.2 Definition of tumor marker

A tumor marker is a substance that is present in or produced by tumor itself, or produced by the host in response to a tumor [6] that can be used to differentiate a tumor from normal tissue or to determine the presence of a tumor based on its measurement in the blood or secretions. Such a substance can be found in cells, tissue, or body fluids [7]. It can be measured qualitatively or quantitatively by chemical, immunological, or molecular biological methods to identify the presence of a cancer [8].

Morphologically, cancer tissue has been recognized by pathologists as resembling fetal tissue more closely than normal adult differentiated tissue. Tumors are graded according to their degree of differentiation: as being well differentiated, poorly differentiated, or anaplastic (without form). Few markers are specific for single individual tumor (tumor-specific markers); most are found with different tumors of the same tissue type (tumor-associated markers). They are present in higher quantities in cancer tissue or in blood of cancer patients than in benign tumors or in the blood of normal subjects.

Tumor markers have been categorized as enzymes, isoenzymes, hormones, and oncofetal antigens, carbohydrate epitopes recognized by monoclonal antibodies, receptors, oncogene product and genetic changes. There are only a handful of well-established tumor markers that are being used by physicians. Many other potential markers are still being under research. Now there are many studies that are trying to find new genes involved in signaling molecules or proteins that "tell" cells to proliferate, invade or metastasize [9].

1.3 Classification of Tumor Markers

Tumor markers may be classified into chemical and genetic tumor Markers. [10]

1.3.1 Chemical tumor markers

Table (1-1) Summarizes the classification of chemical tumor markers according to biochemical characteristics, and their associated malignancy.

Table (1-1) Chemical tumor markers [11]

Marker type	Associated malignancy	Example
Enzymes	Liver	Alcohol dehydrogenase
	Bone, Liver, Leukemia, Sarcoma	Alkaline phosphatase
	Ovarian, lung, trophoplastic, gastrointestinal, seminoma, hodgkin's	Alkaline phosphatase placental
	Pancreas, Various	Amylase
	Colon, Breast	Aryl Sulfatase B
	Colon, Bladder, Gastrointestinal, Various	Galactosyl Transferase
	Lung, (small-cell) neuroblastoma, Carcinoid, melanoma, pancreatic	Neuron-Specific enolase
	Prostate, Various (large bowel, lung, ovarian)	Prostate-specific antigen (PSA) Ribonuclease
	Colorectal, Breast, etc.	Telomerase
	Colon, Breast, Lung	Sialyl Transferenase
Hormone	Gushing·s syndrome, Lung (small cell)	ACTH
	Lung (small cell) adrenal Cortex, deudonal	Antidiuretic hormone
	Medullary thyroid	Calcitonin
	Pituitary adenoma, Renal, Lung, Embryonal, choriocarinoma, Testicular (nonseminomatous)	hCG
	Torophoblastic, Gonads, Lungs, Breast	Human placental lactogen
	Liver, Renal, Breast, Lung, Various	Parathyroid hormone
	Pituitary adenoma, renal, lung, breast.	prolactin
Oncofetal Antigen	Hepato cellular, germ line (non seminoma)	□-feto protein
	Colon	β- oncofetal antigen
	Liver	Carcino fetal ferritin
	Colorectal, Gastrointestinal, Pancreatic, Lung, Breast	CEA
	pancreatic	Pancreatic oncofetal
	Cervical, Lung, Skin, Head& neck (Squamous)	Squamous cell antigen
	Colon, Gastrointestinal, Bladder	Tennesse antigen
Mucin	Ovarian, endometrial, Lung	CA125
	Breast, ovarian	CA15-3

	Breast	CA27-29
	Breast, ovarian	MCA
	Pancreatic, Ovarian, Gastrointestinal, Lung	Du-PAN-2
protein	Multiple Myeloma, β-Cell lymphpoma chronic	β-2 microglobulin
	Insulinoma	C-peptide
	Liver, Lung, Leukemia	Ferritin
	multiple myeloma, Lymphomas	Immunoglobulin
	Pancreatic, Stomach	Pancreas associated antigen
	Trophoplastic, Germ cell	Pregnancy specific protein
	Hepatocellular	Prothrombin precursor
	Ovarian	Tumor associated trypsin inhibitor
Blood Group Related antigen	Pancreatic, Hepatic, Gastrointestinal,	CA19-9
	Pancreatic, Gastrointestinal, Ovarian	CA19-5
	Colon, Pancreatic Gastrointestinal,	CA50
	Ovarian, Breast, Colon, Gastrointestinal,	CA72,4,CA242
Others	Breast	Estrogen&progesterone receptors
	Brain, Various	polyamine
	Bone Metastasis (Breast), (multiple myeloma)	Hydroxy proline
	Neuroblastoma, pheochromocytoma	Catecholamine metabolites
	Gastroitestinal, Lung, Rhenmatoid	Lipid-associated sialic acid

1.3.2 Genetic tumor markers

A simple definition of cancer is "a relatively autonomous growth of tissue". Understanding the cause of autonomous growth would clearly facilitate the search for care. Advance in molecular genetics have provided a better understanding of the genesis of human cancer. The proliferation of normal cell is thought to be regulated by growth – promoting oncogenes and counterbalanced by growth – constraining tumor suppressor genes. The development of cancer appears to involve the activation or altered expression of oncogenes, and the loss or inactivation of tumor suppressor genes.[11]

Oncogenes (cell activation genes) are derived from proto-oncogenes (normal celluler genes) which may be activated by dominant mutations. The type of mutation might be point mutation, insertion, deletion, translocation, or inversion. Most oncogenes are associated with haematological malignancies such as leukemia and to lesser extent, solid tumors. [12]

Suppressor genes (genes involved in the recognition and repair of damaged DNA) have mostly been isolated from solid tumors. p53 tumor suppressor gene is the most frequently mutated gene in human cancer, indicating its important role in the conservation of normal cell cycle progression [13]. One of p53'S essential roles is to arrest the cells in G1 after genotoxic damage, to allow DNA repair prior to DNA replication and cell division. In response to massive DNA damage, p53 triggers the apoptotic cell death pathway [14]. The loss of function of this gene may result in the inability of DNA repair process and may lead to the development of tumorgensis [15].

The exciting promise of using the detection of oncogenes and suppressor genes, for diagnosis, determining the prognosis, and predicting the response to the chemotherapy remains to be realized. Oncogens detection remains an experimental approach to human cancer.

1.4 Ideal Tumor Marker

An ideal tumor marker should be specific for a given type of cancer and sensitive enough to detect small tumors for early diagnosis or during screening, provide an estimation of tumor burden, and serve for monitoring effects of therapy and detecting recurrence of tumors [7]. It can be measured qualitatively or quantatively by chemical, immunological, or molecular biological methods to identify the presence of a cancer [8].

1.5 Clinical Applications of Tumor Markers

Clinical applications of tumor markers depend on specificity and sensitivity. Specificity refers to the detection of specific tumors by specific markers. Sensitivity, in this instance, has to do with detecting all patients with the specific tumor.

The potential uses of tumor markers are [16]:

- Screening in general population.
- Differential diagnosis of symptomatic patients.
- Clinical staging of cancer
- Estimating tumor volume.
- Prognostic indicator for disease progression
- Evaluating success of treatment.
- Detecting response to therapy
- Radioimmunolocalization of tumor marker.
- Determining direction for immunotherapy.

In general tumor markers may be used for diagnosis, prognosis, and monitoring effect of therapy, as well as a target for tumor localization and therapy. Monitoring treatment with tumor markers is an accepted application and generally indicates successful treatment; such monitoring is seen after both invasive and noninvasive treatment.

The use of tumor markers for screening the presence of cancer in asymptomatic individuals in a general population has been limited because most tumor markers are present in normal, benign and cancer tissues and are not specific enough to be used for screening cancer [17]. However if the incidence of cancer is high among certain population, screening is feasible [18]. Potential uses of some tumor markers are summarized in table (1-2).

Table (1-2) Clinical Uses of some tumor markers [19]

Tumor marker	Biochemical properties	Molecular weight	Primary clinical applications
Alpha–fetoprotein	Glycoprotein, 4% carbohydrate;	~70kDa	Diagnosis and monitoring of primary

(AFP)	considerable homology with albumin		hepatocellular carcinoma and germ cell tumors. Prognosis of germ cell tumors.
Cancer antigen 125 (CA125)	Mucin identified by monoclonal antibodies	~200kDa	Monitoring ovarian carcinoma. Prognosis after chemotherapy
Cancer antigen 15-3 (CA15.3)	Mucin identified by monoclonal antibodies	>250 kDa	Monitoring breast cancer
Cancer antigen 72.4 (CA 72.4)	Glycoprotein identified by monoclonal antibodies	~48 kDa	Monitoring gastric carcinoma
Cancer antigen 19-9 (CA19-9)	Glycolipid carring the Lewis a blood group determinate	~1,000 kDa	Monitoring pancreatic carcinoma
Carcinoembri-yonic antigen (CEA)	Family of glycoproteins, 45%-60% carbohydrate	~180 kDa	Monitoring gastrointestinal and other Adenocarcinomas
Estrogen receptor	Nuclear transcription	65 kDa	Predicting response to endocrine therapy in breast cancer
Human chorionic gonadotrophin (hCG)	Glycoprotein hormone consisting of tow non- covalently bound subunits (α and β)	~36 kDa	Diagnosis and monitoring non-seminomatous germ cell tumors, Prognosis of germ cell tumors.
Placental alkaline phosphatase (PLAP)	Heat – stable isoenzyme of alkaline phosphatase	~86 kDa	Monitoring of germ cell tumors (seminomas)
Progesterone receptor	Nuclear transcription factor	A from : 94 kDa B from :120 kDa	Predicting response to endocrine therapy in breast cancer.
Prostate specific antigen (PSA)	Glycoprotein serine protease	~36 kDa	Diagnosis, screening and Monitoring prostatic carcinoma
Tissue polypeptide antigen (TPA)	Fragments of cytokeratin 8,18 and 19	~22 kDa	Monitoring bladder and lung carcinoma
Tissue polypeptide specific antigen (TPS)	Fragments of cytokeratin 18	~22 kDa	Monitoring metastatic breast carcinoma

1.6 Tumors of Ovary

Classification

The pathological conditions of the ovary may be classified as [20, 21]:

1.6.1 Non-neoplastic Functional Cysts

Follicular cyst

Corpus luteum cyst.

Theca lutein and granulose lutein cysts.

Polycystic ovarian disease.

Endometriomatous cysts.

1.6.2 Ovarian Neoplasm's.

The classification of ovarian neoplasm's given in table (1-3), is a simplified version of world health organization (WHO) histological classification, which separates ovarian neoplasm's according to the most probable tissue of origin. [22]

Table (1-3) Derivation of various ovarian neoplasms' and some data on their frequency and age distribution [22]

Origin	Surface Epithelial cells (surface Epithelial – stromal cell tumor)	Germ cell	sex cord - stroma	Metastasis to ovaries
overall frequency	65-70%	15-20%	5-10%	5%
Proportion of malignant ovarian tumors	90%	3-5%	2-3%	5%
Age group affected	20 + years	0-25 + years	All ages	Variable
Types	- Serous tumor - Mucinous tumor - Endometrioid Tumor - Clear cell Tumor - Transitional cell Tumor - Undifferentiated carcinoma	- Teratoma - Dysgerminoma - Endodermal sinus tumor - Chorio carcinoma	- Fibroma - Granulos-theca cell tumor - Sertoli – leydig cell tumor	

1.7 Epithelial Ovarian Tumors

The most common group of ovarian neoplasm originates from the coelomic mesothelium that covers the ovary, which after neoplastic transformation seems to retain the capacity to recapitulate the epithelial components of the mullerian ducts. According to the (WHO) classification of ovarian tumors, surface epithelial-stromal tumors can be divided into serous tumors, mucinous tumors, endometrioid tumors, clear cell tumors, transitional tumors and undifferentiated carcinoma [23, 24,25] table (1-3).

Serous tumor is the most frequent of the ovarian tumors and the most common epithelial ovarian carcinoma, accounting for 40-50% of all such tumors. [26]

According to histopathological classification of ovarian tumors, serous tumors can be classified into. [27]

Benign
- Cystadenoma and papillary cystadenoma.
- Surface papilloma
- Adenfibroma and cyst adenofibroma.

Borderline malignancy (of low malignant potential)
- Cystic tumors and papillary cystic tumor.
- Surface papillary tumor.
- Adenofibroma and cystadenofibroma.

Malignant.
- Adenocarcinoma, papillary adenocarcinoma.
- Cystadenocarcinoma.
- Surface papillary adenocarcinoma.
- Adenocarcinofibroma & cystadenocarcinofibroma.

Evidence is lacking about whether ovarian carcinoma may go through a borderline phase during its development and whether borderline tumors always shift into invasive ovarian carcinoma [28-29].

In the overall spectrum of serous tumors, about 60% are benign, 15% of low malignant potential, and 25% malignant [22]. Benign serous cystadenomas occur slightly more often than benign mucinous tumors, but in their malignant form serous cyst adenocarcinomas are three to four times more common than mucinous cystadenocarcinomas. Serous and mucinous borderline tumors are seen but other types of epithelial tumors of borderline malignancy, such as the variant of Brenner and endometrioid tumors are rare [30].

1.7.1 Incidence

Ovarian cancer is the leading cause of death from gynecological malignancies [31] worldwide, the highest incidence of disease is found in America and northern Europe, the lowest incidence is found in Asia and Latin Amarica[32]. In United States approximately 23000 cases occur annually leading to 13900 death each year [33], rate among blacks are lower than among whites, but rates for women of Chinese and Japanese are higher than rates in their countries of origin [32]. In Iraq, ovarian cancer forms 38% of all gynecological malignancies, it was the seventh most common cancer among females with an incidence of 0.8 per 100,000 woman [34]. It is the most common cancer to occur at an advanced stage [35].

1.7.2 Etiology and Risk Factors of ovarian cancer

Although the exact etiology of ovarian cancer is unknown, there are many risk factors which have been associated with the developing of ovarian cancer, such as Genetic, environmental, hormonal, and nutritional.

1.7.2.1 Genetic factors

The strongest known risk factor for ovarian cancer is family history which is present in about 10-15 % of women who develop the disease [36]. Family history in one relative increased the lifetime probability of ovarian cancer in a 35- years old women from 1.5 to 5%; the probability increased to 7% if she had two relatives with the disease.

The rare familial ovarian cancer syndromes are accounting for less than 1% of ovarian cancer cases. The most common hereditary syndrome is the breast-ovarian cancer syndrome. Most of these families have germ- line mutation in one of the breast cancer susceptibility genes, BRCA-1 [37] or BRCA-2. [38]

1.7.2.2 Increasing Ages

The incidence of ovarian cancer increases with age, the highest proportion of cases is diagnosed in women 50 to 59 of age. In women 50 to 75 years of age, the annual incidence is 50 per 100,000 (adjust for prior oophorectomy), approximately twice the rate in young women [39, 40], while benign tumors occur mostly in young women between the ages of 20-40 years old. [22]

1.7.2.3 Reproductive factors

Several potentially modifiable reproductive factors appear to reduce the risk of ovarian cancer

- Pregnancy reduces the odds of ovarian cancer by 25 to 50 percent [41,42] the decrease in risk is associated with an increasing number of pregnancies.

- Use of the oral contraceptive pill is associated with a 35 % reduction in the risk of ovarian cancer, increasing the duration of use is associated with decreasing risk, [41,42] ten years of use by women with a positive family history can reduce their risk to a level below that for women with no family history who never used oral contraceptives. [43]

- Breast feeding is associated with a more modest effect on risk, reducing the odds of ovarian cancer by 20 % [41,42].

Certain gynecological surgical procedures are also associated with a lower likelihood of ovarian cancer. The risk of ovarian cancer is reduced by about 15% after tubal ligation or hysterectomy with ovarian preservation [41,42]. The protective mechanism of these procedures may relate to impairment of ovarian function, causing an ovulation, or protection from exposure to exogenous carcinogens that enter the peritoneal cavity through the vagina.

Talcum powder may be one of the carcinogen materials, studies have shown that woman who use talcum powder as part of their perineal hygiene are at increased risk. [43] Talc is found in soap powders, and deodorants, and is used in packing of condoms and [30, 44, 45] contraceptive diaphragms, talc might then migrate through vagina to reach the ovaries.

Infertility may increase the risk of ovarian cancer [46, 47]. An increased risk of ovarian cancer has also been reported with infertility treatment, particularly prolonged use of clomiphene citrate. [48]

1.7.3 Staging

Staging of ovarian cancer is based on the finding at the time of surgery and pathological review. Because of the clinically occult spread, surgery is mandatory. The clinical staging of cancer is intended to provide means by which information related to the progress of the disease, the methods and success of treatment modalities is obtained.

Ovarian malignancies are staged according to the international federation of gynecology and obstetrics (FIGO), basing on the finding of surgical exploration[49] see table (1-4).

Table (1-4) Staging of ovarian cancer according to FIGO. ([49])

Stage I
In stage I, cancer is found in one or both of the ovaries. Stage I is divided into
Stage IA: Cancer is found in a single ovary.
Stage IB: Cancer is found in both ovaries
Stage IC: cancer is found in one or both ovaries and one of the following is true:
Cancer is found on the outside surface of one or both ovaries.
The tumor has ruptured the ovary wall.

Cancer cells are found in fluid from the peritoneal cavity (the body cavity that contains most of the organs in the abdomen). The fluid may already be in the peritoneal cavity or it may be added by the doctor to wash the peritoneum (tissue lining the peritoneal cavity).

Stage II
In stage II, cancer is found in one or both ovaries and has spread into other areas of pelvis. Stage II is divided into
   Stage IIA: Cancer has spread to the uterus and / or the fallopian tubes.
   Stage IIB: Cancer has spread to other tissue within the pelvis.
   Stage IIC: cancer has spread to the uterus and/or fallopian tubes and /or other tissue within pelvis and one of the following is true:
   Cancer is found on the outside surface of one or both ovaries.
   The tumor has ruptured the ovary wall.
   Cancer cells are found in fluid from the peritoneal cavity.

Stage III
In stage III, cancer is found in one or both ovaries and has spread to other parts of the abdomen. Cancer has spread to the surface of the liver. Stage III is divided into:
   Stage IIIA: The tumor is found only in the pelvis, but cancer cells have spread to the surface of the peritoneum.
   Stage IIIB: Cancer has spread to the peritoneum but is not larger than 2 centimeters (less than 1 inch) in diameter.
   Stage IIIC: Cancer has spread to the peritoneum and is larger than 2 centimeters in diameter and/or has spread to lymph nodes in the abdomen.

STAGE IV

In stage IV, cancer is found in one or both ovaries and has metastasized (spread) beyond the abdomen to other parts of the body .Cancer is found in the tissues of the liver.

1.7.4 Diagnosis

Ovarian tumors are occasionally detected on pelvis examination, although early stage tumors are rarely found due to deep anatomic location of the ovary. Thus tumors detected by pelvic examination are usually at an advanced stage and associated with poor prognosis [50], more than 56-70% of the patients are diagnosed as having stage III or IV disease. [51]

Tests that examine the ovaries, pelvic area, blood, and ovarian tissue are used to help diagnose ovarian cancer.

These include the following. [49]

- **Pelvic exam**: A procedure to check the uterus, Vagina, ovaries, fallopian tubes, bladder, and rectum to find any abnormality in their shape or size.

- **Ultrasound test**: Transvaginal sonography (TVS) is capable of detecting more than 95% of stage I ovarian cancers, it also detects large numbers of patients with benign disease who subsequently undergo surgery to rule out malignancy, the predictive value was only 1.5%. [52]

- **CA125 Test**: A blood test used to measure the level of CA125 [53], a substance sometimes found in an increased amount in the blood, other body fluids or tissues.

- **Computerized axial tomography (CAT scan)**: A series of detailed pictures of areas inside the body, taken from different angles. This method fails to differentiate benign disease from stage I disease. [54, 55]

- **Intravenous pyelogram**: A series of x-ray of the kidneys, Ureters, and bladder to help determine if cancer has spread outside the ovaries.

- **Biopsy**: Removal of tissue for examination under microscope.

1.7.5 Treatment

There are treatments for all patients with ovarian epithelial cancer. Some treatment are standard, and some are being tested in clinical trials. A treatment clinical trial is a research study meant to help improve current treatments or [49] obtain information on new treatments for patients with cancer.

1.7.5.1 Standard treatment: three kinds of standard treatment are used, these include the following:

Surgery

Most patients have surgery to remove as much of the tumor as possible. Different types of surgery may include

- Hysterectomy (removal of the ovaries, fallopian tubes, and uterus).
- Unilateral Salpingo-oophorectomy (removal of one ovary and one fallopian tube).
- Bilatera salpingo-oophorectomy (removal of both ovaries and both fallopian tubes).
- Omentectomy (partial removal of the lining of the abdominal cavity).
- Lymph node biopsy (removal of the lymphnodes for examination under a microscope to check for cancer cells).

Radiation therapy

Radiation therapy is the use of x- ray or other types of radiation to kill cancer cells and shrink tumors. Radiation therapy may use external or internal radiation.[49]

Chemotherapy

Chemotherapy is the use of drugs to kill cancer cells. Chemotherapy may be taken orally or injected into a vein or muscle. Another way to give chemotherapy is intraperitoneal chemotherapy. With this method, most of the drug remains in the abdomen; this technique is effective in advanced disease with minimal residual disease. [44]

- Biological therapy
- High-dose chemotherapy with bone marrow transplantation.

Biological therapy is the treatment to stimulate the ability of the immune system to fight cancer. Substances made by the body or made in laboratory are used to boost, direct, restore the body's natural defense against disease.

Biological therapy is sometimes called biological response modifier (BRM) therapy or immunotherapy. [49]

Within the last few years, different immunotherapeutic strategies based on immunization with tumor specific antibody constructs or immunogenic peptides have been developed [56, 57]. Alternative concepts include the application of genetically modified tumor cells for the expressions of cytokines or consitimulatory molecules as well as dentritic cells for the effective presentation of immunogenic peptides in the extent of MHC and the activation of cellular immune responses, [57] in this context, ovarian cancer cells express a mutated form of the P53 [58, 59, 60] and/or BRCA1 [61, 62] (Tumor suppressor gene).

Ovarian tumors also over express the CA125 [63] and DF_3/MUCI [64] carcinoma-associated antigens. In addition, these tumors over express the HER_2/neu (c-erbB_2) [65, 66] thus certain targets for immunotherapy of cancer are already known and others although remain undefined presumably exist.

Stage I: Treatment of stage I may include hysterectomy, unilateral or bilateral salping-oophoretomy and omentectomy. It also may include radiation therapy, chemotherapy and clinical trail conservative unilateral salpingo oophorectomy is adequate. It appears that ovarian preservation and women's fertility is safe and reasonable in women of reproductive age.[44, 67]

Stage II: treatment of stage II may include surgery to remove the tumor (hysterectomy, bilateral salpingo-oophorectomy, and omentectomy). Combination with chemotherapy or radiation therapy gives approximately 85-90% five years survival. [44, 68]

Stage III: treatment of stage III may include surgery to remove the tumor (hysterectomy, bilateral salping - oophorectomy, and omentectomy) followed by chemotherapy or chemotherapy followed by second look surgery.

Stage IV: Treatment of stage IV ovarian epithelial cancer is combination chemotherapy with or without surgery to reduce the size of the tumor. Extensive surgery is often insufficient to eliminate the intra-abdominal tumor and response to chemotherapy is only partial in many of these patients[44].

1.8 Ovarian Tumor Markers

Ninety percent of ovarian malignancies are epithelial. [25, 69] There are quantitative and qualitative changes in numerous circulating substances which have been associated with epithelial ovarian cancer. These may reflect an alteration in ovarian function, surface molecular structure or general responses to malignancy.

Expression of specific antigens associated with epithelial ovarian cancer is useful for establishing a diagnosis, classification and providing prognostic information. Monitoring the appropriate antigen titers is very useful in the identification of occult metastasis, monitoring of therapeutic response and detection of asymptomatic recurrence at an early stage. [70, 71, 72]

The antigens defined on ovarian tumors are regarded as tumor-associated rather than tumor-specific [73]. Several tumor markers have been investigated for one or more clinical use in ovarian cancer as shown in table (1-5).

Table (1-5): Tumor markers that have been investigated in ovarian cancer [10].

Marker type		Example
Hormones		Progesterone [74], Estrogene, urinary gonodotrophin fragment.
Enzymes		Placental alkaline phosphatase[75,76] creatine kinase, amylase glactosyl transferase, ribonuclease
Oncofetal antigens		Tissue polypeptide antigen[77] alpha-fetoprotein ,carcinoembryonic antigen(CEA) [78] .
Carbohydrate markers		A:Mucin tumor markers: CA125, CA15-3 B. blood group antigens related cancer marker. CA72-4 [79] .
Genetic markers	Oncogene products	C- erb B-2 amplification HER-2/neu [80]
	Tumor suppressor genes	BRCA1[37] ,BRCA2 [38]

There are several tumor markers that correlate with the incidence of ovarian cancer, but the most important markers are:

1.8.1 CEA

Carcinoembryonic antigen (CEA), one of the onco-fetal proteins, is a cell surface glycoprotein, with a high molecular mass of 150-300 kDa. It is normally expressed in the early embryonic development and tends to disappear with the onset of differentiation of fetal tissue into adult ones. CEA has been studied extensively in ovarian cancer and has been reported to be elevated in 30-65% of epithelial tumors, mainly in patients with advanced stage disease. This antigen has been shown not to correlate well with status of disease. [81]

1.8.2 CA 19.9

CA19.9 is a carbohydrate antigen that is measured by a monoclonal antibody and can be found elevated in only 17-25% of patients with epithelial malignancies [82,83].

1.8.3 CA 15-3

CA15-3 is a mucin-like membrane glycoprotein recognized by a pair of monoclonal antibodies: the murine antibody DF-3 and 115D8 [64]. Distinct epitopes of this high molecular weight antigen (300-400kDa) [84] is the carbohydrate side chain which accounts for about 50% of its structure [85].

CA15.3 is found in adenocarcinoma of breast, lungs, ovaries and pancreas [86, 87]. Its level is elevated in 64% of ovarian cancer, it is most useful tumor marker for breast cancer [88].

1.8.4 IL.6 and IL.10

The interleukins, IL-6 and IL-10, have been shown to be present in very high levels in the ascites and serum of women with advanced stage epithelial cancers [89, 90]. IL-6 correlates well with the stage and status of disease, but is elevated in only about 66% of patients, and its complementarily with CA125 is only modest.

1.8.5 M-CSF

Macrophage colony stimulating factor (M-CSF) has been found to be measurable in the serum of 68% of patients with clinically detectable disease [91,92].

Interestingly, some complementarities with CA125 has been documented. Patients with clinically evident tumor and a negative CA125 (< 35 u.ml^{-1}), 56% had an elevated M-CSF serum level [92].

1.8.6 LSA

Lipid-associated sialic acid (LSA) can be measured in the sera of about 60% of patients with ovarian cancer, mostly those with advanced stage disease. A combination of LSA and CA125 improve sensitivity for detection of advanced disease but does not improve specificity [82].

1.8.7 OVXI

OVXI antigen is a high molecular weight mucin. The antigenic determinate of OVXI antigen was raised by immunization of mice with human ovarian cancer cell line. OVXI antigen is elevated in 67% of patients with clinically evident ovarian cancer who are CA125 negative. The OVXI is elevated however, in only 45% of patients with ovarian cancer. In patients with residual disease at second-look surgery and a negative CA125, 27% had an elevated OVXI level in the serum. [93]

1.8.8 NB 70 K

NB70K antigen appears to be present in most major types of epithelial ovarian cancer, with an apparent molecular weight of 70 kDa [94]. Among sera samples from ovarian cancer patients, elevated NB70K levels were found in 87% of samples that contained elevated CA125 levels. No quantitative correlation was found, however, between levels of NB70K and CA125. [94,95]

1.8.9 TAG 72

Tumors associated glycoprotein (TAG-72) level is elevated in 50% of ovarian carcinoma cases and only in 4% of benign disease cases with the highest level of expression in mucinous cystadenocarcinoma and its measurement may be useful as a confirmatory tumor marker for the presence of ovarian cancer in those patients with elevated CA125 serum levels. Combined TAG-72 and CA-125 test increase the sensitivity for the detection of primary ovarian cancer to 73% with no significant change in specificity [96].

1.9 Cancer Antigen 125(CA125)

1.9.1 Biochemistry

Cancer antigen 125(CA125) was first defined by monoclonal antibody (OC125) more than 20 years ago [53]. It was associated with a family of high molecular weight glycoproteins, that differed from classical mucins by means of carbohydrate conversion(less than 50%) and presence of both N and O linked carbohydrate residues [97,98]. Size exclusion chromatography of native CA125 antigen material from body fluids results in at least two broad peaks of antigen reactivity with approximate relative molecular mass of 200 and >1000 kDa,[99] but lower molecular weight species have also been reported.

Chemical study has revealed sensitivity of CA125 to proteases; low pH, high temperature, and high ionic strength, properties consisted of conformational peptide determinant. However, CA125 activity can also be destroyed with relatively high concentration of periodate and blocked with different lectins, suggesting a close association with carbohydrate. [97]

1.9.2 Structure

Although CA125 biochemical nature has long been elusive, its primary structure was established four years ago, indicating that it is trans-membrane protein with a short intracellular and a giant extracellular domain, the latter is with 22,097 amino acid residues. The extracellular part is composed of an amino-terminal part spanning 12,070 residues [100], followed by more than 60 tandem repeats of 156 amino acid motif and 229-residues linker to trans-membrane domain [101]. Both the amino terminal part and the repeat domains are rich in serine and threeonine residues and are highly glycosylated. The carbohydrate content was estimated to be 24-28%, with O-linked and N-linked glycans [102]. Because highly O-glycosylated repeats are the landmark of the mucin family of glycoproteins, CA125 was also named MUC 16 to reflect the nature of CA125 as a new member of protein family of mucins [103]. The mucin-like repeats contain a domain that was reported to be susceptible to proteolytic cleavage [104]. An additional potential proteolytic cleavage site in CA125 was reported to be located immediately membrane-proximal [101]. Figure (1-1) represents a proposed structure of CA125 antigen.

1.9.3 FUNCTION OF CA125

Although primary structure of CA125 has been elucidated, a functional role for this molecule in physiological context or in cancer remains unknown.

However, a number of publications have pointed out several properties of CA125 that may be of relevance for its biological function.

First, because of its expression in embryonic membranes and adult derivatives of the fetal periderm, CA125 has been suggested to play a role as a lubricant, preventing adhesion of membranes [105]. Anti adhesive properties have also been assigned to other mucins [106].

Second, close analysis of glycans present on CA125 protein revealed the presence of several glycan structures that have been implicated in immune suppression [102] raising the possibility that CA125 might help protect the embryo from maternal immune rejection and play an immunovasive role in ovarian cancer. Furthermore mucin can bind to various sugar-binding molecules, such as galectins [107]. CA125 was found to be a novel counter receptor for galectin-1 [108]. The known cellular responses to the cell-surface recruitment of galectin-1 include a change in proliferation activity, regulation of cell survival and regulation of cell adhesion. Depending both on the cellular context and its local concentration, galectin-1 exerts both inhibitory and stimulatory effects on these processes [109].

Third Gaetje et al. found that CA125 from human peritoneal fluid was shown to enhance the invasiveness of a benign endometriolic cell line EEC145, but it did not affect the invasiveness of a variety of non-endometrioid cell lines, raising the possibility that CA125 plays a role in endometriosis [110].

Recently, Rump et al. in 2004 [111] have demonstrated that mesothelin (a glycoprotein which is present in peritoneal fluid of ovarian cancer patients) [112] is a novel CA125-binding protein and they (CA125 and mesothelin) are co-expressed in advanced grade ovarian adenocarcinoma, which indicates that CA125 might contribute to the metastasis of ovarian cancer to the peritoneum by initiating cell attachment to the mesothelial epithelium via binding to mesothelin.[111]

1.9.4 Expression

CA125 is derived from celomic epithelium (pleura, peritoneum and pericardium), amnion and Mullerian duct during embryonic development. Trace amounts of CA125 are found in adult tissues derived from the epithelial lining of the pleura, peritoneum, pericardium, fallopian tube, endometrium and endocervix [98, 113].

Relative to the expression levels of CA125 found in normal tissues, CA125 is often overexpressed from epithelial ovarian cancer tissue and other tumors of non-gynecological malignances.[53, 114]

Although CA125 is expressed both by normal and tumor cells, cell surface expression and release of soluble proteolytic fragments of CA125 into the extracellular space [115] appear to be associated with the conversion from benign to cancer cells [116].

1.9.5 Developing The CA 125 Assay

The development of an assay for the CA125 tumor marker grows out of attempts of Bast et al [117] which aimed to obtain monoclonal antibodies for serotherapy of patients in ovarian cancer. In this attempt, mice were repeatedly injected with a human ovarian cancer cell line and hybridomas were prepared from immune spleen cells and the P3NS-1 plasmacytoma. From these hybridomas, clones were isolated based on the production of antibodies that bound to the ovarian cancer cell line used for immunization, but not to a B lymphocyte cell line developed for the tumor cell donor. The one hundred twenty-fifth promising clone produced an IgG1 antibody of the desired specificity and was designated as OC (ovarian cancer). [117]

Using immunohistochemical analysis, the OC 125 antibody was found to bind to antigen expressed by approximately 80% of epithelial ovarian cancer as well as by other gynecologic, breast, lung, and colon carcinomas: this antigen was designated as CA (cancer antigen) 125.[117]

The first monoclonal antibody radioimmunoassay for monitoring epithelial ovarian cancer, using OC125 antibody, was reported in 1983 by Bast *et al.* [53]. After that several different formats for the assay have been developed using radiolabeled or enzyme-labeled OC 125 as a probe. Over the last decade, a number of monoclonal antibodies have been developed that react with one or two distinct epitopes on molecules expressing CA125. One of these antibodies, M11, has permitted the development of a second generation assay, CA125II, in which M11 is used to trap antigen, followed by OC125 to detect antigen that has been captured on a solid phase [118].

1.9.6 Clinical Applications of CA125

The best available marker for epithelial ovarian cancer is CA125. The normal range most frequently quoted for CA125 is 0-35 u.ml^{-1}, although 99% of apparently healthy post-menopausal women have levels below 20 u.ml^{-1}. In apparently healthy pre-menopausal women, levels of 100u/ml or higher can occur during menses.[75] Elevation was also observed with the first trimester of normal pregnancy.[119] Although elevated CA125 levels are found in approximately 80% of all patients with epithelial ovarian cancer, high levels are found in only about 50% of stage I disease. [120]

This lack of sensitivity for early disease, and the fact that CA125 can be elevated in multiple benign disease such as endometriosis [121,75], limits the use of CA125 for the diagnosis of early epithelial ovarian cancer. Further limitation is that CA125 can be elevated in adenocarcinomas other than ovarian cancer. Although CA125 can also be elevated in germ cell tumors of ovary [120], the markers of choice for this type of ovarian cancer are $\alpha\beta$-fetoprotein (AFP) and human chorionic gonadotrophin (hCG) and its β-subunite (β-hCG).

1.9.6.1 Screening

The lack of early symptoms means that approximately 70% of the patients with ovarian cancer present with advanced disease. While the overall five- year relative survival rate is of the order of 30%, the survival rate for stage III and IV disease combined is only 10% [122]. In contrast, a five year survival of 90% may be achieved for patients with early stage disease confined to the ovary [123].

As a screening test, the main problems with CA125 are lack of sensitivity for early stage disease (only about 50% of patients with stage I have elevated levels) and lake of specificity. Thus, a single measurement of CA125 is not an adequate screening tool for ovarian cancer [124]. The rate of change in CA125 levels over time appears to be more specific screening method. In one study, the specificity reached 99.9% after redefining a positive test as CA125 concentration greater than 35 u.ml^{-1} was doubles within six months.[124]

CA125, however, in combination with transvaginal ultrasound may have the role in the early detection of ovarian cancer. This screening strategy achieved a specificity of 100%, and an apparent sensitivity of 81.7% [125]. Other reports have found that the use of tumor markers complementary to CA125 (eg. OVX1) is useful to achieve a specificity of 99.9% and an apparent sensitivity of 80%. Measurement of complementary serum markers can be used as primary screening technique followed by transvaginal ultrasongraphy. This could provide cost-effective means of early detection and could significantly decrease the probability of surgical intervention for false-positive test results.[126]

1.9.6.2 Diagnosis

The diagnosis of ovarian cancer is usually carried out by surgery followed by histopathology. However, pre-operative serum levels of CA125 especially in post-menopausal women, may be useful in the differential diagnosis of benign and malignant pelvic masses. Among post menopausal patients with a pelvic mass, a CA125 level greater than 65 $u.ml^{-1}$ has distinguished malignant disease with greater than 90% accuracy. The accuracy of CA125 (cut-off concentration 35 $u.ml^{-1}$) in differentiating between benign and malignant masses was 77%, which was almost identical to accuracy achieved with pelvic examination and Ultrasound (76% and 74% respectively) [127]. The combination of Ultrasound, CA125 and pelvic examination, however, improved the accuracy. Significantly, no cancer was found in any subject in which all three tests were negative. [127]

1.9.6.3 Prognosis (chance of recovery)

The traditional prognostic factors for ovarian cancer include tumor stage, grade, histological type and size of residual tumor after primary debulking (cytoreductive surgery). However multiple studies have shown that CA125 levels after either 1,2 or 3 courses of chemotherapy is one of the strongest available indicators of disease outcome [128].

A prolonged half life for CA125, or decrease in CA125 concentration of less than 7 folds of pretreatment concentration, during the early month of treatment, has been suggested to be an indicator for a poor outcome. CA125 concentration >70 u.ml^{-1} before the third course of chemotherapy was the single most important factor for predicting disease progression at twelve months [128].

1.9.6.4 Monitoring

The most important application of CA125 is in the monitoring of patients with epithelial ovarian cancer. Serial CA125 levels can pre-clinically detect recurrent disease with lead times of 1-17 months (median 3-4 months)[75,120]. Doubling of initially elevated CA125 levels has been associated with disease progression in more than 90% of cases [75]. Furthermore, longitudinal monitoring with this marker has the potential to detect recurrent disease earlier and more cost-effectively than radiological procedures [128]. While early detection of recurrent disease may lead to altered patient management, no study has yet shown that this leads to enhanced survival. The use of CA125 and other markers for monitoring, will attain greater importance, as more effective treatment becomes available for previously - treated ovarian cancer.

1.9.6.5 Treatment

Induction of specific immune responses by vaccination with murine monoclonal anti-idiotypic antibody (Anti-CA125), which imitates the tumor-associated antigen CA125, has a positive influence on the survival of patients with recurrent ovarian carcinoma. Patients subjected to this immunotherapy technique showed increased concentration of human anti mouse antibodies.

Specific anti-anti-idiotypic antibodies, as a marker for induced immunity, were detected in 66% of treated patients. Survival of patients with a positive immune response was 19.9±13.1 months in contrast with 5.3±4.3 months in those patients without detectable Anti CA125-immunity.[129]

The explanation of this specific immuno response caused by vaccination with anti-ioditypic antibody is that the variable antigen binding regions of antibodies (Ab1) contain idiotypic determinants that are immunogenic and induce the formation of so-called anti-idiotypic antibodies (Ab2), some of these antibodies are able to functionally mimic the three dimensional structure of original antigen, thus selective immunization with Ab2 could induce specific immune reaction directed against the original antigen. [129]

Antitumor vaccines were also developed by fusions of tumor associated antigens with dendritic cells. Human ovarian carcinomas express the CA125, HER_2/neu, and MUC1 Tumor associated antigens which are potential targets for the induction of active specific immunotherapy. Fusions of ovarian cancer cells to dentritic cells resulted in the formation of heterokaryons that express the CA125 antigen and dendritic cells-derived costimulatory and adhesion molecules. The fusion cells have been shown to stimulate proliferation of autologous T cell that induce cytolytic T-cell activity and lysis of autologous tumor cells. [130]

Chapter Two

Preliminary studies for the binding of ^{125}I- antiCA125 antibody to the CA125 in Human Sera and homogenates of benign and malignant ovarian tumors.

Abstract

Measurements of the two biochemical tumor markers CA125 and CEA were carried out in serum samples obtained from 30 healthy donors, 34 ovarian cancer patients (20 post-menopausal patients with malignant ovarian tumors (OI) and 14 pre-menopausal patients with ovarian tumors (OII) and 24 ovarian benign patients (OIII) using Immunoradiometric assay (IRMA) technique.

Mean values of CA125 in pre-menopausal patients with benign and malignant ovarian tumors and CEA in pre-menopausal patients with ovarian cancer were found to be significantly higher ($P<0.05$) than their corresponding values in sera of healthy control, while insignificant differences ($P>0.05$) between CEA values in patients with benign tumor and healthy control were found. In comparison between post-menopausal and pre-menopausal patients with ovarian cancer tumor, values of CA125 and CEA in post-menopausal were significantly higher ($P<0.05$) than those found in pre-menopausal group. The tumor marker CA125 shows the best sensitivity 80% for detecting ovarian cancer patients, than CEA, which gave 44% sensitivity. Also CA125 gave the highest specificity 100% for the ability of this marker to exclude normal individuals while CEA gave a specificity of 90%. The mean value of the ratio of CA125 level to CEA level in sera of ovarian cancer patients was found to be 87 in those patients with elevated CA125 concentration.

The binding of CA125 to ^{125}I-anti CA125 antibody in the tissue of benign and malignant ovarian tumors was preliminarily tested. The results showed that the supernatant fraction of the tissue homogenates contains higher CA125 level than the pellet fraction in all studied groups.

The effects of protein concentration, ^{125}I-anti CA125 antibody concentration, pH of the reaction medium, time of reaction and temperature were studied for the binding of CA125 to ^{125}I-anti CA125 antibody, in the tissue homogenates of malignant and benign ovarian tumors. The optimum conditions observed for the binding were as follows:

Optimum protein concentration in tissue homogenate was (225, 150 and 175 µ.ml^{-1}) for (OI, OII and OIII) respectively.

^{125}I-anti CA125 antibody optimum concentration was (450, 360 and 450 µ.ml^{-1}) for (OI, OII and OIII) respectively. Optimum pH was (7.2, 6.2 and 6.4) for (OI, OII and OIII) respectively. The optimum time and temperature was 240 minute at 4°C for all studied groups.

The use of different halides was shown to cause promotion effects on the binding of ^{125}I-anti CA125 antibody to CA125 in groups OI, OII and OIII except I^- in group OI. The studies also show that the use of different mono and divalent cations increases the binding in all groups except NH_4^+ in group OIII.

2.1 Introduction

The role of ovarian tumor markers is to enhance the clinician's ability to provide more effective management of the disease. CA125 was found to be the best available marker for epithelial ovarian cancer. This oncofetal antigen is found in the embryonic coelom epithelium and, later, in the derived fetal tissues. CA125 is not expressed, or barely expressed, on the epithelial tissues of the ovary but is found in serous adenocarcinomas of the ovary from which it is shed and can then be assayed in the blood [131].

CA125 has limited specificity. It has been reported that CA125 is elevated in approximately 1% of healthy women [27], 6-40% of women with benign masses (e.g., uterine fibroids, endometriosis, and pancreatic pseudocyst) [121] and 29% of women with non-gynecologic cancers (e.g., pancreas, lung, stomach, colon and breast) [53,108], while generally reported specificity in screening studies should be about 99% [132]. It has been reported that it may be possible to improve the specificity of CA125 measurement by either selective screening of post – menopausal women [124], modifying the assay technique, measuring other tumor markers beside CA125 [126], persistent elevation of CA125 level over time, or combining CA125 measurement with ultrasound. [125]

Serum CA125 concentration was determined by several methods including Immunoradiometric assay (IRMA) [53], Enzymeimmunoassay (EIA), Immunoflorometric assay (IFMA) [133] and enzyme-linked immunosorbent assay (ELISA) [134]. Today in commercially available CA125 assays, two monoclonal antibodies directed against different protein determinants in the CA125 protein core are used. Such antibodies seem to be less influenced by differences in glycosylation between different individuals and conditions [118].

CA125 has been used in the management of patients with ovarian cancer. It has been evaluated for its ability to determine diagnosis, prognosis, monitor therapy, predict recurrence of disease following curative surgery and treatment of ovarian cancer using immunotherapeutic strategies [135].

The objective of the present study was to evaluate the clinical application of biochemical tumor markers CA125 and CEA in the diagnosis of ovarian cancer. Also, this study was carried out in order to develop an immunoradiometric assay technique to determine optimum condition of ^{125}I-antiCA125 antibody binding with CA125 in ovarian tumor tissue homogenates.

Materials and Methods
2.2 Materials

2.2.1 Chemicals

All chemicals in this study were of analar grade, the specification of these chemicals are tabulated in table (2.1)

Table 2-1: Specification of the Used Chemicals

No.	Chemical	Company
1.	Immunoradiometric kit for CA125 antigen level. Immunoradiometric kit for CEA antigen level.	Immunotech (France)
2.	Tris buffer, Bovine serum albumin, $ZnCl_2$, $CaCl_2$, $MgCl_2$, EDTA, NH_4CL, urea and NaN_3	Fluka (Switzerland)
3.	$CuSO_4.5H_2O$, Na, K –Tartarate, NaOH, HCl, Na_2CO_3, NaF, NaCl, NaBr, NaI, $MnCl_2$, polyethylene glycol 6000 (PEG 6000) and Folin Ciocalteaue reagent	BDH (U.K)
4.	Blue dextran, Sepharose CL-6B	Pharmacia Fine Chemicals (Sweden)

2.2.2 Instruments

Table (2-2) Instruments Used and Companies

Instruments	Company
Gamma counter type 1270 rack Gamma II	LKB
Double Beam spectrophotometer	Shimadzu
pH meter	Pyeunicam
Sartorius analytical balance	Germany
Cooling centrifuge with maximum speed 5000 rpm	Hettich
SM shaker	England
Memmert water bath, Memmert incubator	Germany

2.2.3 Patients

This is a prospective study from November 2002 to September 2004 for 58 women admitted for surgical management of ovarian masses in different gynecological centers in Baghdad and southern Iraq matched with 30 healthy individuals.

Several points were taken into consideration, related to individual used throughout this study which includes the following:

(1) No evidence of liver disease.
(2) Not pregnant.
(3) Un smokers.
(4) Not taken any type of treatment.
(5) No oral contraceptive pill used.
(6) The time of taking the samples out of ministration period.

Patients included in this study were divided into three groups:

Group 1 consisted of 20 post – menopausal patients with ovarian cancer, group 2 consisted of 14 pre menopausal patients with ovarian cancer and group 3 consisted of 24 patients with Benign ovarian tumor. In addition to group 4 consisted of 30 healthy individuals.

The host information of all patients and normal healthy subjects is summarized in table (2-3).

Table (2-3): The host information of ovarian tumors patient and healthy subjects Studied.

Group	Patients	No.	Age	Type of tumor
OI	Post-menopausal malignant ovarian tumor	20	55-72	Serous cystadenocarcinoma
OII	Pre-menopausal malignant ovarian tumor	14	19-45	Serous cystadenocarcinoma
OIII	Benign ovarian tumor	24	22-46	Benign epithelial cyst (serous cystadenoma)
Control	healthy individuals	30	20-50	control

All patients were admitted for the treatment to (Medical City, Baghdad Teaching Hospital), AL- Habbibia General Hospital, Ibn Ghaswan Hospital (Basrah) and AL-Saadun private hospital (Basrah).

All surgical operations of tumor were carried out under the supervision of surgeons Dr. Fouad Al Dahhan, Dr. Luay Edward Kury and Dr. Amal Fatoohi.

2.2.4 Preparation of Blood Samples

Five milliliters of blood sample were obtained from patients by vein puncture just before surgery. Blood samples were left for 20 min at room temperature after coagulation; sera were separated by centrifugation at 1500 g for 10 min. Serum specimens were then frozen at -20°C until time of analysis.

2.2.5 Specimens Collection

The tumor tissues were surgically removed from ovarian tumor patient by either unilateral salpingo oophorectomy or total abdominal hysterectomy with bilateral salpingo oophorectomy. The specimens were cut off and immediately rinsed with ice-cold isotonic saline solution. They were collected individually in plastic receptacles and stored at -20°C until homogenization.

2.2.6 Preparation of phosphate Buffered Saline

Phosphate buffered saline (PBS) 0.1 M, pH 7.2 was prepared as the following:

A: Disodium basic phosphate (0.1 M); 1.419 g Na_2HPO_4 and 0.9 g of NaCl were dissolved in a final volume 100 ml deionized distilled water.

B: Monobasic sodium phosphate (0.1M); 1.1998 g of NaH_2PO_4 and 0.9 g of NaCl were dissolved in a final volume 100 ml deionized distilled water.

Phosphate buffer saline pH 7.2 was prepared by mixing a volume of solution A with appropriate amounts of solution B to obtain the required pH.

2.2.7 Preparation of Ovarian Tumors Tissues Homogenates

The frozen tissue was weighed, sliced finely and scalped in Petri dish standing on ice bath, and then homogenized with three fold volumes of PBS buffer pH 7.2, using manual homogenizer . The homogenate was filtered through four layers of nylon gauze in order to eliminate fibers connective tissues, and then centrifuged at 1500 g for 30 min at 4°C in order to precipitate the remaining intact cells and the intact nucleus. The supernatant fraction at this speed was separated and divided in a liquots and freezed at -20°C until use

2.3 Methods

2.3.1 Determination of protein concentration

Solutions

1. Standard bovine serum albumin (BSA), (0.2 mg/ml) as stock solution.
2. Reagent A: Alkaline carbonate solution (2% Na_2CO_3 in 0.1 N NaOH).
3. Reagent B: copper sulphate- sodium potassium tartarate solution (0.5% $CuSO_4 \cdot 5H_2O$ in 1% Na, K tartarate)
4. Reagent C: Alkaline copper solution, Mixing (50ml of reagent A with 1 ml of reagent B), discard after one day
5. Reagent D: Folin Ciocaltean reagent (1N) was prepared by the dilution of the commercial reagent (2N) with an equal volume of distilled water on the day of use.

Total homogenate protein's content was determined by the method of Lowry [136], using bovine serum albumin (BSA) as the standard solution. The details of the method are according to the following steps:

1. A volume of 1 ml of each of standard BSA (zero, 20, 40, 60, 80, 100, 120, 140, 160, 180, and 200) µg/ml was pipetted in a set of test tubes the experiment was carried out in duplicate.

2. A volume of 100 µl of ovarian tumors homogenate was also pipetted in test tubes and the volumes were made up to 1 ml with distilled water.
3. A volume of 5 ml of reagent C was added to all assay tubes. Then the contents were mixed by vortexing and allowed to stand for 10 min at room temperature.
4. A volume of 0.5 ml of reagent D was added drop by drop with mixing to all assay tubes the mixture was left to stand for 30 min at room temperature.
5. The absorbance of the developing color was read at 600 nm against the appropriate blank.
6. The standard curve was obtained by plotting the absorbance against the corresponding concentrations of standard protein and used to determine the unknown protein concentration of the sample (ovarian tumors homogenate) Fig (2-1)

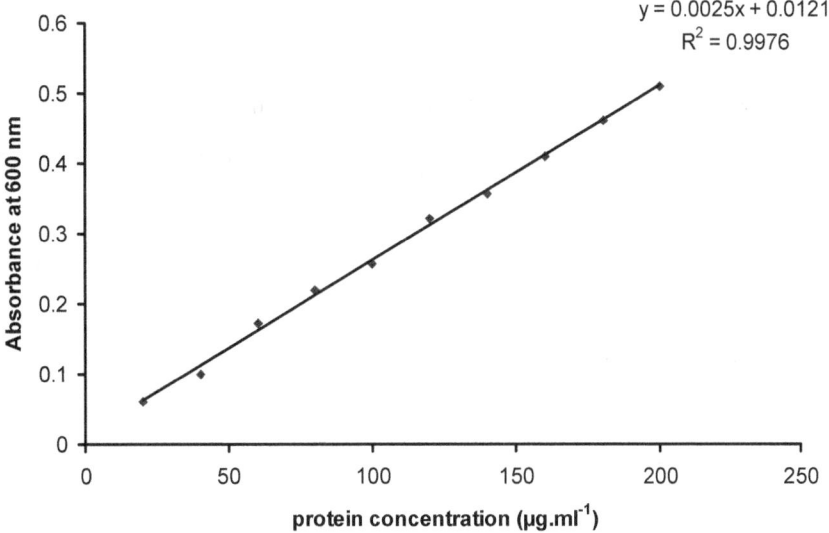

**Figure (2-1) standard curve of protein determination
(All other details are explained in the text)**

2.3.2 Determination of Cancer Antigen CA125 level in Sera of Patient with Benign and Malignant Ovarian Tumors

Serum CA125 levels were measured by immunoradiometric assay kit (IRMA) supplied by Immunotech (France).

IRMA – CA125 is a solid phase two-site "sandwich assay", utilizes to mouse monoclonal antibodies (OC125 and M11) directed against to different epitopes on the CA125 molecule. The M11 antibody is couted on polystyren tube (solid phase) while OC125 antibody is used as tracer after being radiolabelled with iodine 125. The CA125 antigen molecule present in the two antibodies.

Following the formation of the coated antibody/antigen/iodinated antibody sandwich, the unbound tracer is easily remove by a washing step. The radioactivity bound to the solid phase is proportional to the concentration of CA125 present in the sample.

Reagents

The following reagents were equipped with the kit:

1. Tracer: One vial (33 ml) contains less than 480 kBq of ^{125}I- labeled anti-CA125 in liquid form with buffer, BSA, NaN_3 (<0.1%).
2. Coated Tubes: Anti CA125 monoclonal antibody-coated tubes (100 plastic tubes).
3. Standard: 5 vials contain (0, 15, 50, 200 and 500 $u.ml^{-1}$ of human CA125 antigen).
4. Control serum: 1 vial (1.0 ml) of human CA125 in human serum with sodium azide (<0.1%).
5. Washing solution: 1 vial (50 ml): concentrated solution should be diluted with 950 ml distilled water before use.

Procedure

The assay protocol is described in table (2-4).

Table (2-4) IRMA assay protocol of CA125 u.ml^{-1}

	0	15	50	200	500	control	unknown	
							1	2 etc.
coated tubes no.	1,2	3, 4	5,6	7,8	9,10	11,12	13,14	15 etc.
standard (µl)	100	100	100	100	100			
Control or sample (µl)						100	100	100
^{125}I-anti-CA125 antibody* (µl)	300	300	300	300	300	300	300	300
	All tubes were incubated for 4 hrs at 25°C in horizontal shaker.							
	The contents of each tube were aspirated, and tubes were washed twice with 2 ml diluted washing solution except total count tubes.							
	The radioactivity bound in each tube were measured in gamma counter for 1 min.							

* 300 µl of tracer were added to 2 additional tubes to obtain total c.p.m

Note: Samples having concentrations greater than the highest standard were diluted with zero standard before assay.

Calculations

The specific binding of each concentration was measured by dividing the counts of each concentration on the total counts

$$(B/T \%) = \frac{\text{standard or sample mean count}}{\text{total activity mean count}} \times 100$$

The standard curve was generating by plotting the B/T% on vertical axis and the CA125 concentration of the standards on the horizontal axis (u.ml^{-1})

2.3.3 Determination of Cancer Antigen CEA level in Sera of Patient With Benign and Malignant Ovarian Tumors

Serum CEA levels were measured by immunoradiometric assay kit (IRMA) supplied by Immunotech .

Principles of the assay

IRMA – CEA is a solid phase two-site "sandwich assay ", utilizes to mouse monoclonal antibodies directed against to different epitopes on the CEA molecule. The samples or calibrators are incubated in tubes with the first monoclonal antibody in the presence of the second monoclonal antibody labeled with iodine 125.

After incubation, the content of tubes was aspirated and the tubes were rinsed so as to remove ^{125}I- antiCA125 antibody. The bound radioactivity was then determined in gamma counter. The CEA concentration in the samples was obtained by interpolation from the standard curve and was directly proportional to the radioactivity measured.

Reagents

The following reagents were equipped with the kit:

1. Tracer: one vial (22 ml) contains less than 640 kBq of ^{125}I- labeled anti-CEA in liquid form with buffer, BSA, NaN_3 (<0.1%).
2. Coated Tubes: Anti CEA monoclonal antibody-coated tubes (100 plastic tubes).
3. Standard: 5 vials contain (0, 1, 5, 20, 100 and 400) $ng.ml^{-1}$ of human CEA antigen.
4. Control serum: 2 vials contain CEA lyophilized in human serum.

5. Washing solution: 1 vial contains (50 ml): concentrated solution should be diluted with 950 ml distilled water before use.

Procedure

The assay protocol is described in table (2-5).

Table (2-5) IRMA assay protocol of CEA ng.ml^{-1}

	CEA standard in ng.ml^{-1}						Control		Unknown samples	
	0	1	5	20	100	400	Level 1	Level 2	1	2 etc.
coated tubes no.	1, 2	3, 4	5, 6	7, 8	9,10	11, 12	13,14	15,16	17,18	19, etc.
standard (µl)	50	50	50	50	50	50				
Control or sample (µl)							50	50	50	50
^{125}I-anti-CA125 antibody* (µl)	200	200	200	200	200	200	200	200	200	200
	All tubes were incubated for 2 hrs. at 25°C in horizontal shaker.									
	The contents of each tube were aspirated and tubes were washed twice with 2 ml of diluted washing solution except total counts tubes.									
	The radioactivity bound in each tube were measured in gamma counter for 1 min.									

* 200 µl of ^{125}I-antiCEA antibody were added to 2 additional tubes to obtain total count c.p.m

Calculations

The specific binding of each concentration was measured by dividing the counts of each concentration on the total counts

$$(B/T\ \%) = \frac{\text{standard or sample mean count}}{\text{total activity mean count}} \times 100$$

The standard curve was generating by plotting the B/T% on vertical axis and the CEA concentration of the standards on the horizontal axis (ng.ml^{-1})

Figure (2-3): Standard curve of CEA determination in human sera by IRMA method (All details are explained in the text).

2.3.4 Preliminary Test of CA125 Binding to ^{125}I-anti CA125 antibody in Ovarian Tumor Homogenate

Reagents

Tris buffer of 0.05 M, pH 7.4 for binding experiments was prepared according to the following:

Tris (hydroxyl methyl amino methan) 0.6075g, 0.1816g of EDTA, 1g Bovine serum albumin (BSA) and 0.02g sodium azide (NaN_3), were dissolved in 80 ml deionized distilled water and the pH was adjusted with HCl (1M) at pH 7.4 then the solution was completed to 100 ml with deionized distilled water.

Polyethylenglycol (PEG 6000) was prepared by dissolving 2 g in 10ml of Tris buffer (pH = 7.4, 0.05 M).

Procedure

1. Five clean and dry tubes were counted for their background using Gamma counter.

2. Twenty five microliter (450 µg.ml^{-1}) of ^{125}I-anti CA125 antibody (tracer) was added to each of five tubes denoted as

- First tube : Non specific binding without precipitating agent.
- Second tube: Non specific binding with precipitating agent.
- Third tube : Binding without precipitating agent
- Fourth tube : Binding with precipitating agent
- Fifth tube : Total c.p.m (T)

1. Filtrate of homogenate, 50 µl (337 µg) was added to third and fourth tubes.
2. The volume of all tubes was completed to 400 µl using Tris-buffer pH 7.4, 0.05 M except the T tube.
3. The tubes were incubated at 25°C for 4 hrs.
4. After incubation 400 µl of 20% polyethyleneglycol 6000 (PEG 6000) was added to the second and fourth tubes and the incubation was continued for further 30 min.

1. After incubation all tubes were centrifuged at 1500 g for 30 min. at 4°C except (T) tube.
2. The supernatant was aspirated, except (T) tube
3. The radioactivity in each tube was counted using gamma counter for 1 min.
4. The pellet of the homogenate was suspended in 1:3 Tris-buffer pH 7.4, 0.05 M, and the same steps mentioned above were repeated for the suspended pellet to determine the radioactivity of the complex.

Calculations

1. The counts radioactivity in tubes number 2, 1 (expressed in c.p.m.) represents the non specific binding (NSB) with and without using precipitating agent respectively.
2. The counts radioactivity in tubes number 4, 3 (expressed in c.p.m.) represents the sample count with and without using precipitating agent respectively.
3. (Sample counts-non specific binding counts) represents bound fraction (B).
4. The counts radioactivity in the tubes containing ^{125}I-anti CA125 antibody only represents the total counts (T). The (B/T) ratio counted as follows:

$$\frac{B}{T}\% = \frac{\text{Sample counts} - \text{non specific binding counts (NSB)}}{\text{Total counts (T)}} \times 100$$

2.3.5 Factors Affecting the Binding CA125 to ^{125}I-anti CA125 antibody in ovarian tumor Homogenate.

2.3.5.1 Effect of Different Amount of protein concentration of the tumor Homogenate on the Binding of CA125 with ^{125}I-anti CA125 antibody.

Reagents:

All reagents were prepared as described previously in section (2.3.4).

Procedure

1. Twenty five microliters (450 µg.ml^{-1}) of ^{125}I-anti CA125 antibody were read for their radioactivity and added to an increasing amounts of protein (37.5, 75, 150, 175, 225 and 300 µg.ml^{-1}) of the supernatant of (post-

menopausal malignant ovarian tumors "OI", pre-menopausal malignant ovarian tumors "OII", and benign ovarian tumors "OIII").

Then all volums were completed to 400 µl with Tris buffer (0.05M, pH 7.4).

2. The assay tubes were then incubated for 4 hrs at 25°C.
3. At the end of the incubation 400 µl of 20% polyethyleneglycol 6000 (PEG 6000) was added and the incubation was continued for further 0.5hr.
4. At the end of incubation, the assay tubes were centrifuged at 1500 g for 30 min at 4°C.
5. Supernatant was aspirated carefully.
6. The radioactivity of the complex was counted using gamma counter.

Calculations
1. The B/T % was calculated as described in section (2.3.4).
2. The B/T% was plotted against the increasing amount of protein of ovarian tumor homogenate

2.3.5.2 Effect of ^{125}I-anti CA125 antibody concentration on its binding to CA125

Reagents
All reagents were prepared as described previously in section (2.3.4).

Procedure
1. Increasing concentrations of ^{125}I-anti CA125 antibody (90, 180, 270, 360, 450, and 900 µg.ml^{-1}) were read for their radioactivity and then added to homogenate (OI, OII, OIII) containing (225, 150, 175 µg.ml^{-1}) respectively. Then all tubes were completed to 400 µl with Tris-buffer (0.05M, pH 7.4).
2. Steps 2, 3, 4, 5 and 6 mentioned in the experiment (2.3.5.1) were repeated.

Calculations

1. The B/T% was determined using the same mathematical equation mentioned in section (2.3.4).
2. The percent of binding was plotted against ^{125}I-anti CA125 antibody concentrations.

2.3.5.3 The Effect of pH on Binding of CA125 to ^{125}I- anti CA125 antibody

Reagents

All reagents were prepared as mentioned in section (2.3.4), except PEG 6000. PEG 6000 which was prepared in a set of different pHs (6.0-8.0) by dissolving 2 g of PEG 6000 in 10 ml of Tris-buffer of different pHs (6.0-8.0).

Procedure

1. Tracer (450, 360, 450 µg.ml^{-1}) were added to (225, 150, 175 µg.ml^{-1}) of OI, OII and OIII homogenate respectively.
2. Each reaction mixture was completed to 400 µl with Tris-buffer at different pH (6.0-8.0).
3. Steps 2, 3, 4, 5 and 6 of the experiment 2.3.5.1 were repeated.

Calculations

1. Values of B/T % were calculated as described in section (2.3.4)
2. B/T % was plotted against their pH values.

2.3.5.4 Time course of the binding of CA125 with ^{125}I-antiCA125 antibody in
   ovarian tumor homogenate

Reagent

All reagents were prepared according to the experiment in section (2.3.4) except 20% PEG 6000 solution which was prepared according to the optimum pH of each group (i.e. OI, OII and OIII).

Procedure
1. Tracer (450, 360, 450 µg.ml^{-1}) were added to (225, 150, 175 µg.ml^{-1}) of OI, OII and OIII homogenate respectively.
2. Each mixture was completed to 400 µl with Tris-buffer at the optimum pH of each group
3. All tubes were incubated at 25°C at different time intervals (0.5, 1, 1.5, 2, 2.5, 3, 3.5, 4, 4.5, and 5) hrs.
4. Steps 3, 4, 5 and 6 in the experiments (2.3.5.1) were repeated.
5. To determine the time course of CA125 binding to ^{125}I-anti CA125 antibody at different temperatures.

Steps 1, 2, 3, 4 and 5 in this experiment were repeated at different temperature (5, 37 and 45) °C.

Calculations
1. The same mathematical equation mentioned in section (2.3.4) was used to calculate (B/T) % at each time and temperature.
2. The (B/T) % values were plotted against the time of incubation at different temperatures.

2.3.5.5 Effect of Different Halides on the Binding of CA125 to ^{125}I-anti CA125
antibody.

Reagents

1. Tris buffer, that was prepared as described in section (2.3.4), was adjusted to corresponding pH for each group of tissue homogenate.
2. Halides solution was prepared in concentration of (0.01M) in Tris buffer at pH (7.2, 6.2 and 6.4) individually, by dissolving each of 0.021 gm of NaF, 0.0292 gm of NaCl, 0.0515 gm of NaBr, and 0.075 gm of NaI in final volume of 50 ml of Tris buffer and the pH was adjusted.
3. The ovarian tumor homogenates were prepared as described in section (2.2.7), except phosphate buffer was used instead of phosphate buffer saline at the same pH and concentration was used as homogenizer buffer.

Procedure

1. Tracer (450, 360, 450 µg.ml^{-1}) were added to (225, 150, 175 µg.ml^{-1}) of protein of (OI, OII and OIII) homogenate respectively.
2. Fifty micro liters of the following halides (0.01 M) (NaI, NaBr, NaCl and NaF) were added in each assay tube. (A sample without the addition of any salt was used as a control).
3. The volume of the mixture was completed to 400 µl with Tris-buffer at the optimum pH of each group.
4. The assay tubes were then incubated for 240 minute at 5°C for all studied groups.
5. Steps 3, 4, 5 and 6 mentioned in section (2.3.5.1) were repeated.

Calculations

1. The values of (B/T) % were calculated as described in section (2.3.4).
2. (B/T) % was plotted against the halide type.

2.3.5.6 *Effect of Monovalent and Divalent Cation on the binding*

Reagents
1. Tris buffer was prepared as described in section (2.3.4) was adjusted to corresponding pH for each group of tissue homogenate.
2. Monovalent and divalent cations salts were prepared in concentration of (0.025M) in Tris buffer at pH (7.2, 6.2 and 6.4) individually, by dissolving each of 0.0931 gm of KCl, 0.0668 gm of NH_4Cl, 0.2541 gm of $MgCl_2.6H_2O$, 0.1388 gm of $CaCl_2.2H_2O$, 0.2474 gm of $MnCl_2\ 4H_2O$, 0.315 gm of $CuSO_4.5H_2O$ and 0.1703 gm of $ZnCl_2$) in a final volume 50 ml of Tris and the pH was adjusted.

Procedure
1. Step (1) of effect of halide experiment was repeated.
2. Fifty micro liters of (0.25 M) of the following monovalent and divalent cations (KCl, NH_4Cl, $MgCl_2\ 6H_2O$, $CaCl_2.2H_2O$, $MnCl_2.4H_2O$, $CuSO_4.5H_2O$ and $ZnCl_2$) were added to each group of tissue homogenate.
3. Steps 3, 4, 5, and 6 in effect of halide experiment were repeated.

Calculations
1. The values of (B/T) % were calculated as described in section (2.3.4).
2. B/T % was plotted against each monovalent and divalent cations.

2.4. Result and Discussion

Three groups of ovarian tumors were included in this study. These groups were classified according to the type of ovarian tumors (benign and malignant) and the malignant ovarian tumors were again classified into sub groups (pre-menopausal and post-menopausal). Each type was examined histologically according to WHO classification system.

Homogenization of tissue samples was carried out in cold medium (4^0C) to avoid protein denaturation and to decrease the proteolytic enzymes activity. The filtration of the tissue homogenate through several layers of nylon gauze was used to remove any suspended piece of unhomogenized fragments and blood vessels, while the centrifugation of homogenate at 1500 g removed the unruptured cells and intact nuclei of ruptured cells.

2.4.1 Determination of Cancer Antigen CA125 level in Sera of Patient with Benign and Malignant Ovarian Tumors

CA125 levels in sera were measured with an Immunoradiometeric assay (IRMA) in three groups of ovarian tumors matched with one group of control subjects. Group I consisted of twenty post-menopausal patients with malignant ovarian tumors, group II consisted of fourteen pre-menopausal patients with malignant ovarian tumors and group III consisted of twenty four pre-menopausal patients with benign ovarian tumors.

The data of CA125 measurements in normal healthy individuals, benign ovarian tumors and malignant ovarian tumors will be presented separately.

Normal controls

Low levels of CA125 were observed in the sera of 30 apparently healthy women used as a control (Table 2-4). The mean CA125 levels (±SD) in this group was (11.9 ± 6.6 u.ml^{-1}) with an upper normal value of 35 u.ml^{-1}.

Table (2-6): Sera CA125 levels (u.ml^{-1}) in patients with benign and malignant ovarian tumors compared to the control group

Group	Patients	No.	Age range	CA125 assay u.ml^{-1}			P values
				Range	Median	mean ± SD	
OI	Post-menopausal malignant ovarian tumor	20	55-72	12-2300	288	512± 621	P<0.05
OII	Pre-menopausal malignant ovarian tumor	14	19-45	10-610	161	212± 200	P<0.05
OIII	Benign ovarian tumor	24	22-46	5-50	13	19.7± 13.93	P<0.05
Control	Healthy individuals	30	20-50	3-28	11	12.9± 6.6	

P – value ≤ 0.05 is consider significant.

A positive scoring or an abnormal level was indicated by those values of CA125 which exceeded the 35u.ml^{-1} limited [53]. All normal controls had CA125 concentration lower than 35u.ml^{-1} suggesting a test specificity of 100% for the ability of this marker to exclude normal individuals.

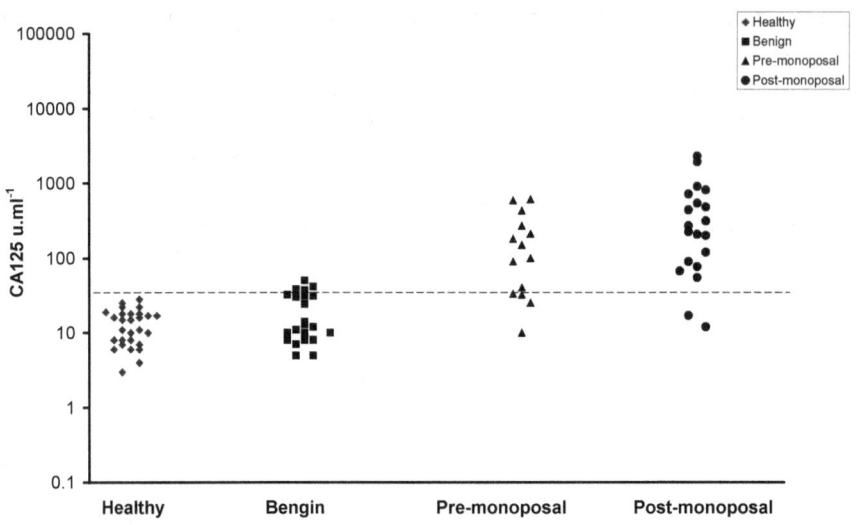

Figure (2-4): Distribution of CA125 value over different groups of patients and healthy individuals.
(All other details are explained in the text).

Benign ovarian tumor

Figure (2.4) shows that of 24 samples of patients with histological confirmed benign ovarian cases, four had level of CA125 above the cutoff value $>35 u.ml^{-1}$ (about 16%). The mean level of CA125 antigen (19.7±13.93) observed in these patients (Table 2-6) was significantly different from normal controls ($P<0.05$). Fleurn et al [137] explained why most benign cases have CA125 level below $35 u.ml^{-1}$ as that in benign ovarian tumor there might be an effective barrier between the antigen-producing neoplastic cells and the serum. Such barriers may play a role in the distribution of tumor antigens over various body compartments whereas in malignant tumors infiltrative growth lead to the release of antigen into the circulation [137].

Another explanation suggests that peritoneum serves as a barrier for high molecular weight tumor antigens, and lag in the transfer of CA125 from Cyst fluid through the cyst wall might be increased by the high molecular weight of this glycoprotein which has been estimated to exceed 200 kDa [137].

Slight elevation of CA125 serum levels in few patients with benign ovarian tumors may be explained by the observations of Bast et al which assumed that high antigen levels in cyst fluid might be able to establish a concentration gradient favouring diffusion of antigen into the lymph vessels and veins of the ovary[117].

Ovarian Cancer

The data in table (2-6) show that the mean serum value ±SD of CA125 in pre-menopausal malignant ovarian tumor patients (212 ± 200 u.ml^{-1}), was significantly higher than that in healthy control or patients with benign ovarian tumor. These results are in agreement with that found by AL-Barazanji [138] who obtained the same results using Mini VIDAS CA125 II kit.

Result in table (2-6) also indicates that there is significant difference between mean serum value ±SD of CA125 in post-menopausal ovarian cancer patients (512 ± 621 u.ml^{-1}) and that found in pre-menopausal ovarian cancer patients ($P<0.05$) that is the same finding of Malkasione et al study [139].

Data in table (2-6) indicate that determination of CA125 serum levels may be useful as a prognostic factor in the differentiation between malignant and benign ovarian cancer especially in postmenopausal patients. These results were in agreement with the observations reported by other investigators which suggested that among postmenopausal patients with pelvic mass, CA125 level greater than 65u.ml^{-1} indicated the presence of malignant disease with greater than 90% accuracy [134].

In table (2-7) the percentage of positive scoring of CA125 is presented in relation to menopausal status of ovarian cancer women. The post menopausal patients gave the highest percentage 90% of CA125 positive scoring, in comparison to the pre- menopausal patients with 71% sensitivity.

Table (2-7): positively of CA125 in relation to menopausal status

Menopausal state	No. of patients	No. of elevated CA125 level	% Patients with elevated CA125
Pre- menopausal	14	10	71
Post- menopausal	20	18	90

2.4.2 Determination of CEA level in sera of ovarian tumor patients

Tumor markers complementary to CA125 were mentioned as a useful method to improve the specificity of CA125 assay. A specificity of 99.6% and sensitivity of 80% were reported to be achieved using OVXI antigen as a complementary tumor marker to CA125 in the diagnosis of ovarian cancer. [126] CEA levels have been reported to be elevated in a high percentage of ovarian cancer cases (30-65%).[53] High ratio of CA125 to CEA in serum was suggested to be a useful method to differentiate ovarian from non-ovarian malignant diseases when both sera contain increased CA125 concentrations. [140]

Normal Controls

Low levels of serum CEA were observed in normal women (n=30) who had a mean value (±SD) 1.2±0.82 ng.ml^{-1} with the cut off value of 3.0 ng.ml^{-1} (Table 2-8), and a percentage specificity of 90%. These values are close to those obtained by other investigators. [141, 142]

Table (2-8): Sera CEA Levels (ng.ml^{-1}) in Patients with Benign and Malignant Ovarian Tumors Compared to the Control Group.

Group	Patients	No.	Age range	CEA assay ng.ml^{-1}			P values
				Range	Median	mean ± SD	
OI	Post-menopausal malignant ovarian tumor	20	55-72	0.9-15	2.8	4.1± 3.66	P<0.05
OII	Pre-menopausal malignant ovarian tumor	14	19-45	0.8-10	2.85	3.39± 2.35	P<0.05
OIII	Benign ovarian tumor	24	22-46	0.5-5.5	1.45	1.6 ± 1.37	P>0.05
Control	Healthy individuals	30	20-50	0.3-3.6	0.9	1.2± 0.82	

P – value ≤ 0.05 is consider significant.

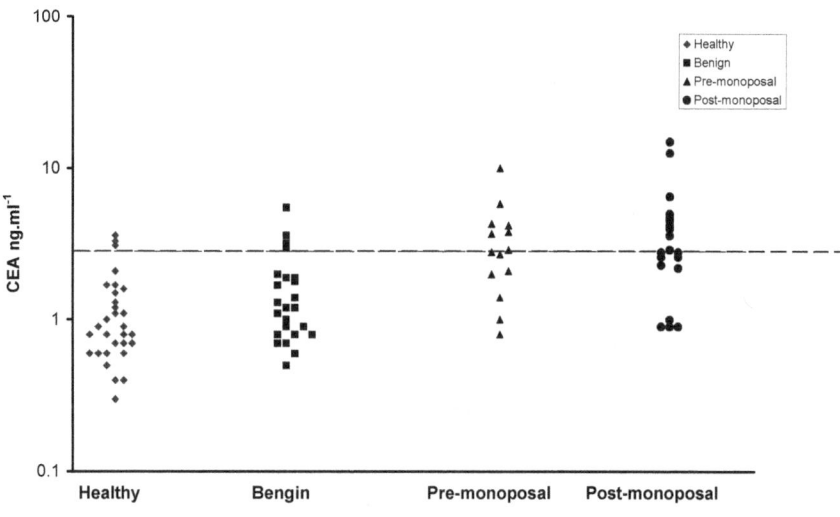

Figure (2-5): Distribution of CEA value over different groups of patients and healthy individuals.
(All other details are explained in the text).

Benign Ovarian Tumor

Of 24 samples from patients with histologically confirmed benign ovarian cases(Fig 2-5), four of them had CEA >3.0 ng.ml^{-1}. The other 20 patients gave CEA value <3.0 ng.ml^{-1}, which is not significantly different from normal controls (P>0.05).

Ovarian Cancer

The data in table (2-8) show that the mean serum value (±SD) of CEA in pre-menopausal patients with ovarian cancer is (3.39±2.35 ng.ml^{-1}) which is significantly higher (P<0.05) than their correspondent values in sera of healthy and that in patient with benign tumors, while there were insignificant differences (P>0.05) between CEA values in patients with benign tumor in comparison to their values in healthy control.

Table (2.9) shows that the rate of positive scoring was found not remarkably affected by menopausal states. It was 45% in post-menopausal states in comparison to 43% in pre-menopausal states.

The sensitivity of CEA tumor marker was found 44%, which is lower than that found by Donaldson et al. (60%) that may be due to different cell types included in each study. [143]

Table (2-9): positively of CEA in relation to menopausal status

Menopausal state	No. of patients	No. of elevated CEA level	% Patients with elevated CEA
Pre- menopausal	14	6	43
Post- menopausal	20	9	45

2.4.3 Determination of the ratio of CA125 level to CEA level in Sera of ovarian cancer patients

Of 34 samples from patients with histologically confirmed malignant ovarian cases, 29 samples contain increased CA125 concentration (85%). High ratio of CA125 level to CEA level in sera of patients with increased CA125 concentration were found 87, in comparison to 0.94 for non-ovarian malignances (colorectal, breast, lung, and pancreatic carcinomas), reported by James et al. [140]

This observation confirms the results found by James et al. which suggest that high ratio could be used to differentiate ovarian from non ovarian malignant diseases when both sera contain increased CA125 concentration, and that will really improve the specificity of the CA125 test for ovarian cancer.

2.4.4 Preliminary test of the binding of CA125 to ^{125}I-anti CA125 antibody in Ovarian tumor homogenate.

This part of the work was carried out to check the assay method in order to be able to find out the optimum conditions for CA125 binding to its specific antibody in our studied women. Supernatant and pellet formed at speed 1500 g in the three groups of human ovarian tumor homogenate (benign ovarian tumor, pre and post-menopausal malignant ovarian tumors) were used in this experiment. Table (2-10) shows the results of the preliminary test for the binding.

Table (2-10): Incidence of CA125 in Supernatant and Pellet fractions in the three fferent Ovarian homogenate

Group	B/T %							
	supernatant				Pellet			
	NSB$^-$	(NSB)$^+$	B$^-$	B$^+$	NSB$^-$	(NSB)$^+$	B$^-$	B$^+$
Post-menopausal (OI)	1.2	1.21	2.1	12.2	1.25	1.19	1.9	4
Pre-menopausal (OII)	1.07	1.1	1.1	5.3	1.1	1.1	1.13	1.6
Benign(OIII)	1.17	1.2	1.7	3	1.7	1.18	1.15	1.1

NSB$^-$: nonspecific binding in absence of precipitating agent.
(NSB)$^+$: non specific binding in presence of precipitating agent.
B$^-$: binding in absence of precipitating agent.
B$^+$: binding in presence of precipitating agent.

The results reveal that the supernatant fraction contains higher CA125 content than the pellet fraction according to the (B/T%) values, therefore the pellet fraction was discarded. Complex (^{125}I-antiCA125 antibody/CA125) formed did not precipitate in the absence of the precipitating agent . So it is necessary to use (20% PEG 6000) in the reaction mixture to precipitate this complex .

2.4.5 Factors Affect of ^{125}I-anti CA125 antibody binding to CA125 in ovarian tumor homogenates

2.4.5.1 The Effect of different amounts of protein concentration of the tumor homogenate on the binding with ^{125}I- anti CA125 antibody.

To obtain the optimum concentration of homogenates for the binding of CA125 with ^{125}I-anti CA125 antibody, the supernatant of the homogenate containing increasing amounts of CA125 were incubated with a fixed amount of ^{125}I-anti CA125 antibody, according to the details in section (2.3.5.1).

Figure (2-6) represents the quantities precipitation curve in which the amount of (^{125}I-antiCA125 antibody/CA125) complex in three groups (benign ovarian tumors, pre-and post-menopausal ovarian tumors) was plotted as a function of CA125 concentration.

The results revealed that the binding of CA125 to ^{125}I-antiCA125 antibody increases with increasing CA125 homogenate until a point of maximum binding was reached, thus the increase in protein concentration which would increase the number of binding sites until the saturation state. After this point as the amount of CA125 increased the amount of complex formed diminished that means the reaction behaves according to Hook effect which has ascending and descending phases at low and high antigen concentration [144]. The decrease in binding after reaching the maximum binding may be due to the conformational changes in CA125 and ^{125}I-antiCA125 antibody [145].

According to the results obtained in this experiment the amount of (225, 150, 175 µg.ml^{-1}) of tissue homogenate in groups OI, OII and OIII respectively were used in all subsequent experiments.

Figure (2-6): The effect of protein concentration on the binding of CA125 to its ^{125}I-antiCA125 antibody in ovarian tumors homogenates OI, OII and OIII (All other details are explained in the text).

2.4.5.2 *Effect Of ^{125}I-antiCA125 antibody concentration on the binding to CA125.*

The experiment was carried out in the presence of fixed amount of protein concentration of the homogenate and increasing concentration of ^{125}I-antiCA125 antibody.

The results are illustrated in figure (2-7) which represents ^{125}I-antiCA125 antibody binding with supernatant fraction of the three studied groups. As shown in figure (2-7) it is obvious that the amount of (^{125}I-antiCA125 antibody/CA125) complex rises gradually, and then the ovarian tumor protein was saturated with ^{125}I-antiCA125 antibody. When the amount of antibody is in moderate excess, the probability of cross-linking of ^{125}I-antiCA125 antibody to CA125 in the incubation mixture is more likely, and hence large complex formation is favoured then the maximum B/T percent was detected. After that the binding percent decreased as the amount of ^{125}I-antiCA125 antibody increased, the reason is that all antigenic sites covered with antibody and complex formation is inhibited [146].

According to the results obtained in this experiment the amount of (450, 360, 450, µg.ml^{-1}) of ^{125}I-antiCA125 antibody in the three studied groups (OI, OII and OIII) respectively were used in all subsequent experiments.

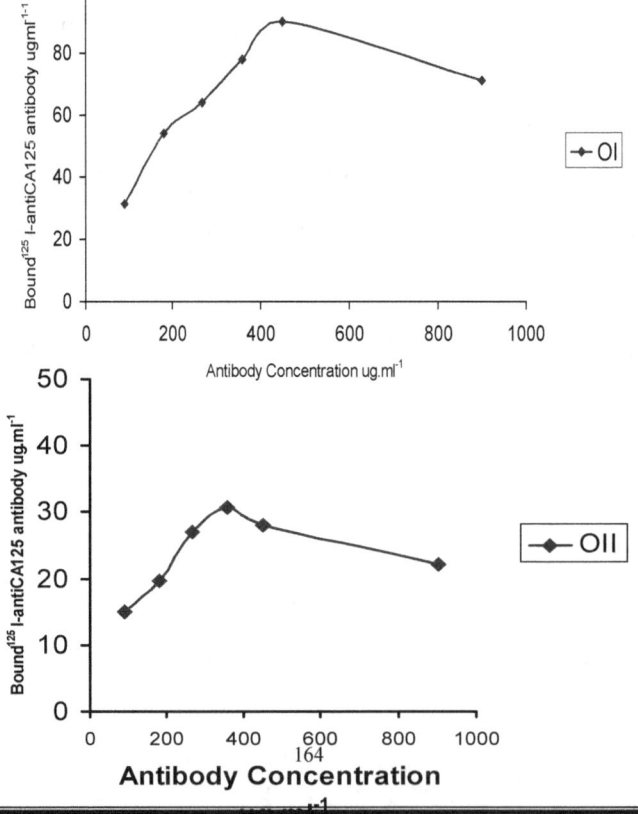

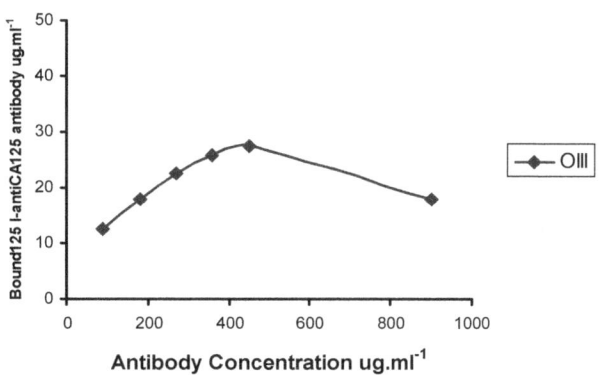

Figure (2-7): The effect of ^{125}I-antiCA125 antibody concentration on the binding with CA125 Antigen in ovarian tumors homogenates OI, OII and OIII (All other details are explained in the text).

2.4.5.3 Effect of pH on binding of CA125 with ^{125}I-anti CA125 antibody

Figure (2-8) shows the value of the binding of CA125 to ^{125}I-anti CA125 antibody in the three studied groups (OI, OII and OIII) at different pH values. Maximum value of the binding occurs at pH 7.2 for the binding of post-menopausal malignant ovarian tumors with ^{125}I-anti CA125 antibody and pH 6.2, pH 6.4 for OII and OIII groups respectively, these results are in agreement with many protocols developed to detect CA125 antigen in serum samples using immunoradiometric assay at optimum reaction pH around 6.0 [53, 97, 133]. These results indicate that the binding was pH dependent and the shift in the pH of the environment may affect the properties of CA125 molecules involved in the binding, this effect may include protonation deprotonation processes occurring within the possible ionizable groups of the amino acids present in the binding domain of these molecules [147]. In addition, ^{125}I-antiCA125 antibody itself may have ionizable groups and only at a certain pH the antibody will have ionic form where it can bind to CA125.[148]

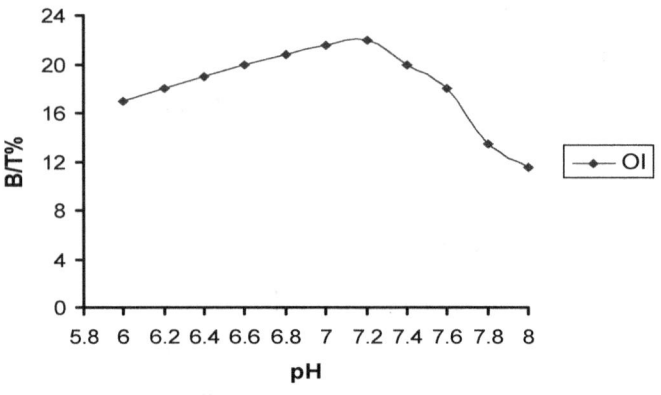

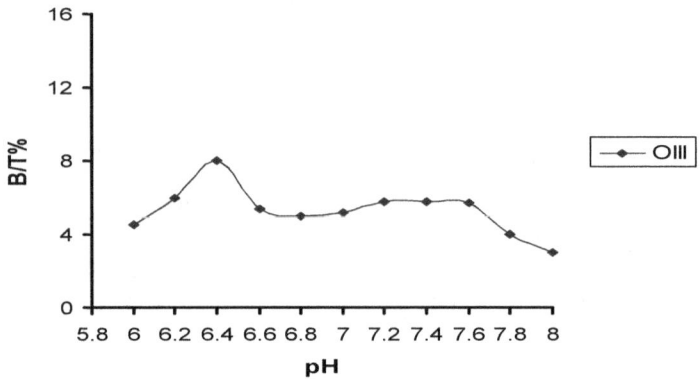

Figure (2-8): The effect of pH on the binding with CA125 to its ^{125}I-anti CA125 antibody in ovarian tumors homogenates OI, OII and OIII (All other details are explained in the text).

2.4.5.4 Time course of the binding of CA125 to ^{125}I-antiCA125 antibody in ovarian tumor homogenate

Figure (2-9) shows the time course of binding of CA125 to ^{125}I-antiCA125 antibody at different temperatures (5, 20, 37 and 45°C). The maximum binding occurred at 5°C after incubation for 4 hrs in crude fractions of post and pre menopausal malignant ovarian tumor and at 5°C after incubation for 4.5 hrs for benign ovarian tumor homogenate, in these states it seems that the energy is enough to overcome the energy barrier and give maximum binding[149].

The results indicate that ^{125}I-antiCA125 antibody binding to crude fraction of CA125 is temperature and time dependent process.

The decrease in the binding as temperature increase may be due to either degradation of CA125 or irreversible dissociation of the (^{125}I-antiCA125 antibody/CA125) complex at higher temperature, denaturation and destruction tertiary structure may occur leading to conformational changes and loss of activity.

The results obtained in these experiments were used in all subsequent experiments.

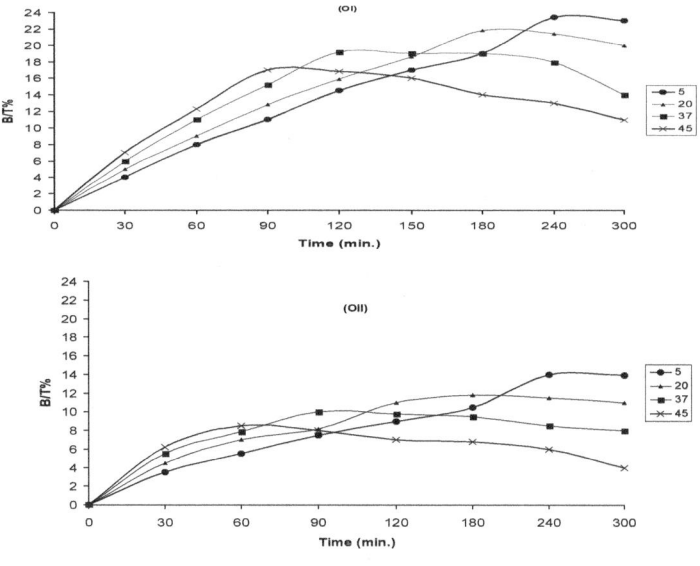

(2-9)

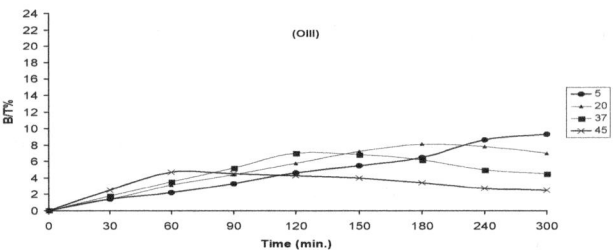

Time course of binding of CA125 to its ^{125}I-antiCA125 antibody in ovarian tumors homogenates OI, OII and OIII (All other details are explained in the text).

2.4.5.5 The Effect of Different Halides on the Binding

Figure (2-10) shows the effect of different sodium halides (i.e NaF, NaCl, NaBr, and NaI) at 0.01 M concentration on the binding of ^{125}I-antiCA125 antibody with CA125 in benign ovarian tumors and pre and post-menopausal malignant ovarian tumors.

It seemed that the sodium halides promoted the binding according to the following order:

NaI < NaBr < NaCl < NaF

The order corresponds to the decreasing ionic radius and increasing radius of hydration presumably, the lesser degree of hydration permits greater interaction of the salt with an ionic group located in the antigen or antibody. [11]

Melander and Horvath [150] reported that the capacity of the halides salt was due to the influence of hydrophobic interaction and dependence on the molal surface tension increment (MSTI), the halides with higher MSTI strengthens the hydrophobic interaction, while halide with lower MTSI values reverses this effect.

The magnitude of surface-tension increment depends on the interaction of salt ions with the surrounding water. High – lytropic series salts (kosmotropes) interact with water strongly; water molecules surrounding the salt ions are more structured relative to bulk water. Low-lyotropic series salts (chaotropes) break the structure of the surrounding water molecules (relative to the bulk water) as a result of the large size of the ion and its weak interaction with water. [151]

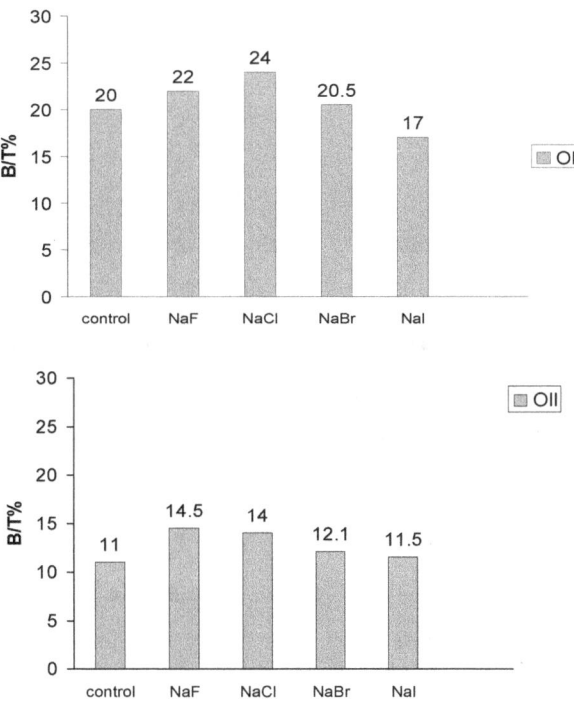

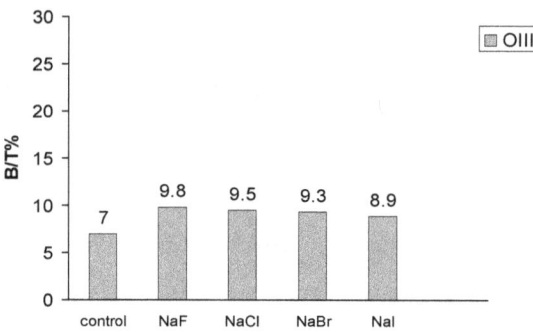

(2-10): The effect of different halides on the binding of CA125 to its ^{125}I-antiCA125 antibody in ovarian tumors homogenates OI, OII and OIII (All other details are explained in the text).

2.4.5.6 The Effect of Monovalent and Divalent Cations on the binding.

The effect of different salts on the extent of binding of ^{125}I-antiCA125 antibody to CA125 in benign ovarian tumors, post and pre-menopausal malignant ovarian tumors are shown in figures (2-11) and (2-12).

The result indicates that the presence of divalent cations (i.e. $MgCl_2.6H_2O$, $CaCl_2$, $MnCl_2.4H_2O$, $CuSO_4.5H_2O$ and $ZnCl_2$) at 25mM concentration increases the binding in different ratios in comparison to the control as shown in figure (2-11). Cu(II) increases the binding more than other divalent cations for the three tissues homogenates the reason may be due to electrostatic interactions.

In general, the mechanism by which these salts effect protein-protein interactions is not completely clear, one hypothesis assumes that salt may alter the nature of the hydrophobic forces controlling the stabilization of protein-protein complex formed and these vary depending on the nature of the interacting groups [152]. Results illustrated in figure (2-11) suggested that these salts may provide some conformational changes in the CA125 and charge groups of the binding domain of the antibody and antigen molecules.[153]

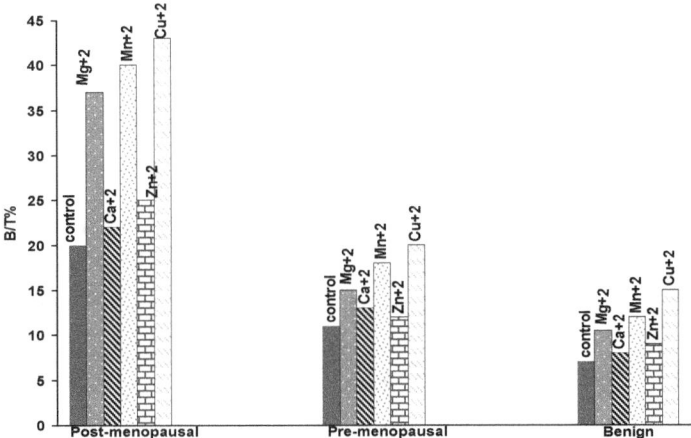

Figure (2-11): Effect of different divalent cations on the binding of ^{125}I-anti CA125 antibody with CA125 in ovarian tumors homogenates OI.OII and OIII (All other details are explained in the text).

Figure (2-12) illustrated the effect of monovalent cations (KCl and NH$_4$Cl) on the binding of ^{125}I-antiCA125 antibody to its antigen. KCl at 25 mM concentration was shown to increase the binding of the three tissues homogenates. While NH$_4$Cl at the same concentration seemed to increase the binding of post and pre-menopausal malignant ovarian tumor homogenates and slightly inhibited the binding 0f benign ovarian tumor which may be due to the presupposition that the lesser degree of hydration permits greater interaction of the salt with an ionic group located in the antibody combining site and then inhibits the complex formation. [11]

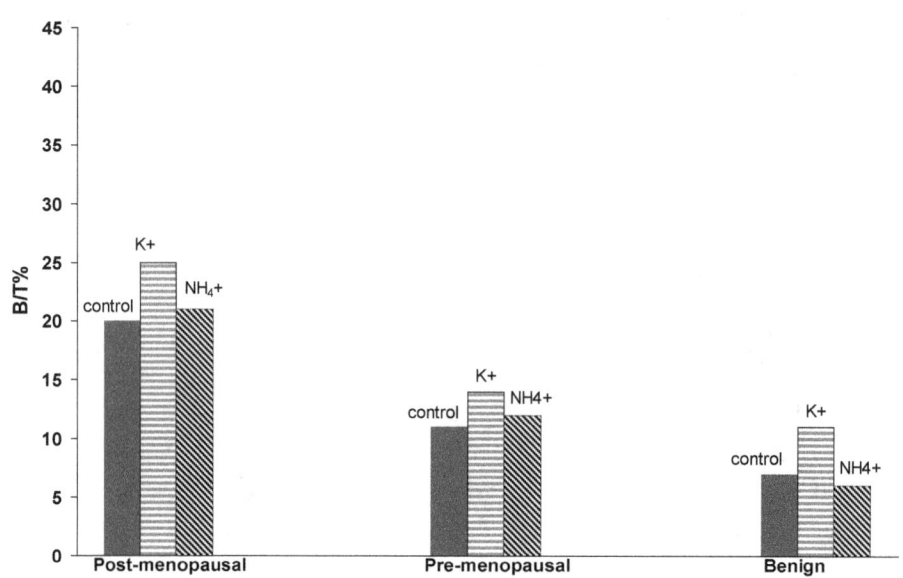

Figure (2-12): Effect of different monovalent cations on the binding of ^{125}I-antiCA125 antibody with CA125 in ovarian tumors homogenates OI, OII and OIII.
(All other details are explained in the text).

Chapter Three

Chromatographic purification of CA125 by Gel Filtration and Binding Characterization to Its Specific Antibody.

Abstract

Cancer antigen CA125 was partially purified from homogenate of malignant ovarian tumor by Gel filtration chromatography technique.

The results revealed presence of two forms of CA125 antigen (BI) and (BII) with molecular weight 670 and 100 KD respectively. (BI) form possesses a high affinity for the binding to its antibody ^{125}I-antiCA125 in comparison to (BII) form.

The elution volume (Ve) and the K_{av} values for elution of CA125 from Sepharose CL-6B column were calculated. The experiments of optimum conditions of binding between the two forms of CA125 antigen and ^{125}I-anti CA125 antibody were determined.

3.1 Introduction

CA125 antigen has been characterized as a high molecular weight glycoprotein aggregate with notable size heterogeneity ranged from 200 - 1000 kDa.

Many authors tried to isolate and purify CA125 from different sources like sera of ovarian carcinoma patients [94], ovarian cancer cell line (OVCA433) [97] and human milk, using size exclusion chromatography, affinity chromatography, gel electrophoresis and buoyant density ultracentrifugation techniques [97]. Another study found that CA125 antigen isolated from amoniotic fluid using gel filtration and anion exchange chromatography was composed of two subunits of approximately 240 and 180 kDa as detected by iodine 125-lablled OC125 monoclonal antibody. [154]

In this present study, post-menopausal malignant ovarian tumor tissue was used as a source for partial purification of CA125. The factors affecting the binding of partial purified CA125 to ^{125}I-antiCA125 antibody was also studied.

Materials and methods
3.2 Materials

3.2.1 Chemicals

All chemicals and reagents mentioned in section (2.2.1) were used in the experiments of this chapter.

3.2.2 Instruments

All instruments mentioned in section (2.2.2) were also used in the experiments of this chapter.

3.2.3 Patients

The tissues homogenates of post-menopausal patients with ovarian cancer (OI) were used in the following experiments.

3.3 Methods

3.3.1 Partial Purification of CA125 by Sepharose CL-6B Column.

3.3.1.1 Preparation of the Column

The dimensions of the column were chosen according to the following equation. [155]

$$\text{Diameter} = \sqrt[3]{\frac{m}{10}}$$

Where m = amount of protein in mg.

L = 30 x diameter

L = length of the column.

3.3.1.2 Preparation of the Buffer

Tris-HCl buffer of 0.05M, pH=7.2 containing 0.02% Sodium azide was prepared as mentioned previously in section (2.3.4).

3.3.1.3 Preparation of the Gel

Sepharose CL-6B gel was prepared by allowing the pre-swollen gel to swell again in Tris-buffer (0.05M pH 7.2) then left to settle and the excess of buffer was decanted. The step was repeated several times. The gel was degassed using evacuation pump and slurry was left for 24 hrs to equilibrate with buffer.[97]

The swollen gel was suspended and carefully poured into a vertical glass column (1.0x27cm) down the wall using a glass rod. After the gel has settled, the column was equilibrated with Tris-buffer for 24 hrs.

3.3.1.4 Void Volume Determination

The void volume of the column was determined by using blue dextran 2000 at a concentration of 2mg.ml^{-1} dissolved in Tris-buffer pH 7.2, and then the elution was carried out with the same buffer at a flow rate of 12 ml /1 hr at 10°C.

Fractions of 1 ml were collected and their absorbance was measured at 600 nm. Figure (3.1) shows the elution profile of blue dextran 2000. The volume of the buffer required to elute the blue dextran, which represents the void volume, was (10ml).

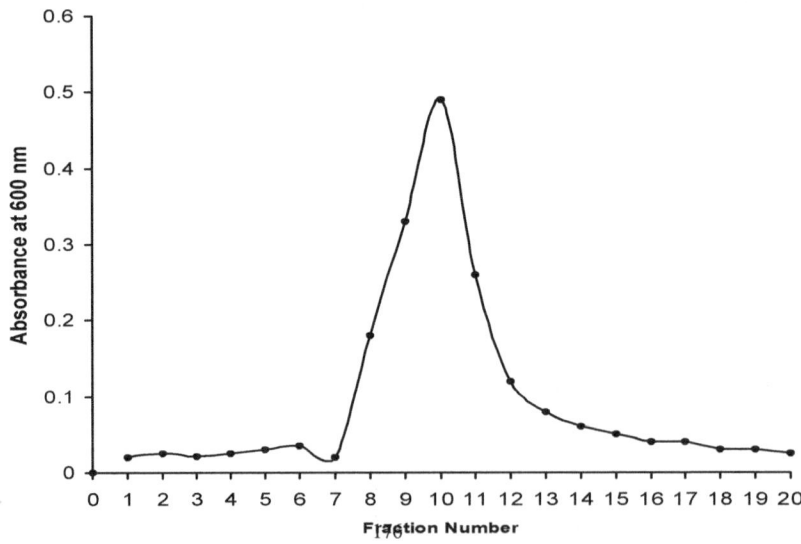

Figure (3-1): The elution profile of blue dextran 2000 using sepharose CL-6B gel, 12 ml/hr flow rate, Tris-buffer pH 7.2 and 10°C. (All other details are explained in the text).

3.3.1.5 Determination of the Molecular Weight by Gel Filtration Chromatography:

Pharmacia calibration kit for determination of M.wt by gel filtration was used. The kit comprises highly purified proteins individually packed. Each protein was reconstituted in 1.0 ml. Tris buffer pH 7.2. The standard proteins and their M.wt are detailed in table (3.1).

Table (3-1): Standard proteins and their molecular weights (All other details are explained in the text).

Protein	M.wt kDa	Conc.mg.ml^{-1}
Thyroglobulin	669	5.0
Ferritin	440	1.0
Catalase	232	5.0
Aldolase	158	5.0

Procedure

The same sepharose CL-6B column used in this section (3.3.1) was calibrated for molecular weight determination. Standard protein solutions were prepared according to the manufacturer instruction, then applied through two portions (0.5ml/portion), thyroglobulin and catalase in the first, Ferritin and Aldolase in the second. Elution was carried out with Tris buffer pH 7.2 at a flow rate 12 ml/hr at 10°C. The absorbencies of the fractions collected were measured at 280 nm to evaluate the elution volume (Ve) of the standard proteins.

Calculations

The Kav of the proteins eluted were determined using the following equation [156]

$$Kav = \frac{Ve - V_O}{Vt - V_O}$$

Where:

V_0 = void volume

V_e = Elution volume

V_t = Total gel bed volume, which was calculated according o the following:

$$V_t = \left(\frac{d}{2}\right)^2 \times 3.14 \times h \qquad (d=1.0 \text{ cm}, h= 27 \text{ cm})$$

The calibration curve of Kav against log M.wt of the proteins was plotted.

3.3.1.6 Separation of CA125 from Malignant postmenopausal Ovarian Tumor

Homogenate

Tris-buffer (0.05M, pH7.2) containing 0.02% Sodium azide was prepared as described previously in section (2.3.4.).

Procedure

The sample of tissue homogenate (500μl) containing approximately 7.8mg protein was applied to the surface of the gel, equilibrated with Tris-buffer 0.05M, pH 7.2 the sample was eluted using the same buffer with flow rate of 12ml/hr and fractions volume of 1ml each were collected. Gel filtration was carried out at 10°C and the absorbance of each fraction was measured at 280 nm.

The fractions that contained CA125 antigen was identified by the assay method as follows:

1-   Twenty five micro liters (450 µg.ml^{-1}) of ^{125}I-antiCA125 antibody was added to 100µl of each fraction number of post-menopausal malignant ovarian tumor homogenate. Then all tubes were completed to 400µl with Tris-buffer (0.05M, pH 7.2).

2-   Steps 2, 3, 4, 5, and 6 mentioned in experiment (2.3.5.1) were repeated.

Calculations

1-   The absorbance of each fraction was determined at 280 nm.

2-   The value of B/T ratio for the eluted fractions was calculated as mentioned in section 2.3.4.

3-   The values of B/T ratio and the absorbencies at 280nm were plotted against the fraction number.

3.3.1.7 Dialysis for Concentration

After preparing dialysis tube, the fractions that contained high level of the binding activity were pooled and concentrated by dialyzing against sucrose at 4°C for 3hrs to get the required concentration to be used in the next experiments.

3.4 Determination of the optimum Reaction Conditions for the Binding of the partially purified CA125 antigen to ^{125}I-antiCA125 antibody.

The optimum reaction conditions for the binding of partially purified CA125 to its ^{125}I-antiCA125 antibody were studied using the same experiments mentioned for the factors affecting the binding in chapter 2.

3.5 Results and Discussion

3.5.1. Partial Purification of CA125

Partial purification of CA125 was performed by gel exclusion chromatography technique. Post-menopausal malignant ovarian tumor homogenate (OI) was applied to sepharose CL-6B (1.0x27cm) column. The void volume (Vo) of this column was (10ml) as predicted from the elution profile of the blue dextran figure (3-1).

Figure (3-2) shows the elution profile for (OI) homogenate after measuring the absorbance of collected fractions at 280 nm. It gave three main peaks separated according to their molecular weight, their fractions number were 10, 19 and 28.

The binding reaction that was carried out for the collected fractions gave two peaks (BI&BII) at fraction number 11 and the fraction number 21 for BI & BII respectively, as shown in figure (3-2). The resultant fractions containing the binding activity of CA125 were collected, pooled and concentrated then subjected to protein determination as described in section (2.3.1).

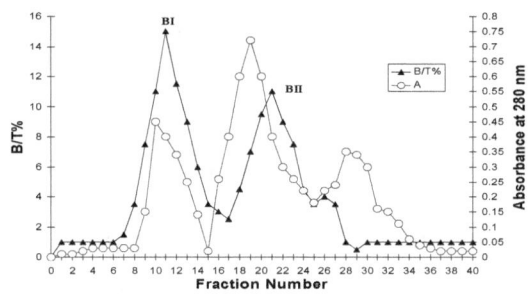

**Figure (3-2): The elution profile of human CA125 from post-menopausal malignant ovarian tumor using sepharose CL-6B gel, 12ml/hr flow rate, Tris-buffer pH 7.2, at 10°C.(All other details are

explained in the text).

Different standard proteins of known molecular weights were used to determine the molecular weight of the isolated antigens. The elution volumes (Ve) of standard proteins are shown in figure (3-3). The Kav values for these standard proteins were calculated by using the formula represented in section (3.3.1.4) and the calibration curve was plotted between Kav values of the standard proteins versus their logarithmic molecular weight as shown in figure (3-4).

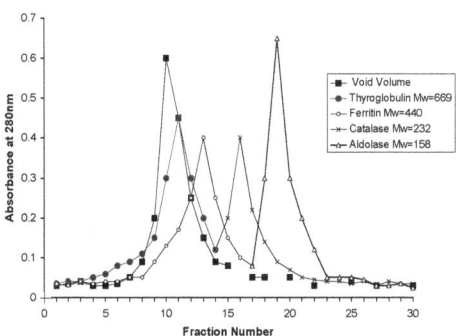

Figure (3-3) The elution profile of standard proteins using sepharose CL-6B
gel, 12 ml/hr flow rate, Tris-buffer pH 7.2, at 10°C. (All other details are explained in the text.

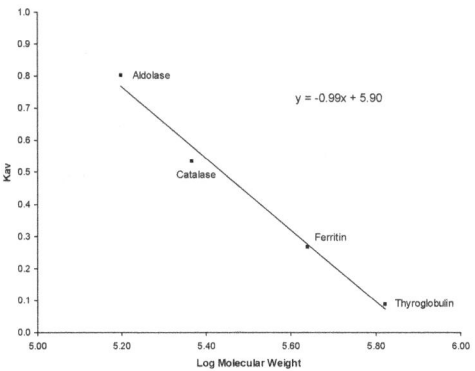

Figure (3-4) Calibration curve for determination of M.wt by gel filtration chromatography (All other details are explained in the text).

The straight line equation generated from this plot (figure 3.4) was used for the determination of the molecular weight of partially purified CA125. The results shows that both forms have high molecular weight where the first BI has 670 kDa and the second (BII) has 100 kDa. These results may be explained according to the idea that the lower molecular weight antigen (BII) is considered a breakdown product of a high molecular weight species and therefore contains the same antigenic determinants [154,157]. On the other hand high molecular antigen (BI) may be explained according to that CA125 has high molecular mass aggregate. The size exclusion of native CA125 from body fluids gave at least two broad peaks reactivity of 200 and > 1000kDa molecular weight. [99]

3.5.2 Determination of the Optimum Reaction Conditions for the Binding of Partially Purified CA125 to ^{125}I- antiCA125 antibody

3.5.2.1. Optimum protein concentration

Figure (3-5) shows the effect of increasing amount of partially purified CA125 (BI & BII) to fixed amount of ^{125}I-anti CA125-antibody to produce (^{125}I-antiCA125 antibody/ CA125) complex. The shape of the curve is similar to that obtained for the crude CA125, the figure shows that the amount of partially purified CA125 needed to reach maximum binding with ^{125}I-antiCA125-antibody as 90, 110 µg.ml^{-1} which is less than the amount needed for crude extract (225 µg.ml^{-1}).

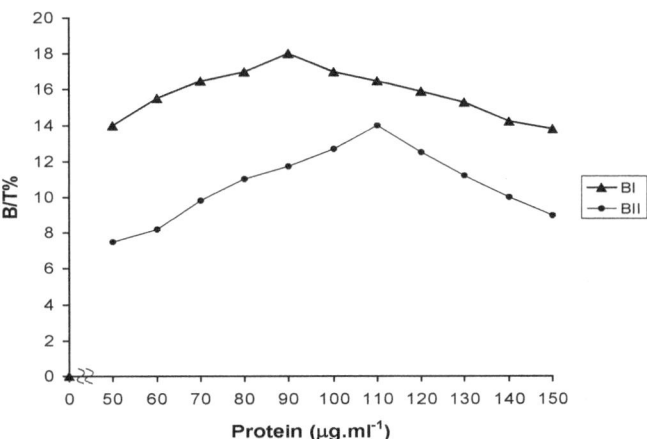

Figure (3-5): The effect of protein concentration on the binding of ^{125}I-anti CA125 antibody with partially purified CA125 (BI and BII) (All other details are explained in the text).

3.5.2.2. Optimum ^{125}I- anti CA125-antibody Concentration.

Figure (3-6) illustrates the effect of increasing ^{125}I-antiCA125 antibody concentration on the binding with partially purified forms of CA125 (BI & BII). The maximum binding obtained when 360 µg.ml^{-1} for (BI) and 450 µg.ml^{-1} for (BII) were used. From these result it was found that partially purified CA125 (BI) form was saturated with small concentration of ^{125}I-antiCA125 antibody than those required for BII. Thus it was concluded that BI has higher affinities at low concentrations toward ^{125}I-antiCA125 antibody than BII.

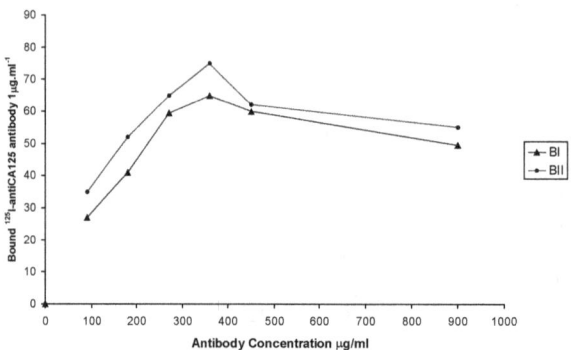

Figure (3-6): The effect of ^{125}I-antiCA125 antibody concentration on the binding with partially purified CA125 (BI and BII)(All other details are explained in the text).

3.5.2.3. Optimum pH

Figure (3-7) shows the effect of pH on binding of ^{125}I-antiCA125 antibody to partially purified CA125 (BI&BII) of post-menopausal malignant ovarian tumor homogenate. The results revealed that the optimum pH for (BI) and (BII) was 6.8 and 7.2 respectively. These results indicate that the binding was pH dependent and the differences in the optimum pHs may suggest the differences in the binding sites of these partially purified antigens [158].

3.5.2.4 The time course of the binding of partially purified CA125 (BI &BII)

to ^{125}I- antiCA125 antibody.

The optimum time and temperature for partially purified CA125 (BI and BII) was studied. Figures (3-8) and (3-9) show that the (BI) form antigen binds to its specific antibody in highest state after 180 min at 5°C, while BII form reach the maximum binding after 210 min at 5°C.

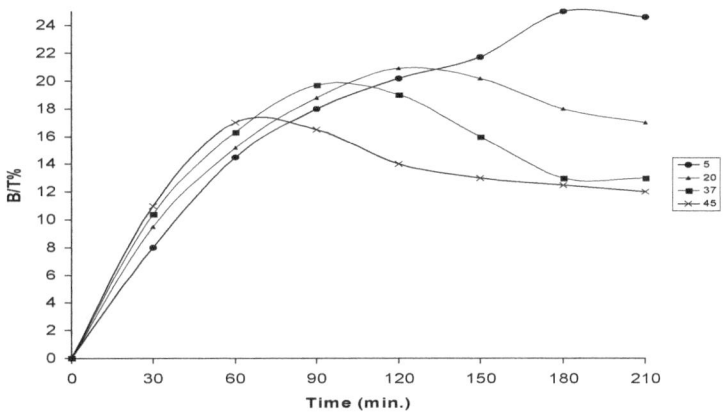

Figure (3-8): Time course of binding of ^{125}I-antiCA125 antibody with partially purified CA125 (BI) (All details are explained in the text).

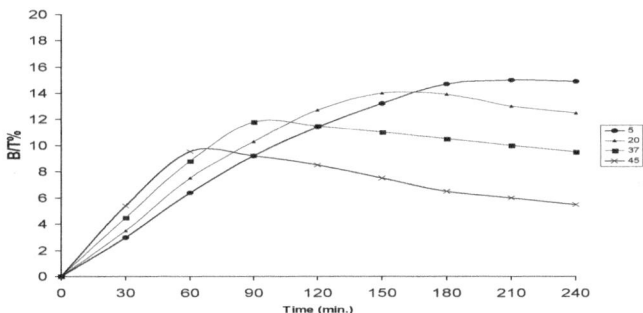

Figure(3-9): Time course of binding of ^{125}I-antiCA125 antibody with partially purified CA125 (BII)(All details are explained in the text).

In comparison with crude homogenate, the time was shortened for both BI & BII from 240 minutes for the crude homogenate to 180 and 210 minutes for BI & BII respectively. A possible explanation for the fast kinetics of complex formation with partial purified antigen may be due to losing of inhibitory factors, by exclusive gel filtration process. This in turn affects the rate of complex formation between CA125 and its specific antibody

Chapter Four

Kinetic & Thermodynamic Studies of the Binding of CA125 with ^{125}I-antiCA125 antibody in Ovarian Tumor Homogenates

Abstract

Kinetic and thermodynamic parameters associated with the binding of ^{125}I-anti125 antibody to crude CA125 of benign, post and pre-menopausal malignant ovarian tumors and with partially purified CA125 (BI) and (BII) forms of post-menopausal malignant ovarian tumor were carried out using different rate equations. Then the order of the reactions were tested. It was showed that the reaction in all groups follow second rate law. In addition, the kinetic parameters K_a, K_d, k_{+1}, k_{-1}, $t_{1/2}$ of association and dissociation were determined at 5, 20, 37 and 45°C. In all studied groups the affinity constant (K_a) and maximum binding capacity (B_{max}) decrease and their rate constant (k_{+1}) values increase with increasing temperature. Scatchared plots of all groups showed no curvature in the plotted lines, where the data obeyed the straight line equation suggested that the CA125 has a single binding site or more than one site with identical affinities. The thermodynamics of the binding of ^{125}I-antiCA125 antibody with CA125 for all groups were studied using Van't Hoff and Arrhenius equations, the thermodynamic parameters of standard state ($\Delta H°$, $\Delta G°$ and $\Delta S°$) were determined. The data showed that the binding reactions were exothermic ($\Delta H°<0$) and spontaneous ($\Delta G°<0$) and the binding reactions were entropically and enthalpically driven ($\Delta S°>0$ and $\Delta H°<0$). Arrhenius plot indicated that there was a linear- relationship between log k_{+1} and 1/T. The transition state thermodynamic parameters (Ea, ΔH^*, ΔG^* and ΔS^*) for the formation of (^{125}I-anti CA125 antibody/CA125) were determined.

Kinetic & Thermodynamic Studies of the Binding of CA125 with ^{125}I-antiCA125 antibody in Ovarian Tumor Homogenates

4.1 Introduction

Molecular interactions involve cooperative, independent and contiguous binding regions. Molecular interaction generates dynamic structural changes, which increase the complexity of these interactions. The rate of the reaction and equilibrium conditions is the algebraic sum of the energies involved in reversible macromolecular interactions [160]. The specific reaction between antibody and antigen, as a type of these interactions, is usually driven by electrostatic forces between oppositely charged amino acids, hydrogen bonding, and hydrophobic interactions. The equilibrium reaction termed "biospecific interaction" is characterized by the affinity of the reaction to form Antibody- Antigen complex. [161]

The analysis of temperature dependence of kinetic and equilibrium constants allows determination of the energetic of binding. The changes in Gibes free energy, enthalpy and entropy that are associated with the binding of antibody to its antigen can be calculated mathematically using such constant [162].

In other words, thermodynamic measurements of reactions interactions under equilibrium conditions provide information about differences between the initial and final states of each reactant, while kinetics studies supplement the information on the differences between these states and an intermediate activated complex state, (i.e. the pathway taken by the reactants to reach the final product).[163,164]

The elucidation of biomolecular interactions is of steadily increasing importance. Exact knowledge of the principles governing the strengths and formation of molecular interaction is of highest importance for a huge number of applications in widely different areas, such as : The design of new drugs, the understanding of cross-reactions of antibodies used in medical diagnosis or medical treatment, the improvement of our understanding in diseases, the understanding and regulation of biocatalytic activity, the understanding cell-cell communication and cell differentiation, ...etc.

In this chapter, the basic mathematical analysis was described and used to explain the mechanism, through kinetics and thermodynamic, of binding of CA125 antibody to its CA125 antigen in benign, post-and pre-menopausal malignant ovarian tumor homogenates and to its partially purified forms (BI) and (BII) to form (^{125}I-antiCA125 antibody/CA125) complex.

Materials and Methods
4.2 Materials

4.2.1 Chemicals

All chemicals and reagents mentioned in section (2.2.1) were used in the experiments of this chapter.

4.2.2 Instruments

All instruments mentioned in section (2.2.2) were also used in the experiments of this chapter.

4.3 Methods

4.3.1. Kinetic Studies

4.3.1.1 Time course of Binding

A. The time course of the binding of ^{125}I-antiCA125 antibody with CA125 in ovarian tumor homogenate

Reagents

All reagents were prepared according to section (2.3.4) except 20% PEG6000 which was prepared according to the optimum pH of each group.

Procedure

1. Tracer (450, 360 and 450) µg.ml^{-1} were added to (225, 150 and 175 µg.ml^{-1} protein) of OI, OII and OIII respectively.
2. Each mixture was completed to 400µl with Tris-buffer at the optimum pH of each group.
3. All tubes were incubated at 5°C at different time intervals (30, 60, 90, 120, 150, 210, 240, 270 and 300) minutes.
4. Steps 3, 4, 5, and 6 in the section (2.3.5.1.) were repeated.
5. To determine the time course of CA125 binding to ^{125}I-antiCA125 antibody at different temperatures. Steps 1, 2, 3 and, 4 in this experiment were repeated at (20, 37 and 45°C).

Calculations

The B/T% values were calculated as described in section (2.3.4.) and plotted against incubation time at different temperatures.

B. The time course of binding of ^{125}I-antiCA125 antibody with partially purified forms (BI) and BII of malignant ovarian tumor.

Reagent

All reagents were prepared according to the section (2.3.3.) except for 20% PEG 6000 which was prepared according to optimum pH of each group.

Procedure

1. Tracer (360 and 450) µg.ml^{-1} were added to 90 and 110 µg.ml^{-1} protein) of BI and BII respectively.
2. Each mixture was completed to 400µl with Tris-buffer at optimum pH of each group.

3. The (^{125}I-antiCA125 antibody/CA125) complex for each group were estimated by following steps 3 and 4 in section 4.3.1.1.A

4. The experiment was repeated at different temperatures (20, 37 and 45°C).

Calculations

The B/T% values were calculated as described in section (2.3.4) and plotted against incubation time at different temperatures.

4.3.1.2. Determination of Kinetic parameters

A. Determination of the affinity constant (K_d) and maximal binding capacity (B_{max}) of ^{125}I-antiCA125 antibody associated with CA125 in ovarian tumor homogenates.

1. Increasing volumes (4, 8, 12, 16 and 20 μl) of ^{125}I-antiCA125 antibody containing (72, 144, 216, 288, and 360 μg.ml^{-1} protein) respectively was added to each (150 μg.ml^{-1}) of pre-menopausal malignant ovarian tumor homogenate. Then the final reaction volume was completed to 400μl with the same buffer.

2. All tubes were incubated at 5°C for 240 minutes.

3. The (^{125}I-antiCA125 antibody/CA125) complex was estimated by following the steps 3, 4, 5, and 6 in the section (2.3.5.1.)

4. The previous steps were performed at different temperature (20, 37 and 45°C).

5. The experiment was repeated using increasing volumes (5, 10, 15, 20 and 25μl) of ^{125}I-antiCA125 antibody containing (90, 180, 270, 360 and 450) μg.ml^{-1} protein respectively, were added to (225 and 175) μg.ml^{-1} of each of the post-menopausal malignant ovarian tumor homogenate and benign ovarian tumor homogenate respectively, instead of pre-menopausal ovarian tumor homogenate (in step 1 above). Tris-buffer at optimum pH of each

group was used to complete the volume of the reaction and to prepare 20% PEG 6000.

6. The times of incubation needed to get the equilibrium state for all cases are reported in table (4-1).

Table (4-1): The time of incubation for Benign and malignant post and pre-menopausal ovarian tumor homogenates at different temperature.

Temp. °C	Time		
	Post. Menopausal malignant ovarian tumor homogenate	Pre-menopausal malignant ovarian tumor homogenate	Benign ovarian tumor homogenate
5	240	240	270
20	180	150	180
37	120	90	120
45	90	60	60

Calculations

1. The B/F ratio was computed for each tube, where:

B: is the bound radioactivity (mean counts in c.p.m.) which represent the formation of (^{125}I-antiCA125 antibody/CA125) complex.

F: is the free radioactivity (mean counts in c.p.m.), which represents the (unbound or unreacted), ^{125}I-antiCA125 antibody.

T : is the total activity (mean counts in c.p.m.)

F : T (total counts)-B (bound radioactivity)

2. The concentration of (^{125}I-antiCA125 antibody/CA125) complex in mg.ml^{-1} which found after time (t) was calculated from the following equation:

$$B\ (mg.ml^{-1}) = \frac{B(c.p.m.)}{T(c.p.m.)} \times \text{concentration of } ^{125}\text{I - antiCA125 antibody}$$

in incubation medium in mg.ml^{-1}

3. The affinity constant and maximal binding capacity was determined according to scatchared equation [165].

$$\frac{B}{F} = \frac{1}{K_d} \times (B_{max} - B)$$

$$K_a = \frac{1}{K_d}$$

Where K_a = affinity constant

K_d = dissociation constant

B_{max} = maximal binding capacity

4. The plot of B/F ratio Vs. the B values in mg.ml^{-1} gives a linear relationship. The value of affinity constant of the binding (K_a) at each temperature can be calculated from the slope of the straight line, while the value of the total concentration of CA125 (B_{max}) in ovarian tumor homogenate of each group was calculated from the intercept of the x-axis.

B. Determination of the affinity constant (K_a) and maximal binding capacity (B_{max}) of ^{125}I-antiCA125 antibody associated with partially purified CA125 (BI) and (BII) of post-menopausal ovarian tumor homogenate.

1. Increasing volume (4, 8, 12, 16 and 20 µl) of ^{125}I-antiCA125 antibody containing (72, 144, 216, 288 and 360) µg.ml^{-1} protein respectively were each added to (90 µg.ml^{-1}) of partially purified CA125 (BI) form. Then final reaction volume was completed to 400 µl with the same buffer.

2. All tubes were incubated at 5°C for 180 minute

3. The (^{125}I-antiCA125 antibody/CA125) complex was estimated by following the steps 3, 4, 5, and 6 in the section (2.3.5.1).

4. The previous steps were performed at different temperature (20, 37 and 45°C).

5. The experiment was repeated using increasing volumes (5, 10, 15, 20 and 25µl) of ^{125}I-antiCA125 antibody containing (90, 180, 270, 360 and 450µg protein) respectively were each added to (110 µg) of partially purified CA125 of post-menopausal ovarian tumor homogenate (BII) form instead of (BI) (in

step 1 above). Tris-buffer at pH = 6.8 was used to complete the volume of the reaction and to prepare 20% PEG6000.

6. The times of incubation needed to get the equilibrium state for both cases are reported in table (4-2).

Table (4-2): The time of incubation for partially purified CA125 of postmenopausal ovarian tumor homogenate at different temperatures.

Temp.°C	Time min.	
	Partially purified CA125 (BI) form	Partially purified CA125 (BII) form
5	180	210
20	120	150
37	90	90
45	60	60

Calculations

The method outlined in experiment (4.3.1.2A) was followed exactly to out line the values of K_a and B_{max} at each temperature.

4.3.2 The thermodynamic Studies

4.3.2.1 The thermodynamic studies of the interaction of ^{125}I-antiCA125 antibody with CA125 in ovarian tumor homogenates.

The same steps mentioned in section (4.3.1.1. A) and (4.3.1.2. A) were performed using protein fraction of Benign, malignant post-menopausal and pre-menopausal ovarian tumor homogenates.

Calculations

1. The thermodynamic parameters of standard state were obtained from Van't Hoff plot, the values of the natural logarithm of equilibrium constant (affinity constant K_a) obtained at different temperatures were plotted against

the reciprocal values of the absolute temperature in kelvin (1/T), according to the following equation:

$$\ln K_a = \frac{\Delta S°}{R} - \frac{\Delta H°}{RT}$$

Where:

$\Delta H°$ = The enthalpy change of the standard state.

$\Delta S°$ = The entropy change of the standard state.

R = The gas constant (8.314 J.K^{-1}.mol^{-1})

ΔH value was obtained from the slope of the linear relationship of the plot.

The change in Gibbs free energy of the standard state ($\Delta G°$) was obtained from the following equation:

$\Delta G° = -RT \ln K_a$

where K_a is the affinity constant, while the standard state entropy ($\Delta S°$) change was obtained from.

$$\Delta S° = \frac{\Delta H° - \Delta G°}{T}$$

2. The thermodynamic parameters of the transition state were obtained from Arrhenius plot of $\ln k_{+1}$ values against (1/T) values, that given a linear relationship according to the following equation

$$\ln k_{+1} = \ln A - \left[\frac{Ea}{RT}\right]$$

Where:

A: Arrhenius constant.

The value of the activation energy (Ea) of the binding reaction can be determined from the slope of the straight line.

The enthalpy of transition state ΔH^* was obtained from

$\Delta H^* = Ea - RT$

Transition state of free energy change ΔG^* is calculated from the following equation

$$\Delta G^* = -RT \ln k_{+1} + RT \ln \frac{KT}{h}$$

where K and h were boltzman and Blank's constants which are equal to $(1.38 \times 10^{-23} \text{ J.K}^{-1})$, $(6.62 \times 10^{-34} \text{ J.sec}^{-1})$ respectively.

The change in entropy of the transition state ΔS^* was calculated from the following equation:

$$\Delta S^* = \frac{\Delta H^* - \Delta G^*}{T}$$

4.3.2.2 The thermodynamic studies of the interaction of ^{125}I-antiCA125 antibody with partially purified CA125 (BI) and (BII) of post-menopausal ovarian tumor homogenate.

The experiment was performed as described in section (4.3.1.1.B) and (4.3.1.2.B) using partially purified CA125 (BI) and (BII) forms of malignant post – menopausal ovarian tumor homogenate.

Calculations

The method outlined in the experiment (4.3.2.1.) was followed exactly for estimating the thermodynamic parameters of the standard and transition state.

4.4. Results and Discussion

4.4.1 Determination of kinetic parameters of CA125 Associated with ^{125}I-antiCA125 antibody.

The time course of (^{125}I-antiCA125 antibody/CA125) complex formation was carried out to describe the kinetic parameters of the binding. The simplest proposed model representing this interaction is:

$$^{125}I\text{-antiCA125 antibody} + CA125 \xrightleftharpoons{k_{+1}} [^{125}I\text{-antiCA125 antibody/CA125}]$$

Where

k_{+1}: is the association rate of ^{125}I-antiCA125 antibody to CA125.

k_{-1}: is the dissociation rate of ^{125}I-antiCA125 antibody/CA125) complex formed.

At equilibrium

$$K_a = \frac{\left[^{125}\text{I - antiCA125 antibody / CA125}\right]}{\left[^{125}\text{I - antiCA125 antibody}\right]\left[\text{CA125}\right]} \quad \ldots\ldots (1)$$

$$K_d = \frac{\left[^{125}\text{I - antiCA125 antibody}\right]\left[\text{CA125}\right]}{\left[^{125}\text{I - antiCA125 antibody / CA125}\right]} \quad \ldots\ldots (2)$$

Thus:

$$K_a = \frac{1}{K_d} = \frac{k_{+1}}{k_{-1}} \quad \ldots\ldots (3)$$

The value of K_a and maximal binding capacity (B_{max}) were calculated from scatchared plot at four different temperatures for all studied groups [OI, OII, OIII and partially purified CA125 (BI & BII) of malignant post-menopausal ovarian tumor homogenate. The experiment was carried out at the optimum conditions that were obtained in previous experiments and was repeated at different temperatures (20, 37 and 45°C).

Scatchared plots were analyzed according to their linearity as shown in figures (4.1 A, B and C) and (4.2.A & B), all groups showed no curvature in the plotted lines where the data obeyed the straight line equation, indicating that CA125 has a single binding site or more than one site with identical affinities.

Table (4.3) shows that the affinity constant (K_a) and (B_{max}) depended on the type of tumor (benign or malignant) and on the temperature. K_a decreases with the increased temperature in all studied groups. The highest value of K_a occurred in OI group at 5°C, it is about (5.432 mg.ml^{-1}) which suggest the highest affinity for binding among the two rest groups. The increase in temperature may affect the protein conformation which leads to decrease the affinity of binding. On the other hand, determination of (B_{max}) of

CA125 to each type of tissue homogenate shows similar result for K_a value, it is temperature depended, B_{max} decreased with increasing temperature.

The results in table (4-4) also reveal that there is a decrease in K_a and B_{max} values for partially purified CA125 (BI) and (BII) forms with increasing temperature. K_a for BI and BII was (7.092 mg^{-1}.ml and 3.333 mg^{-1}.ml at 5°C respectively, while it was 3.20 mg^{-1}.ml and 2.080 mg.ml^{-1} at 45°C for the two groups respectively. In comparison of K_a and B_{max} values for BI and BII, BI show higher affinity and lower binding capacity than BII.

In general, it can be concluded that partially purified CA125 (BI) form interacts with its specific antibody with higher affinity than the interaction of crude CA125 antigen.

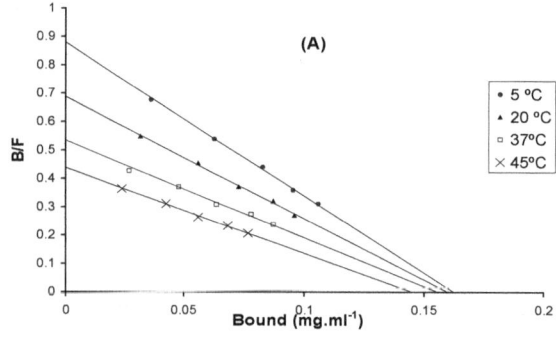

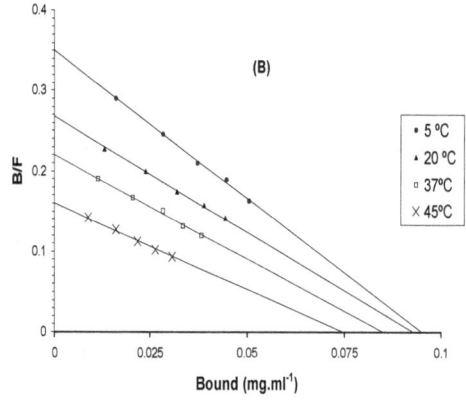

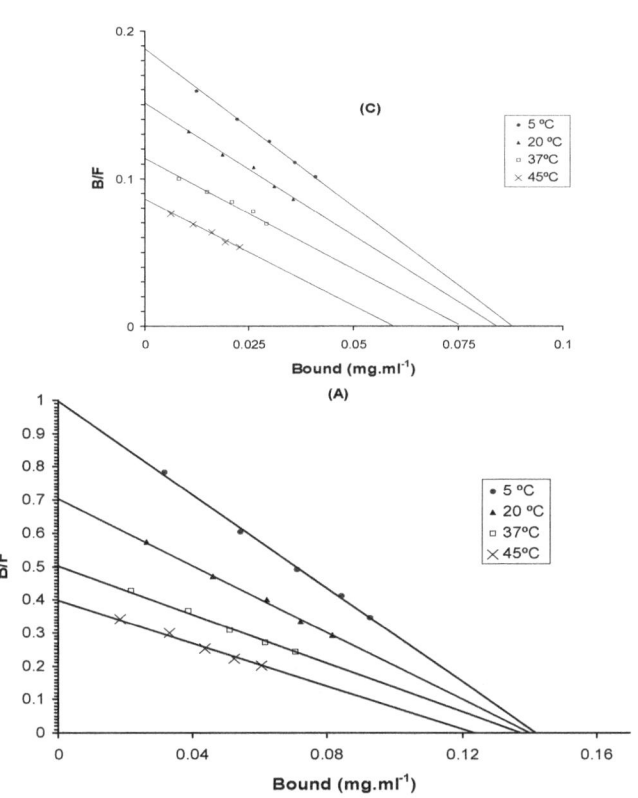

Figure(4-1): Scatchard Plot for, A)OI, B)OII, C) OIII at different temperatures. (All other details are explained in the text).

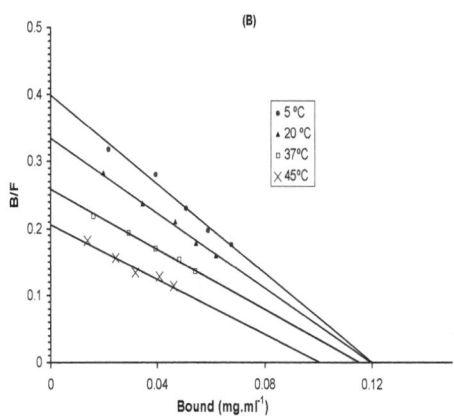

Figure (4-2): Scatchard Plot for partially purified CA 125, A) BI, B) BII, at different temperatures. (All other details are explained in the text).

Table 4-3: Association, dissociation constants and maximal binding capacity of the binding of ^{125}I-antibody CA125 antibody to CA125 antigen in ovarian tumor homogenates at different temperatures

Temperature °C	K_a (mg^{-1}.ml)	K_d (mg.ml^{-1})	B_{max} (mg.ml^{-1})
Malignant post-menopausal ovarian tumor			
5	5.432	0.184	0.162
20	4.367	0.228	0.158
37	3.419	0.292	0.155
45	3.034	0.329	0.145
Malignant pre-menopausal ovarian tumor			
2	3.684	0.271	0.095
20	3.027	0.330	0.092
37	2.588	0.386	0.085
45	2.133	0.468	0.075
Benign ovarian tumor			
5	2.148	0.465	0.087
20	1.800	0.555	0.083
37	1.554	0.643	0.074
45	1.433	0.697	0.060

Association, dissociation constants and maximal binding capacity of the binding of ^{125}I-antiCA125 antibody to partially purified CA125 BI and BII of malignant post-menopausal ovarian tumor homogenates at different temperatures.

Temperature °C	K_a mg^{-1}.ml	K_d (mg.ml^{-1})	B_{max} (mg.ml^{-1})
			Partially purified (BI)
5	7.092	0.141	0.141
20	5.000	0.200	0.140
37	3.676	0.272	0.137
45	3.2	0.312	0.125
Partially purified (BII)			
2	3.333	0.300	0.120
20	2.750	0.363	0.120
37	2.263	0.441	0.110
45	2.080	0.480	0.100

However the time course data could be used to determine the reaction order of CA125 binding to its specific antibody using the graphical method. Attempts were carried out using pseudo first order and second order graphs.

For second order graph the following equations [163] were used

$$\ln [AbAg]_e \left[\frac{[Ab]_T - [AbAg]_t [AbAg]_e / [Ag]_T}{[Ab]_T ([AbAg]_e - [AbAg]_t)} \right] = k_{+1} t \left[\frac{[Ab]_T [Ag]_T - [AbAg]_e}{[AbAg]_e} \right] \quad ...4$$

Where:

K_{+1}: is the association rate constant.

$[AbAg]_e$: is the concentration of (^{125}I-antibodyCA125 antibody/CA125)complex formed at equilibrium.

$[AbAg]_t$: is the concentration of (^{125}I-antibodyCA125 antibody/CA125)complex after time t.

$[Ab]_T$: is the initial antibody concentration at time 0.

$[Ag]_T$: is the initial antigen concentration at time 0.

Or by using another second order kinetic equation from:

$$\frac{1}{[Ab]_T - [Ag]_T} \ln \left(\frac{[Ab]_T - [AbAg]_t}{[Ag]_T - [AbAg]_t} \right) = K_{+1} t + \frac{1}{[Ab]_T - [Ag]_T} \ln \frac{[Ab]_T}{[Ag]_T} \quad ....5$$

For first order graph as the percent of binding was in some cases small [166] and must be labeled antibody remains free and only small fractions binds even at equilibrium, ie. $[Ab]_T \gg [AbAg]_e$

Thus

$$[Ab]_T \gg \frac{[AbAg]_t [AbAg]_e}{[Ag]_T}$$

So the following equation could be used in order to fit the pseudo-first order kinetics:

$$\ln \frac{[AbAg]_e}{[AbAg]_e - [AbAg]_t} = K_{+1} \cdot t \frac{[Ab]_T [Ag]_T}{[AbAg]_e} \quad ....6$$

On the other hand figure (4-3 A, B &C) and (4-4 A&B) show the plot of

$$\frac{1}{[Ab]_T - [Ag]_T} \ln\left(\frac{[Ab]_T - [AbAg]_t}{[Ag]_T - [AbAg]_t}\right)$$

Against time give a straight line for all studies groups OI, OII, OIII and partially purified CA125 (BI and BII form). The association rate constant k_{+1} was determined at each temperature from the slope of the plot.

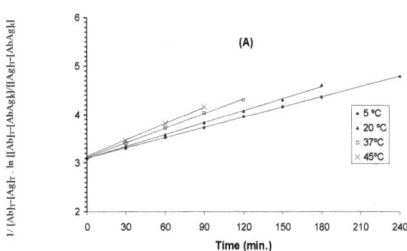

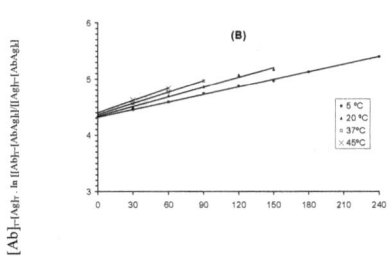

Figure (4-3): Kinetics of the binding of ^{125}I-anti CA125 antibody to CA125 of
A: Malignant post-menopausal ovarian tumor homogenate.
B: Malignant pre-menopausal ovarian tumor homogenate.
C: Benign ovarian tumor homogenate. At different temperature using second order rate law (All other details are explained in the text).

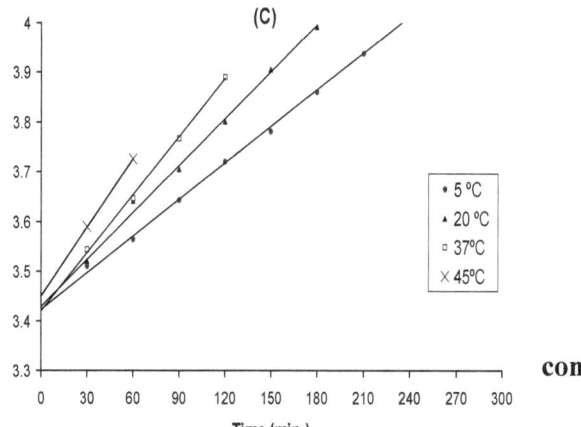

Figure (4-3) continued

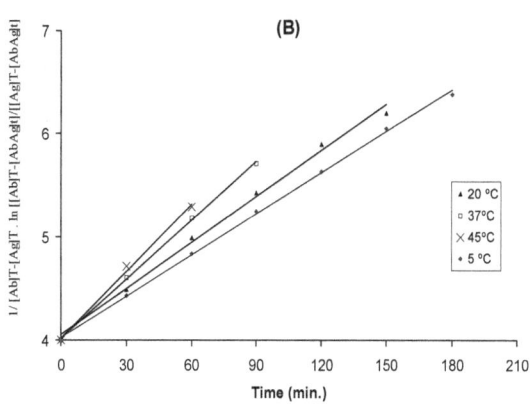

Figure (4-4): Kinetics of the binding of ^{125}I-anti CA125 antibody with partially purified CA125 BI and BII from malignant post- menopausal ovarian tumor homogenate. At different temperature using second order rate law
(All other details are explained in the text).

Kinetic parameters for all studied groups (OI, OII, OIII, BI and BII) were illustrated in tables (4-5) and (4-6). The value of k_{+1} indicates that highest rate of association of CA125 with ^{125}I-antiCA125 antibody occurs at 45°C, whereas the lowest rate occurs at 5°C. Thus when the reaction temperature was increased from 5 °C to 45°C, the values of the association constant increased approximately (1.6, 1.6, 1.8, 1.3 and 1.6 folds) in group OI, OI, OIII, BI and BII respectively.

According to k_{+1} values, the rate of reaction in OI is faster than in OII and OIII which may relate to the origin of CA125 tumor marker.

Table (4-6) also shows that reaction rate of the interaction of partially purified CA125 to ^{125}I-antiCA125 antibody is faster than that in crude CA125 (OI group). The increase in reaction rate is associated with decrease in the reaction time from 240 min. for crude antigen to 180 min and 210 min for BI and BII respectively.

The value of k_{-1} was also determined from the values of K_a (equation 3), which has been estimated at the four temperatures investigated. The results showed that k_{-1} increased with elevation of temperature. The increase in k_{-1} value was about 2.8 folds for all studied groups when the temperature increased from 5 °C to 45 °C.

Table (4-5): Kinetic parameters for the binding of ^{125}I-antibodyCA125 antibody with CA125 in ovarian tumor homogenates at different temperatures using second order rate law (All other details are explained in the text).

Temperature °C	k_{+1} (mg^{-1}.ml.min^{-1})	k_{-1} x10^{-3} (min^{-1})	$t_{1/2ass}$ (min)	$t_{1/2\ diss}$ (min)
Malignant post-menopausal ovarian tumor				
5	0.0070	1.288	93	538
20	0.0083	1.900	72	364
37	0.0101	2.954	52	235
45	0.0110	3.625	36	191
Malignant pre-menopausal ovarian tumor				
5	0.004410	1.1970	81	578
20	0.005580	1.8434	51	375
37	0.006722	2.5973	27	26
45	0.007250	3.3989	18	203
Benign ovarian tumor				
5	0.002470	1.150	123	602
20	0.003172	1.7622	84	393
37	0.003925	2.5257	60	274
45	0.004510	3.1447	27	220

Table (4-6): Kinetic parameters for the binding of ^{125}I-antibodyCA125 antibody to partially purified CA125 BI and BII form of malignant post-menopausal ovarian tumor homogenate at different temperature using second order rate law. (All other details are explained in the text).

Temperature °C	k_{+1} (mg^{-1}.ml.min^{-1})	k_{-1} x10^{-3} (min^{-1})	$t_{1/2ass}$ (min)	$t_{1/2\ diss}$ (min)
Partially purified (BI)				
5	0.04500	6.3450	48	109
20	0.04965	9.9300	35	74
37	0.05620	15.288	27	45
45	0.05937	18.550	24	37
Partially purified (BII)				
5	0.01356	4.0680	72	170

20	0.01583	5.7560	55	120
37	0.01860	8.2450	38	84
45	0.02266	10.894	25	63

4.4.2. The thermodynamic studies of the interaction of ^{125}I-antiCA125 antibody with CA125.

4.4.2.1 Thermodynamic parameters of standard state

Figures (4-5 and 4-6) represents the dependence of equilibrium constant (affinity constant) for binding of ^{125}I-antiCA125 antibody to crude CA125 of benign, pre-and post-menopausal and partially purified CA125 in ovarian tumor homogenates on the temperature (Van't Hoff plot).

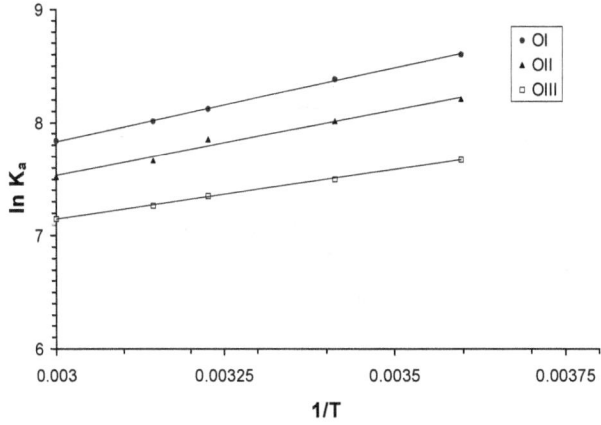

Figure (4-5): Van't Hoff plot for the binding of CA125 to ^{125}I-antiCA125 antibody in ovarian tumor homogenates at different temperature for OI, OII and OIII (All other details are explained in the text)

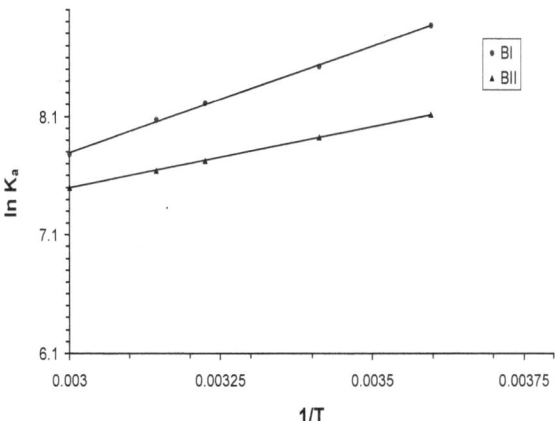

Figure (4-6): Van't Hoff plot for the binding of partially purified CA125 with ^{125}I-antiCA125 antibody at different temperatures (All other details are explained in the text).

Tables (4-7 and 4-8) summarize the calculated thermodynamic parameters for all studied groups (OI, OII, OII, BI and BII) respectively. The results obtained revealed that ΔH^0 in general has small negative value for all groups; their negative sign suggested an exothermic CA125-^{125}I-antiCA125 antibody interaction reaction.

The other values of thermodynamic parameters of the standard state such as $\Delta G°$ and $\Delta S°$ at four temperatures, are summarized in the same tables (4-7 and 4-8).

A high value of positive $\Delta S°$ suggests that the reaction spontaneity was entropically driven.

The high negative value of $\Delta G°$ reflects the stability of complex, hence, the high affinity of the reactants. The high negative values of $\Delta G°$ for the binding reaction are controlled by high positively $\Delta S°$ and low negatively $\Delta H°$. [167] so our CA125-^{125}I-antiCA125 antibody interaction system is characterized by the contribution of $\Delta S°$ and $\Delta H°$ to the stability of the complex formed.

The high value of positive $\Delta S°$ suggests that the reaction was entropically driven and indicates that the hydrophobic interactions are essentially important in stabilizing the complex [168], while the small negative $\Delta H°$ value may indicate favorable interactions between groups within both CA125 and ^{125}I-antiCA125 antibody. These include the non covalent interactions which are fundamentally electrostatic in nature such as charge-charge interactions which occur in both CA125 and ^{125}I-antiCA125 antibody, other types of interactions include charge-dipole, dipole-dipole, charge induced dipole, dipole induced dipole and hydrogen bond. The sum of all types of these interactions can yield sum stabilization to the folded structure of the complex. So the negative value of $\Delta G°$ showed that the overall reaction was energetically favorable in the direction of complex formation.

able (4-7): Thermodynamic parameters for standard state of the binding of ^{125}I-antiCA125 antibody with CA125 in ovarian tumor homogenates at different temperatures.
(All other details are explained in the text).

Temperature$°C$	$\Delta H°(KJ.mol^{-1})$	$\Delta G°(KJ.mol^{-1})$	$\Delta S°(J.mol^{-1} K^{-1})$
Malignant post-menopausal ovarian tumor			
5	-10.808	-19.877	32.622
20	-10.808	-20.416	32.791
37	-10.808	-20.928	32.645
45	-10.808	-21.177	32.6069
Malignant pre-menopausal ovarian tumor			
5	-9.342	-18.978	34.616
20	-9.342	-19.524	34.750
37	-9.342	-20.232	35.125
45	-9.342	20.267	34.355
Benign ovarian tumor			

5	-7.407	-17.732	37.140
20	-7.407	-18.270	37.075
37	-7.407	-18.938	37.196
45	-7.407	-19.2128	37.125

Table(4-8): Thermodynamic parameters for standard state of the binding of ^{125}I-antiCA125 antibody with partially purified CA125 at different temperatures.
(All other details are explained in the text)

Temperature ^{0}C	ΔH^o(KJ.mol^{-1})	ΔG^o(KJ.mol^{-1})	ΔS^o(J.mol^{-1} K^{-1})
Partially purified BI			
5	-15.121	-20.491	19.316
20	-15.121	-20.754	19.225
37	-15.121	-21.157	19.470
45	-15.121	-21.335	19.540
Partially purified BII			
5	-8.507	-18.746	36.830
20	-8.507	-19.290	36.802
37	-8.507	-19.904	36.764
45	-8.507	-20.199	36.767

4.4.2.2. Thermodynamic Parameters of Transition State

According to the transition state theory, the interaction of CA125 to CA125 antibody to form the final product proceeds through the formation of an activated complex (transition state).

CA125+CA125 antibody ⟶ [CA125…CA125antibody] ⟶ CA125-CA125antibody

An activated complex   Final product
(Transition state)

Arrhenius equation and the kinetic constants have been used to determine thermodynamic parameters of the transition state (Ea, ΔH^*, ΔS^* and ΔG^*).

Figure (4-7) and (4-8 A&B) shows Arrhenius plots of ln k_{+1} against 1/T values. The slope of the straight line represents the activation energy Ea. Tables (4-9) and (4-10) show the values of thermodynamic parameters of the transition state of all studied groups (OI, OII, OIII, BI and BII). OIII group showed the highest Ea value, which reflects the high energy required to overcome the energy barrier of transition state for the formation of (^{125}I-antiCA125 antibody-CA125) complex in comparison to the rest groups. On the other hand the value of activation energy is in accordance with the high positive values of ΔG^*, which indicates that the formation of an activated complex (^{125}I-antiCA125 antibody…CA125) is a non spontaneous process and required a lot of energy (equal to Ea) to overcome the transition state energy barrier and giving the final product .Also the positive values of ΔG^* is mainly attributed to the decrease in entropy of the transition state ($\Delta S^* < 0$) in addition, the positive value of ΔH^* in all groups shows that the heat content of the activated complex is more than that of isolated species.[169]

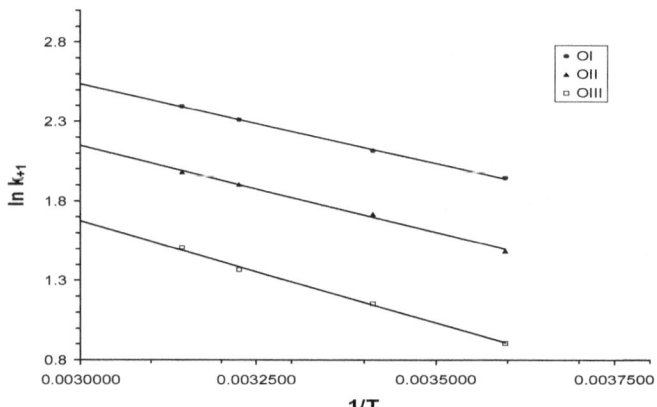

Figure (4-7): Arrhenius plot of the binding of ^{125}I-antiCA125 antibody with its CA125 in ovarian tumor homogenates for OI, OII and OIII. (All other details are explained in the text).

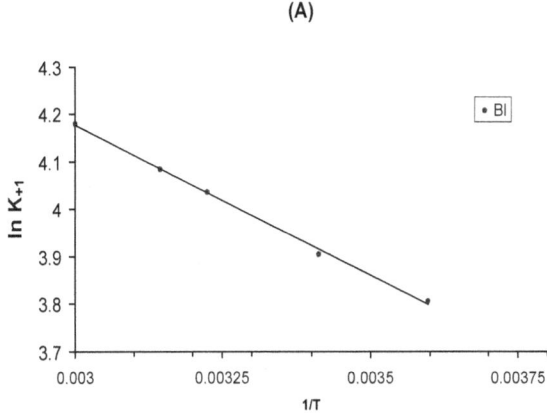

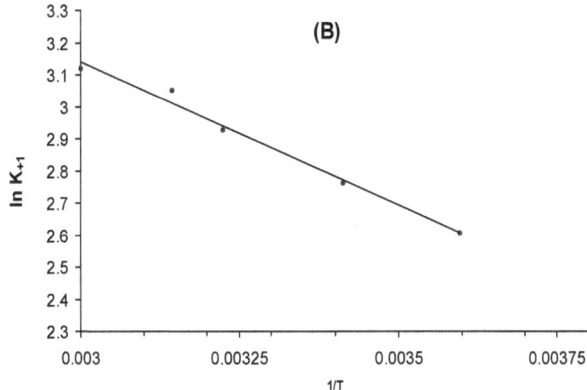

Figure (4-8): Arrhenius plot for the binding of ^{125}I-antiCA125 antibody with partially purified CA125 A) BI, B) BII. (All other details are explained in the text).

Table (4-9): Thermodynamic parameters for the transition state for the binding of ^{125}I-antiCA125 antibody to CA125 in ovarian tumor homogenates at different temperatures. (All details are explained in the text).

Temperature °C	Ea(KJ.mol^{-1})	ΔH^*(KJ.mol^{-1})	ΔG^* (KJ.mol^{-1})	ΔS^*(J.mol^{-1}.K^{-1})
Malignant post – menopausal ovarian tumor				
5	8.132	5.820	63.418	-207.187
20	8.132	5.696	66.561	-207.730
37	8.132	5.554	70.053	-208.061
45	8.132	5.489	71.713	-208.251
Malignant pre – menopausal ovarian tumor				
5	9.287	6.978	64.486	-206.863
20	9.287	6.851	67.528	-207.088
37	9.287	6.710	71.113	-207.751
45	9.287	6.644	72.790	-208.006
Benign				
5	10.640	8.325	65.825	-206.820
20	10.640	8.204	68.903	-207.163
37	10.640	8.063	73.498	-207.854
45	10.640	7.997	75.044	-207.777

Table (4-10): Thermodynamic parameters for the transition state for the binding of ^{125}I-antiCA125 antibody to partially purified CA125 at different temperatures. (All other details are explained in the text).

Temperature °C	Ea(KJ.mol^{-1})	ΔH^*(KJ.mol^{-1})	ΔG^* (KJ.mol^{-1})	ΔS^*(J.mol^{-1}.K^{-1})
Partially purified BI				
5	5.430	3.119	59.118	-201.435
20	5.430	2.994	62.220	-202.136
37	5.430	2.853	65.640	-202.538
45	5.430	2.787	67.255	-202.729
Partially purified BII				
5	7.156	4.845	61.890	-205.197
20	7.156	4.720	65.004	-205.747
37	7.156	4.579	68.482	-206.138
45	7.156	4.513	69.802	-205.311

The values of thermodynamic parameters of the binding reaction gave an overall idea about the nature of forces that regulate the formation of complex. Comparisons of the values of transition state with those of standard state led us to choose a thermodynamic model shown in figure (4-9).

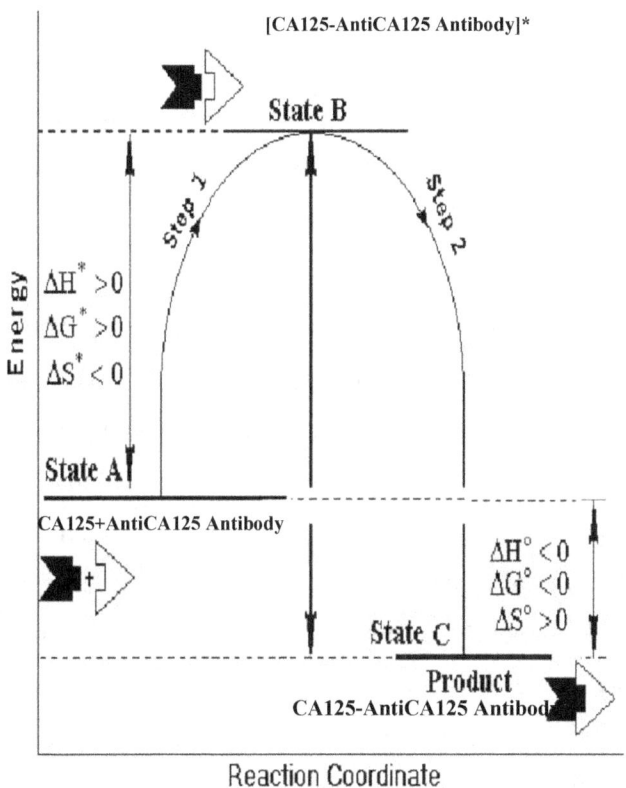

Figure (4-9): General energy diagram and thermodynamic Model applied to the interaction of ^{125}I-anti antibody to CA125 of ovarian human homogenates.

This model proposes that the formation of the (^{125}I-antiCA125 antibody/CA125) complex undergoes three thermodynamic state [170]. The thermodynamic state A represents the initial energy level of ^{125}I-AntiCA125Antibody and its CA125. In the thermodynamic state B, the two species had come together and mutually penetrated their hydration sphere to form a partially immobilized hydrophobically associated species. Thermodynamic state C represents the fully interacting complex (^{125}I-antiCA125 antibody/CA125).

In step 1 of the reaction, the binding of ^{125}I-AntiCA125Antibody to CA125 was associated with positive ΔG^* value. This indicates that the initial step of the reaction requires input of energy for the system. The negative entropy change ΔS^* for this step of reaction reflects the change of the ^{125}I-antiCA125 antibody/CA125 transition complex to more ordered structure. In step 2, the activated complex participates further interactions, giving the fully interacting complex (^{125}I-antiCA125 antibody/CA125).

It is proposed that the formations of a (^{125}I-antiCA125 antibody/CA125) complex occurs in these two steps, the first step stabilized by hydrophobic interactions and the second step, as a consequence of hydrophobic interactions, stabilized by short-range interactions such as electrostatic (ionic) interactions, hydrogen bonding, and Vander Waals' interactions which become possible due to the juxtapositioning of appropriate amino acid residues. Although these short-range interactions probably cannot maintain the integrity of the ^{125}I-antiCA125 antibody/CA125 complex in the absence of the hydrophobic interactions, they are probably responsible for strengthening the stability of the complex. [171]

Hydrophobic interactions contribute to the stability of the complex via high positive excited entropy change ($\Delta S^* > 0$), while electrostatic interactions , hydrogen bonding and Vander Waals' interactions contribute to the stability of the complex via high negative change in entropy ($\Delta S^* < 0$) [171,172].

The thermodynamic data from this study indicates that the binding of ^{125}I-antiCA125 antibody to its CA125 are mainly entropically driven and come in agreement with the concept that hydrophobic and short-range interactions have an important role in the binding of ^{125}I-antiCA125 antibody to its CA125antigen.

Chapter Five

Spectroscopic Studies On Isolated (^{125}I-anti CA125 antibody/CA125) Complex

Abstract

Spectroscopic studies in the ultraviolet region were carried out to characterize the (^{125}I-antiCA125 antibody/CA125) complex of partially purified CA125 antigen (BI and BII) forms which are partially purified from malignant ovarian tumor homogenates.

Gel filtration technique was used to separate ^{125}I-anti CA125 antibody bound to partially purified CA125 (BI and BII) from unbound (free) ^{125}I-antiCA125 antibody. Factors affecting the absorption properties of the two types of complexes such as pH, solvent polarity (solvent perturbation technique), spectrophotometeric pH titration and thermal stability in the presence of different concentration of sodium chloride have been studied.

The spectroscopic pH titration curves for complex of partially purified CA125 (BI) and (BII) for histidine residue gave pk$_a$ of 6.5 and 7.2 respectively, while 11.4 and 11.2 for tyrosine residue respectively. Also, it was showed that 60% of histidine and 36.8% of tyrosine residues are located on the surface of complex of (BII) antigen while these residues were 80% and 25% on the surface of complex of (BI).

5.1 Introduction

Spectrophotometry is one of the most valuable analytical techniques available to biochemists. Unknown compounds may be identified by their characteristic absorption spectra in the ultraviolet, visible or infrared. The wave length that is absorbed and efficiency of absorption depend on both the structure and environment of the molecule.

The most uses of spectroscopic technique in biochemistry employ UV region spectrum. Proteins absorb U.V light at approximately 280 nm due to the presence of tryptophane, tyrosine and (to a lesser extent) phenylalanine residues within their structure, while the absorption of UV light at (215-230) is due to the presence of the polypeptide chain backbone and histidyl residues [173].

The electronic transitions for these chromophors come from n ⟶ π* and π ⟶ π*. Change in the charge and the environment of these chromophors can lead to alteration in the absorption spectrum, and the conformational changes of a protein may also involve environmental change in its chromophoric groups.[174] A large number of environmental factors produce detectable changes in λ_{max}. Among these factors is the pHs of the solvent which determines the ionization state of ionizable chromophore. Also the solvent polarity affects the chromophore electronic transition where the λ_{max} for n- π* transition occurs at shorter wavelength in polar solvents (H_2O, Alcohol) than in longer wavelength. The shift may or may not be accompanied by a change in intensity of spectrum. [175, 176] Thus absorbance measurements can give an idea of location of particular amino acid in protein structure.

Although several new Immunochemical techniques were developed to study antigen/antibody interactions [173, 177], U.V spectra remain as one of the most important methods in immunology because it provides a sensitive and quantitative measurements for the study of antibody structure and its specific ligand binding. [178]

Very limited work concerning physical properties of CA125 specially those related to U.V spectroscopy has been done, such as the studies on CA125 in breast cancer by Haider [179] and In colorectal cancer by Al-Jobory [180]. Also the U.V studies on interaction of CA125 with its specific antibody are not wide spread. Hence, the goal of this chapter is to study the spectroscopic behaviour at the region of U.V of the partially purified CA125 and its complex formed with ^{125}I-antiCA125 antibody at different conditions.

Material and Methods
5.2 Materials

5.2.1 Chemicals

All chemicals and reagents mentioned in section (2.2.1) have been used in the experiments of this chapter.

5.2.2. Instruments

All instruments mentioned in section (2.2.2) have been used in the experiments of this chapter.

5.2.3. Buffers and Reagents

Buffers and reagents mentioned in section (2.3.4) are used in this chapter. Other additional solutions are indicated in each experiment.

5.3 Methods

5.3.1. Gel filtration technique for separation of free and bound ^{125}I- antiCA125 antibody.

5.3.1.1. Preparation of the column.

The dimensions of the column were (1x27cm) chosen according to the equation in section (3.3.1.1).

5.3.1.2. Preparation of the Gel and determination of void volume.

The sepharose CL-6B was used to separate free and bound ^{125}I-antiCA125 antibody,[157] and was prepared as mentioned in section (3.3.1.3) the void volume was determined and found to be 10.ml.

5.3.1.3. Separation procedure of (^{125}I-anti CA125 antibody / CA125) complex.

A. Partially purified CA125 (BI) form with ^{125}I-anti CA125 antibody.

6. Two hundred micro liter from partially purified CA125(BI) antigen in section (3.3.1.5) (360 µg.ml^{-1}) was incubated with 80 µl of ^{125}I-anti CA125 antibody (1440 µg.ml^{-1}), and the reaction was completed to final volume of 600 µl with Tris-buffer (0.05 M, pH 6.8). The tubes were incubated for 180 min at 5°C.

7. At the end of the incubation, the mixture was applied to the surface of a sepharose CL-6B column equilibrated with Tris-buffer 0.05M, pH 6.8. Elution was carried out using the same buffer to separate CA125 bound to ^{125}I-anti CA125 antibody from unbound antigen with flow rate 12ml.hr^{-1}.

8. The radioactivity of each fraction was counted in gamma counter for 1min.

Calculations

Radioactivity (c.p.m) for each fraction was plotted against the fraction number.

B. Partially Purified CA125 (BII) form with ^{125}I-antiCA125 antibody.

1. One hundred and eighty micro liter (440 µg.ml^{-1}) from partially purified CA125 antigen (BII form) in section (3.3.1.5) was incubated with 100 µl of ^{125}I-antiCA125 antibody (1800 µg.ml^{-1}) and the reaction was completed to final volume of 600 µl with Tris-buffer (0.05M pH 7.2). The tubes were incubated for 210 min. at 5°C.

2. At the end of the incubation, the mixture was applied to the surface of a sepharose CL-6B column equilibrated with Tris-buffer 0.05M pH 7.2. The elution was carried out using the same buffer to separate CA125 bound to ^{125}I-antiCA125 antibody from unbound antigen with flow rate 12 ml.hr^{-1}.

3. The radioactivity for each fraction was counted in gamma counter for 1 min.

4. 80 µl of ^{125}I-antiCA125 antibody was completed to 600 µl with Tris-buffer (0.05M pH 7.2), then this volume was applied to the surface of the column in step 2, and step 2 and 3 were repeated.

Calculations

Radioactivity (c.p.m) for each fraction was plotted against the fraction number.

5.3.2. The U.V Spectrum of (^{125}I-anti CA125 antibody/ CA125) Complex, ^{125}I-antiCA25 antibody and Partially Purified CA125.

5.3.2.1. The U.V Spectrum of (^{125}I-anti CA125 antibody / CA125) Complex

The gel filtration profile in section (5.3.1.3 A & B) gave two peaks. The fractions under each peak were pooled and the absorption spectrum was scanned in U.V region against the appropriate blank in reference beam.

5.3.2.2. The UV Spectrum of ^{125}I- anti CA125 antibody.

Twenty five micro litter of ^{125}I-anti CA125 antibody was mixed with 475 µl of Tris (0.05M pH 7.2) and placed in 0.5 cm^3 cuvette. The absorption spectrum was scanned in the UV region against appropriate blank in the reference beam.

5.3.2.3. The UV Spectrum of partially Purified CA125

Two hundred micro litter from partially purified CA125 antigen (BI) was mixed with 300µl of Tris pH 6.8 and placed in 0.5cm^3 cuvette. The absorption spectrum was scanned in UV region against appropriate blank in the reference beam. The same procedure was repeated for partially purified CA125 antigen (BII) using 100 micro liter of (BII) and 400µl Tris-buffer pH7.2 for dilution.

5.3.3. Factors Affecting the Absorption Properties of (^{125}I-anti CA125antibody / CA125) Complex.

5.3.3.1. The pH Effect on the Complex

Reagents

1. KCl-HCl buffer (pH) was prepared as follows

Solution A: Potassium chloride (0.1M), 0.788 gm was dissolved in a final volume of 100ml deionized distilled water.

Solution B: Hydrochloric acid (0.1 N)

The required pH (3.0) was prepared by mixing 50ml of solution A with an appropriate amount of solution B to obtain the required pH, and then the volume was made up to 100ml with deionized distilled water.

2. Citrate-phosphate buffer at different pH was prepared as follows.

Solution A: citric acid (0.05M): 0.9605 gm of citric acid dissolved in 100ml deionizer distilled water.

Solution B: Dibasic sodium phosphate (0.1M): 1.4198gm of Na_2HPO_4 was dissolved in a final volume of 100ml deionized destilled water.

Working buffer pH (4 and 6) was prepared by mixing a volume of solution A with appropriate amount of solution B to obtain the required pH in a final volume of 100ml.

3. Tris buffer at different pH values was prepared as follows:

Solution A: Tris (hydroxyl methyl amino methan) (0.1M): 1.215gm was dissolved in a final volume of 100ml of deionized distilled water.

Solution B: Hydrochloric acid (0.1N)

The required pH (7 and 8) was prepared by mixing 50ml of solution A with appropriate amount of solution B to obtain the required pH, and then the volume was made up to 100ml with deionzied distilled water.

4. Glycine – NaOH buffer was prepared as follows:

Solution A: Glycine (0.1M): 0.7505gm $C_2H_5NO_2$ was dissolved in a final volume of 100ml deionized distilled water.

Solution B: Sodium hydroxide (0.1M):0.4gm NaOH was dissolved in a final volume of 100ml deionized distilled water.

Working buffer pH (9 – 12) was prepared by mixing 50ml of solution A with appropriate amount of solution B to obtain the required pH, then the volume was made up to 100ml with deionized distilled water.

Procedure

One hundred micro liter of pooled fractions under the first peak in (Fig 5-1A) and Fig (5-1 B) which represent (^{125}I-antiCA125 antibody / CA125) complex of BI and BII respectively were completed to 500 µl with different buffers at different pH values (3, 4, 9 and 12) individually then each sample tube was scanned in UV region against a buffer blank at each pH.

5.3.3.2. Effect of Solvent Polarity on UV Spectra of Complex.

The effect of 20% ethanol, and the same amount of ethylene glycol, glycerol and DMSO on the complex was studied.

One hundred micro liter of (^{125}I-antiCA125 antibody/CA125) complex of BI and BII [pooled fractions under the first peak in figure (5–1–A) and (5–1–B)] were mixed with 100 µl of either ethanol, ethylene glycol, glycerol and DMSO) separately. The volume was completed to 500 µl with Tris pH 6.8 and pH 7.2 for complex of BI and BII respectively. The absorbance of each sample was scanned immediately in the UV region (200–350 nm) against blank reference contains 20% appropriate solvent.

5.3.3.3. Spectrophotometric pH Titration of complex

A Series of complexes from of BI and BII (100µl) were completed to 500µl with buffer at pH ranging from 8 to 12. The absorbance of each sample was measured at 295 nm and the absorbance of λ_{max} at each pH value was plotted versus the corresponding pH. Other series of the same complex (100µl) were completed to 500 µl with buffers ranging from 4 to 8. The maximum absorbance of each sample was measured at 211nm and the absorbance of λ_{max} at each pH values was plotted against the corresponding pH.

5.3.3.4. The Effect of NaCl Concentration on the thermal Stability of the complex by UV spectral studies.

Reagents

Buffers used in thermal stability studies of complex of BI and BII were prepared as follows:-

Twenty percent ethylene glycol buffer was prepared by mixing 20ml of ethylene glycol and 80ml of Tris-buffer pH 6.8. NaCl (0.01M) in 20% ethylene glycol buffer was prepared by dissolving 0.05844 gm of NaCl in 100 ml of 20% ethylene glycol buffer, while NaCl (0.1M) in 20% ethylene glycol buffer was prepared by dissolving 0.5844 gm of NaCl in 100ml of 20% ethylene glycol buffer.

20% Ethylene glycol buffer in Tris buffer pH 7.2 was also prepared and used to prepare (0.01M) NaCl and (0.1M) NaCl solution.

Procedure

One hundred micro litter of complex of BI and BII were completed to final volume 500µl with (0.01M) NaCl in 20% ethylene glycol buffers pH 6.8 and pH 7.2 for complex of BI and BII respectively. Each mixture was placed in 0.5cm cuvette in the sample beam and the buffer at the adjusted pH in the reference beam. The absorption was measured at the wavelength of (292 and 295 nm) at different temperatures 20, 30, 40, 50, 60, 70, 80. The experiment was repeated for each complex with another solution (0.1M NaCl in 20% ethylene glycol) at 292 and 295 nm.

5.3.3.5. The Effect of Urea, KCl and Urea - KCl mixture on the spectrum of the complex.

Reagent

1. Eight molar urea was prepared by dissolving 24.02 gram of urea in the final volume of 50 ml of Tris pH 6.8

2. KCl (0.03M) was prepared by dissolving 0.2737 gram of the salt in the final volume of 50 ml of corresponding buffer.
3. 8M urea and 0.03 M KCl solutions were also prepared using Tris pH 7.2 buffers.

Procedure

One hundred micro liters of complex of BI and BII were pipetted in a set of three tubes. The volume was completed to 500 µl with Tris buffer pH 6.8 for complex of BI and Tris pH 7.2 for complex of BII contains either 0.03M KCl, 8M Urea or mixture 1:1 of both 0.03M KCl and 8M urea respectively. Then each Sample was placed in 0.5cm cuvette in the sample beam and the buffer at the same pH in the presence of the same salt in the reference beam.

The absorption of each sample was scanned immediately in the area of (200 – 350 nm).

5.4. Results and Discussion

5.4.1. Gel Filtration Technique for Separation of Free and Bound ^{125}I- anti CA125 antibody

Figures (5-1 A & B) show the results of gel filtration technique to separate ^{125}I-anti CA125 antibody bound to partially purified CA125 (BI) and (BII) forms respectively. The elution profile in figure (5-1A) revealed two peaks: the first peak with low retention time at fraction number 10 (high molecular weight) represent the complex of partial purified CA125 (BI) with ^{125}I-anti CA125 antibody bound to ^{125}I-antiCA125 antibody, while the second peak at fraction number 19 represents the unbound (free) ^{125}I-anti CA125 antibody. The elution profile in figure (5-1B) also revealed two peaks: the first peak at fraction number 15 represent the complex of partial purified CA125 (BII) bound to ^{125}I-anti CA125 antibody, while the second peak at fraction number 19 represents the unbound (free) ^{125}I-anti CA125 antibody.

The elution profile for the label antiCA125antibody is shown in Figure (5-2) in which one peak appeared in the same position of second peak of Figure (5-1A&B) which represents the unbound ^{125}I-antiCA125 antibody. The resultant fractions under the first peak in figures (5-1A) or (5-1B) were collected and pooled.

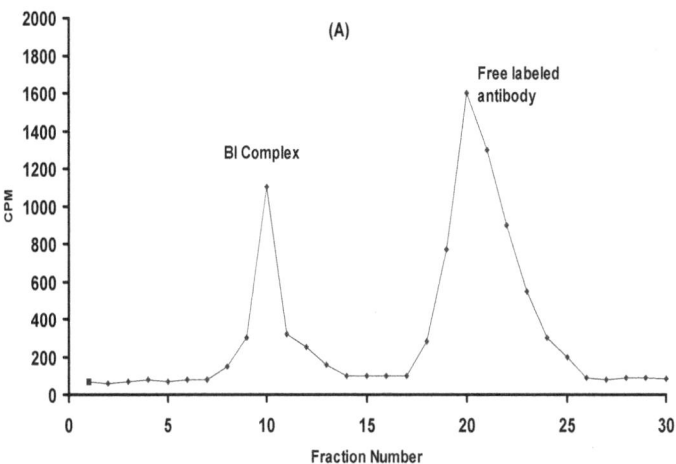

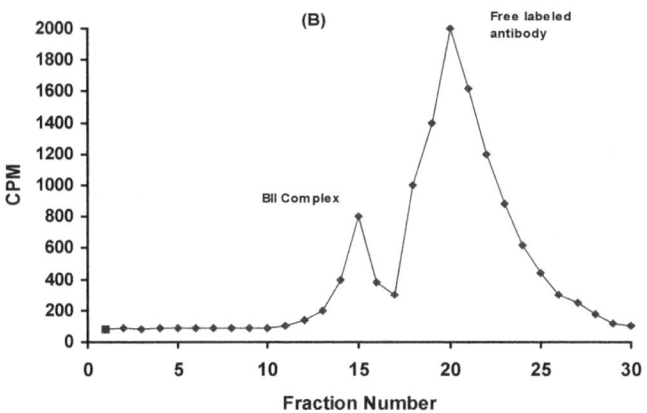

Figure(5-1) The elution profile of the isolated complex (^{125}I-antiCA125 antibody/CA125) and free antibody in
(A) Partially purified CA125 antigen (BI)
(B) Partially purified CA125 antigen (BII) using sepharose CL-6B gel. (All other details are explained in the text)

5.4.2. The UV Spectra of Partially purified CA125, anti CA125 antibody and (^{125}I-antiCA125 antibody/CA125) complex molecules.

The ultraviolet absorption spectra of protein in the regions 250 to 300 nm are contributed from tyrosyl, tryptophan and (to a less extent) phenylalanine residues, but at shorter wavelengths; the contributions come from other groups such as histidyl residues and the peptide bond. The absorbance at lower wave lengths is directly related to the amount of polypeptide material and is usually considerably more sensitive than at 280nm. Absorbance at 215-230nm is useful for monitoring peptides may not contain tryptophan or tyrosine [173].

The UV spectra of partially purified CA125 (BI) and (BII), ^{125}I-antiCA125 antibody and (^{125}I-antiCA125 antibody/CA125) complex were scanned from 200-350nm to determine the absorption spectra and the alteration in the UV spectra as a result of their interaction.

5.4.2.1. The UV Spectrum of Partially Purified CA125.

Figure (5-3) and (5-4) shows the UV spectra of partially purified CA125 (BI) and (BII) respectively. The spectrum of (BI) antigen consisted of two peaks; a large one at 220 nm and smaller at 278nm, while the UV spectrum of BI antigen shows two peaks at 212 and 270nm as shown in table 5-1.

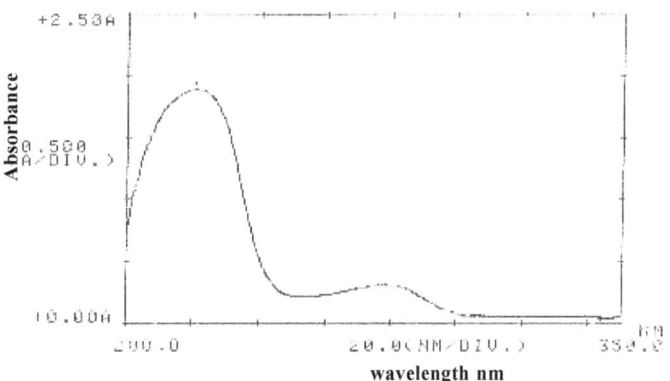

Figure (5-3): UV Spectrum of partially purified CA125 (BI) (All other details are explained in the text).

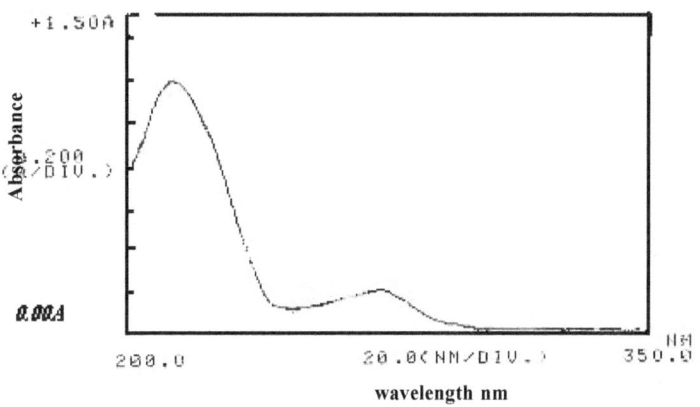

Figure (5-4): UV Spectrum of partially purified CA125 (BII) (All other details are explained in the text).

As a result it seemed that each form of CA125 antigen (BI and BII) has a characteristic spectrum and can be identified by its peaks, the first peak at (220 or 212 nm) could be due to the amide group in polypeptide bond of CA125 molecule with contribution of the histidyl residues. While the second peak (at 278 or 270) is assigned to tyrosyl residue.

5.4.2.2. The UV spectrum of ^{125}I- anti CA125 antibody.

The UV spectrum of ^{125}I-anti CA125 antibody has shown in figure (5-5). The spectrum consisted of two obvious peaks. The first peak at 225nm is assigned to the amide groups in the poly peptide bond with contribution of histidyl residues[173] while the small peak at 278nm is assigned to tyrosyl residue.

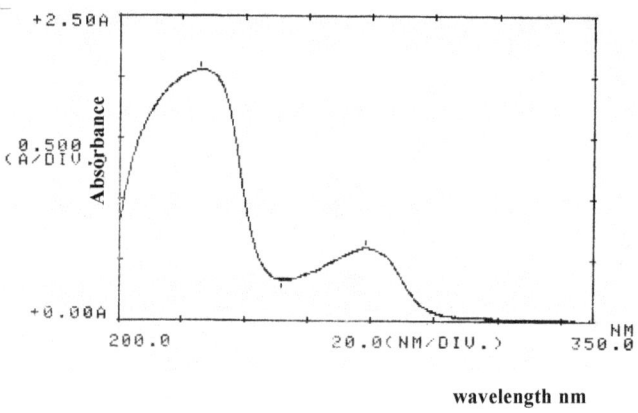

wavelength nm

Figure (5-5): UV spectrum of ^{125}I-antiCA125 antibody (All other details are explained in the test).

5.4.2.3. The UV spectrum of (^{125}I-anti CA125 antibody / CA125) complex.

Figure (5-6 and 5-7) shows the spectra of partially purified CA125 antigen (BI) and (BII) bound to ^{125}I-antiCA125 antibody respectively. The spectra of both complexes consisted of one peak at (214 or 208 nm) for the complex of BI and BII of CA125 antigen respectively shown as shown is table (5-1).

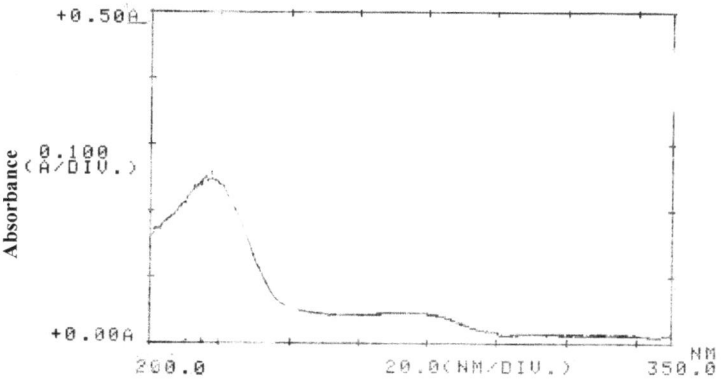

Figure (5-6): UV spectrum of CA125 (BI)/ ^{125}I-antiCA125 antibody complex. (All details are explained in the text).

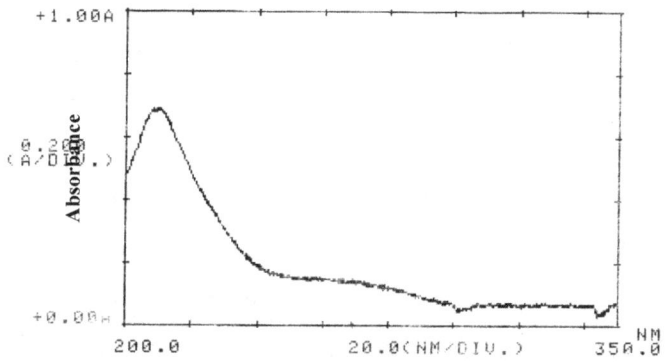

Figure (5-7): UV spectrum of CA125 (BII)/ ^{125}I-antiCA125 antibody complex (All details are explained in the text)

The strong absorption of these peaks (214 or 208 nm) arises from electronic transition in the peptide backbone itself and is therefore sensitive to backbone conformation [181]. There was disappearance of tyrosine peaks in both complexes. These changes are due to fitting of antibody to its antigen to form (^{125}I-Anti CA125 Antibody/CA125) complex. This result is in agreement with Seinerman etal observation who found that the surface of protein interactions was polar as well and the complex formation lead to the burial of charged and polar residues. [182]

Table (5-1): The λ_{max} of (^{125}I-antiCA125 antibody/CA125) Complex, partially purified CA125 and unbound (free) ^{125}I-anti CA125 antibody. (ALL other details are explained in the text).

No.	Fractions	BI λ_{max} (nm)	BII λ_{max} (nm)
1	Partially purified CA125	220,278	212,270
2	^{125}I-antiCA125 antibody	225,278	225,278
3	^{125}I-antiCA125 antibody /CA125) complex	214	208

5.4.3. Factors Affecting the Absorption Properties of (^{125}I-antiCA125 antibody/CA125) Complex of BI and BII Antigen.

5.4.3.1. The Effect of pH on the complex.

The pH of the solvent determines the ionization state of ionizable chromophore in the protein molecule.[181] Table (5-2) shows the λ_{max} values of isolated (^{125}I-antiCA125 antibody /CA125) complex of BI and BII at different pH (3, 4, 9 and 12). At an acidic pH 3 both complexes of BI or BII have one maximum wavelength at (205 or 202 nm) respectively compare to the UV spectra of partially purified CA125 antigen (BI) and (BII) or the spectra of ^{125}I-anti CA125 antibody.

It seems that in acid region there was a blue shift in λ_{max} from (214 or 208 nm) in neutral pH to (205 or 202) in acidic pH for both complexes of (BI) and (BII) respectively. The blue shift is due to the increasing of hydrogen bond formed in the presence of highly positively charged state [183].

When the pH value was increased from neutral to pH 9, there was also only one maximum wavelength found in the spectra of both complexes with the increase in λ_{max} value from (214 or 208) to (223 or 220) for complex of BI and BII respectively. At pH 12 two λ_{max} were obtained for each complex.

λ_{max1} and λ_{max2} of complex of (BI) were at (225, 284nm) respectively whereas λ_{max1} and λ_{max2} of complex of BII were (223, 282nm) respectively.

These results indicate that tyrosine residue in both complexes molecules at neutral pH are located in a way that a small part of it is on the surface of the protein molecule while a large part of these residues is buried but at high pH = 12 the protein becomes denatured (unfolded) and the internal tyrosine has become exposed to the solvent and absorb light. A red shift observed in absorption of these tyrosine residues is certainly related to the ionization of side chain of the tyrosine and this led to the availability of the lone pair on the oxygen atom to happen easier and at lower energy level (red shift).

Table (5-2): The effect of different pH on λ_{max} value of (^{125}I-anti CA125 antibody/CA125) complex. (All details are explained in the text).

pH	λ_{max} (^{125}I-antiCA125 antibody / CA125) (BI complex)	(^{125}I-antiCA125 antibody / CA125) (BII complex)
3	205	202
4	212	207
7	214	208
9	224	221
12	225, 284	223, 282

5.4.3.2. The Effect of solvent polarity on the UV spectrum of the complex

The determination of whether an amino acid is internal or external by measuring the spectra of a protein in polar and non-polar solvent is called the solvent perturbation method. In fact, proteins are rarely studied in completely non-polar solvents. However, significant solvent effects can be induced by the use of a mixture of water and substance of a reduced polarity such as ethanol, ethylene glycol, glycerol and dimethylsulfoxide [144].

Several spectral changes were obtained in the presence of these perturbants, like the alteration of the peak position and intensities of protein spectrum, and the appearance of new chromophores on the surface of protein molecule. These chromophores were embedded in an interior region of the protein in the absence of the solvent. One of the main assumptions of the solvent perturbation technique is that solvents alter the peak position and intensities by altering the energy and probability of electronic transitions.[184-185] In reality the preferential solvation is caused not only by the perturbant interaction with chromophor itself, but also with the group adjacent to the chromophor in the protein.

Table (5-3) shows the effect of different solvents on the (^{125}I-antiCA125 antibody/CA125) complex of (BI) and (BII) form. It was found that (λ_{max} 214 or 208 nm) shown in previous experiments for complex of BI or BII respectively, was shifted to longer wavelength (red sheft) in the presence of ethanol, ethylene glycol and glycerol at a concentration of (20%). These shifts are attributed to the amide group in polypeptide bond with contribution of histidyl residues inter molecular hydrogen bonding between amide group of polypeptide bond in the complex molecule and the solvent may cause these shifts the intermolecular hydrogen bonding increase as the concentration of the solution increase and additional bands start to appear at longer or shorter wavelength [186]. The contribution of histidyl residues in the observed spectra λ_{max1} is difficult to detect because of the overlapping of its absorbance with that of peptide bond.[176] Table (5-3) shows that the spectrum of both protein complexes are is sensitive to change in the polarity of the solvent which may indicate that high percent of histidine residues is located on the surface of the protein molecule.

In the presence of DMSO (20%) there was an increase in λ_{max1} from (214 or 208) to 242 nm for both complexes and new λ_{max} at (284, 282 nm) appeared which belongs to complexes of BI and BII respectively. The new peaks are related to tyrosyl residues. The appearance of λ_{max} of tyrosine residue is related to the perturbing solvent which makes the possibility for the presence of this residue to the surface of the protein structure.

Table 5-3: The effect of solvent polarity on λ_{max} of (^{125}I-antiCA125 antibody / CA125) complex
(All other details are explained in the text)

Solvent 20% of	(^{125}I-antiCA125 antibody/CA125) (BI)		(^{125}I-antiCA125 antibody/CA125) (BII)	
	$\lambda\ max_1$	$\lambda\ max_2$	$\lambda\ max_1$	$\lambda\ max_2$
Ethanol	222	-	219	-
Ethylen glycol	217	-	215	-
Glycerol	223	-	221	-
DMSO	242	284	242	282

5.4.3.3. Spectrophotometric pH Titration of the Complex.

Spectrophotometric pH titration is the following of the changes in absorbance of the chromofor with increasing pH [144]. Many studies of protein structure require the determination of Pk_a values for protein dissociation from ionizable amino acid side chains, because these values give an indication of the location of the amino acid in the protein. This can often be done spectrophotometricaly because dissociation often changes the spectrum of one of the chromophores, the observation of tyrosine dissociation was performed by measuring the absorption at 295 nm (λ_{max} for the ionized form of tyrosine), and the observation of histidine dissociation was carried out by measuring the absorption at 211 nm

The titration curve of (^{125}I-antiCA125 antibody/CA125) complex of (BI) and (BII) for both tyrosyl and histidyl residues are illustrated in figure (5-8 A&B) respectively. Figure (5-8A) shows that the Pk_a for tyrosine is 11.4 for

(^{125}I-Anti CA125 Antibody / CA125) complex of (BI), while the Pk$_a$ for tyrosine is 11.2 for (^{125}I-antiCA125 antibody / CA125) complex of (BII) form. From the same curves it could be concluded that about (36.8%) and (25%) of tyrosyl residues are located on the surface of protein complex of BI and BII respectively. The other residues are buried interiorly in a polar environment of protein complex of both forms of CA125 antigen. A large arise in the absorbance was observed at high pH because protein complexes become denatured.

Figure (5-8B) shows that Pk$_a$ values of histidine residues in complex from BI and BII antigen are (6.5) and (7.2) respectively. Also from these curves it was found that (80%) histidyl residues are located on the surface of the complex of BI antigen, while (60%) located on the surface of the complex of BII antigen. the other histidine residues are buried interior the protein complex of both antigens.

These results are in agreement with those found in solvent perturbation experiment in section (5.4.3.2.) for the percent of histidine residue on the surface of protein complex molecule.

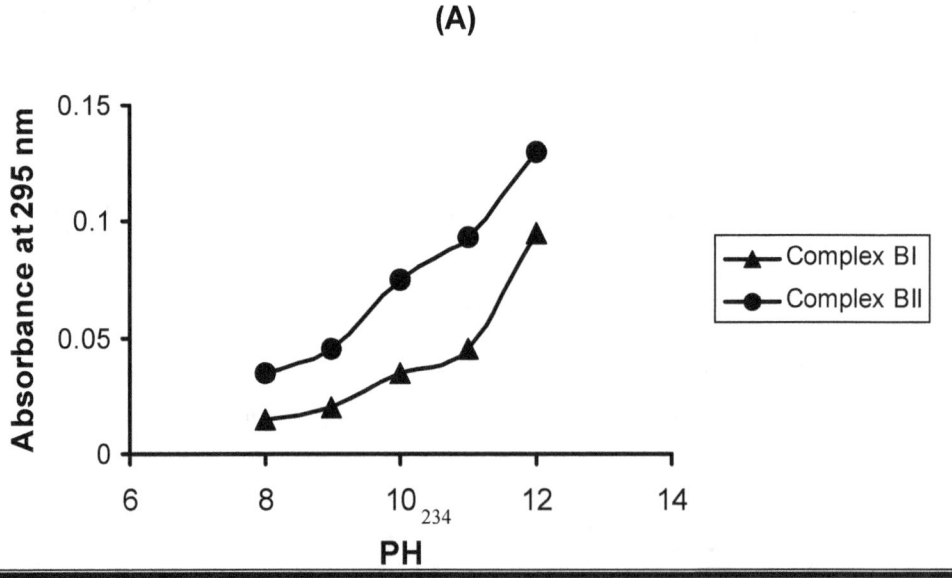

(A)

**Figure (5-8): Spectrophotometric pH titration of (^{125}I-antiCA125 antibody/CA125) complex from BI and BII antigen.
A=for tyrosine, (B) for Histidine.
(All other details are explained in the text).**

5.4.3.4. The effect of NaCl concentration on the thermal stability of the complex by UV spectral studies.

The effect of the different concentration of NaCl on the thermal stability of (^{125}I-antiCA125 antibody/CA125) complex of BI and BII of partially purified CA125 antigen was examined in this experiment. The values of absorbance at λ_{max} (292, 295 nm) for tryptophyl and tyrosyl residues respectively, in two different concentrations of NaCl 0.01 M and 0.1 M in 20% ethylene glycol buffer are shown in figure (5-9A&B) and (5-10A&B).

As shown in figure (5-9A&B) the internal tryptophane and tyrosine are completely exposed to the solvent at 60°C in the presence of 0.01 M NaCl in both complexes of BI and BII. The increment in the absorbance of both tryptophyl and tyrosine residues with increasing temperature could be due to those buried chromophores becomes exposed to the solvent during thermal denaturation [187].

Figure (5-10 A&B) shows that in presence of 0.1 M NaCl, the absorbance of both tryptophan and tyrosine reach higher value at 70°C for both complexes of (BI) and (BI), therefore higher concentration of NaCl causes more stabilization for protein complex.

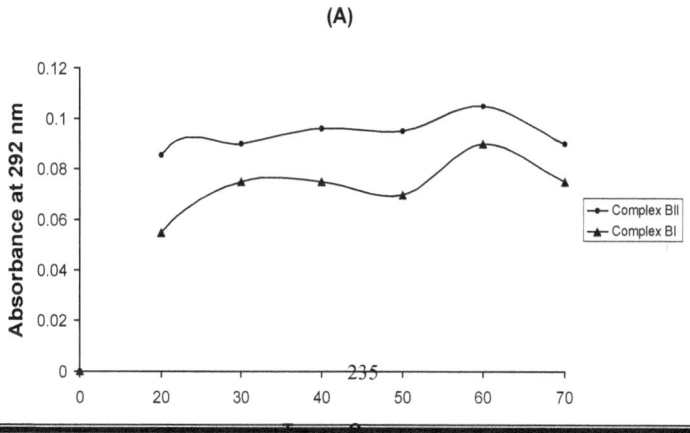

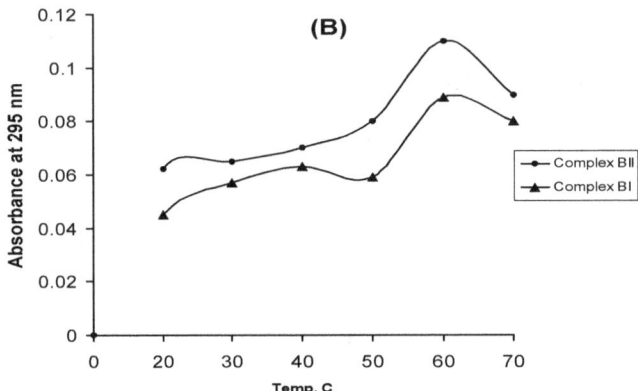

Figure (5-9): Thermal stability curve for complex of BI and BII
(A) at λ_{max} 292 in presence of 0.01M NaCl,
(B) at λ_{max} 295 in the presence of 0.01M NaCl.
(All other details are explained in the text).

The decrease of the absorbance in presence of 0.1M NaCl as compared with that in 0.01M NaCl could be due to salt concentration. Each protein in solution containing salts will collect around it a counter ion atmosphere enriched in oppositely charged small ion, (chloride ion and sodium ion), and such a cloud of ions will tend to screen the protein, the larger the concentration of small ion present, the more effective this electrostatic screening will be, and decrement in the absorption intensity will be observed (181).

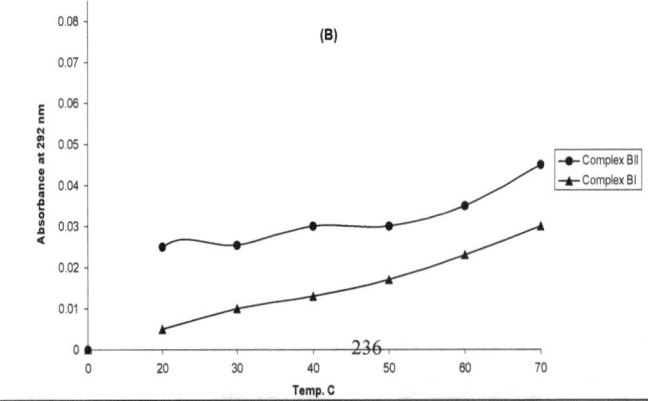

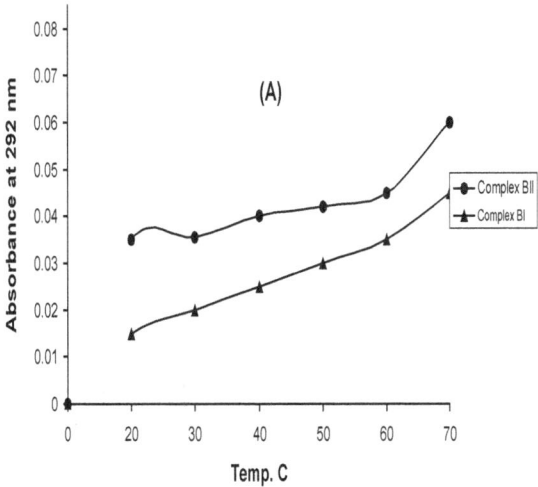

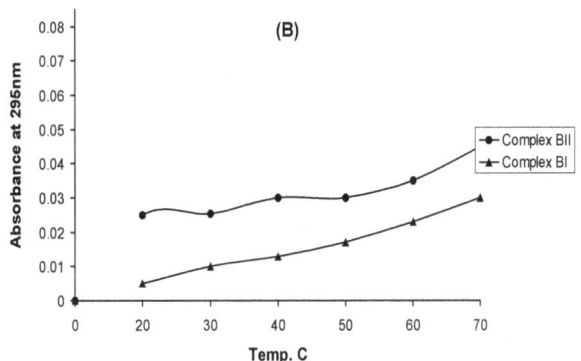

Figure (5-10 A&B): Thermal stability curve for complex of BI and BII:
(A) at λ_{max} 292 in presence of 0.1M NaCl,
(B) at λ_{max} 295 in presence of 0.1M NaCl.
(All other details are explained in the text).

5.4.3.5. Effect of Urea, KCl and (Urea- KCl) Mixture on the Spectrum of the Complex

Table (5-4) shows the effect of 8M urea, 0.03M KCl and a mixture of 1:1 of 8 M urea and 0.03 M KCl on λ_{max} of the complexes of both forms of partially purified CA125 antigen. Comparing the values of λ_{max} of these molecules obtained in the absence of urea or KCl (table 5-1) with those obtained in the presence of 8M urea in table (5-4), it seems that there was a significant red shift in λ_{max1} of poly peptide bond from (215 or 208nm) to λ_{max} (223 or 221 nm) for complex from BI and BII antigen respectively. While there is no λ_{max2} peak assign for aromatic amino acid, i.e. tyrosine residue in both complexes. These results indicate that the molecule solvated with urea (dipole –dipole interaction) and produce a red - shift and new chromofore come to the surface .The red shift is due to the intermolecular hydrogen bonding between the oxygen of the amide group and the solvent [176]. When 0.03M KCl was used, there was a slight blue shift (3-1nm) in λ_{max1} of polypeptide bond in the complex of BI and BII antigen respectively such blue shift can arise by introducing positive (K^+) or negative (Cl^-) charges near the chromophore (the amide group, which might interact with π – electron system of the amide group [174].

When a mixture of 1: 1 of 8M urea and 0.03 M KCl was used, there was a significant red shift in λ_{max}, (215 or 208) to λ_{max} (221 or 218nm) in complex of BI and BII respectively. The same shift in λ_{max} was observed when 8M urea was used alone with each complex. This means that the shift caused by mixture due to the effect of urea but not to 0.03M KCl. Solvent perturbation or denaturation of protein produces many changes in absorption near 230 nm and 280 nm, they are usually about ten times greater near 230nm than at 280nm when the native and the denatured protein are compared. [2] Some of these changes in absorption may be produced by the change in $n – \pi^*$ absorption of poly peptide bond in protein either because of a change in their geometrical arrangement or because of environment changes [181].

Table (5-4): The effect of 8M Urea, 0.03M KCl and mixture (Urea-KCl) on the λ_{max} of complex UV spectrum (All other details are explained in the text).

Solvent	λ_{max} (nm)	
	complex of BI	complex of BII
Urea 8M	223	221
KCl 0.03M	211	207
Urea-KCl Mixture 1:1	221	218

References

1. White A, Handler PH, and Smith E. **Principles of Biochemistry**; 5th Ed; Mc Gray-Hill. 1972; pp.812.

2. Ablev GI. **Alpha-feto protein in ontogenesis and its association with malignant tumors**. Adv Cancer Res 1971; 14:292.

3. Gold P, and Freeman SO .**Demonstration of tumor –specific antigen in human** colonic carcinoma by immunological tolerance absorption technique J Exp Med 1965; 121:439-450.

4. Kohler G, and Milstein. **Continuous cultures of fused cells secreting antibody of predefined specificity Nature** 1975; 257(5517):495-497.

5. Kreuzer H and Massay A. **Recombinant DNA and Biotechnology;** ASM press comp, USA, 1996, chapter 24, pp. 190-198.

6. Hayes DF, Bast R, Desch CE, Fritsche H, Kemeny NE, et al . **A tumor marker utility grading system (TMUGS). A framework to evaluate clinical utility of tumor markers.** Nati Cancer Inst 1996; 88:1456.

7. Bates S E and Longo D L .**Use of serum tumor markers in cancer diagnosis and management.** Semin Oncol. 1987(2)102.

8. Stearns V, Yamauchi H, and Hayes DF. **Circulating tumor markers in breast cancer: Accepted utility and novel prospects.** Breast Cancer Research and treatment. 1998; 52:239-259.

9. Costa J, and Cordon CC. **Cancer Diagnosis: Molecular Pathology; in: cancer principles and practice of oncology**; 6th ed.; De Vita V.T., Hellman S., Rosenberg Eds. Lippincott Williams and Wilkins. 2001; pp.641-657.

10. Anderson SC, and Cockayne S. **Clinical Chemistry**; **concepts and applications**; An HB. Jint .ed; Philadelphia; W.B. Saunders company; 1993; chapter 16, pp.322-330.

11. Moossa AR, Schempff SC, and Robson MC. **Comprehensive Textbook of Oncology**; 2nd ed.; Eds. Baltimopre, Williams & Wilkins, 1991; pp.225-

238.

12. Haber D and Fearon E. **The promise of cancer genetics**. Lancet, 1998; 351:SII1.

13. Orr-weaver TL and Weinberg RA. **A checkpoint on the road to cancer.** Nature 1998; 392:223-224.

14. Brown JM, and Wouters BG. **Apoptosis, p53 and tumor cell sensitivity to anticancer antigen. Cancer Res** 1999; 59: 1391-1399.

15. Kastan MB, Onyekwere O, Sidransky D, Vogelstein B, and Graig RW. **Participation of p53 in the cellular response to DNA damage**. Cancer Res.; 1991; 51: 6304.

16. Wu J. **Diagnosis and management of cancer using serologic tumor markers. In; Clinical Diagnosis and Management by Laboratory Methods**; 20th ed.; J.B. Henry Ed. W.B. Saunders Company; 2001; pp.1028-1042.

17. David W. **Immunoassay Hand Book**; 2nd ed.; U.K. Nature Publishing Group, 2001; chapter 63, pp.635-662.

18. Zurawski VR, Broderick SF, Pickens P, et al. **CA125 levels in group of non hosptalised women: relevance for the early detection of ovarian cancer.** Obstet Gynecol 1987; 69:606-611.

19. **European Group of Tumor Markers (EGTM).** http://www.med.uni.muenchen.de/egtm/detail/4.htm .

20. Thomas j, Nowak A, and Gordon H. **Essential of Pathophysiology**; 2nd ed. WcB Mc Graw-Hill; 1999; pp. 501-504.

21. Eric V Mackay, Norman A Beischer, Lloyd W Cox, and Carl wood. **Illustrated text book of Gynecology**; W.B. Saunders Company 1983, p. 282.

22. Cotran RC, Kumor V, and Collins T. **Robbins Pathologic Basis of Disease**; 6th ed.; WB Saunders Company; 1999; pp.1068-1069.

23. Carol Mattson Porth; **Pathophysiology**; 4th ed.; J. B. Lippincott company Philadelphia; 1994, p.749.

24. Fuys Woodruff J D; **Pathology: Practical Gynecologic Oncology**; 2nd ed.; Williams and Wilkins Company; 1995; p.1079.
25. Kristensen GB and Trope C. **Epithelial ovarian carcinoma.** Lancet 1997; 349:113-117.
26. Scott JR, Disaia PJ, Hammond CB, and Spellacy WN. **Danforth's Obstetrics and Gynecology**; 8th ed.,; Lippincott Williams & Willkins ; 1999; pp 678-695.
27. Rosa J. **Ackerman's Surgical Pathology**; 8th ed. Atimes Mirror Company; 1996; p1474.
28. Caroline Van Haaften and Cinda M Boyer. **Epithelial ovarian tumors in the reproductive age group: Age is not an independent prognostic factore.** Cancer 1996; 77: 1131.
29. Karlan BY and Platt LD. **The current status of ultrasound and color Doppler imaging in screening for ovarian cancer** .Gynecol Oncol. 1994; 55:528
30. Charles R Whitefield; **Dewhurst's text Book of Obstetrics and Gynecology**; 5th ed.; Black well science; 1995; PP.759-774.
31. Tiernery JR, Mcphee SJ, and Oapadakis Mia.; **Current Medical Diagnosis & Treatment**; 38th ed.; Appelton & Lange; 1999; P. 718.
32. Parkin DM, Whelan SL, Ferlay J, Raymond L, and Young J. **Cancer incidence in five continents**; vol VII Lyon: International Agency for Research on cancer 1997 (IARC scientific Publication No. 143).
33. Greenlee RT, Hill-Harmon MB, Murray T, and Thun M. **Cancer statistics.** CA Cancer J. Clin 2001; 51:15.
34. **Iraqi cancer registry** 1995-1997.
35. Piver MS, Baker TR, Piedmote M, and Sandecki AM .**Epidemiology and etiology of ovarian cancer.** Seminars in Oncology 1991; 18 (3): 177-185.
36. Kerlikowske K, Brown JS, and Grady DG. **Should women with familial ovarian cancer undergo prophylactic oophorectomy?** Obstet Gynecol;

1992; 80:700.

37. Serova O, Montagna M, Torchard D, et al. **A high incidence of BRAC1 mutations in 20 breast-ovarian cancer families.** Am J. Hum. Genet; 1996; 58:42

38. Wooster R, Bignell G, Lancaster J et al. **Identification of breast cancer susceptibility gene BRAC2.** Nature 1995; 378: 789.

39. Gillis CR, Hole DJ, still RM, Davis J, and Kaye SB. **Medical audit, cancer registration and survival in ovarian cancar.** Lancet 991; 337: 611-612.

40. Yancik R, Ries LG, and Yates JW. **An analysis of surveillance, epidemiology, and end results program data.** Is J Obstet Gynecol 1966; 154:636-47?

41. Whittermore AS, Harris R, and Itnyre J. **Characteristics relating to ovarian cancer risk: Collaborative analysis of twelveU.S.case-controlstudies .II Invasive epithelial ovarian cancers in white women.** Am. J. Epidemiol 1992; 136: 1184.

42. Gross TP and Schlesselman JJ. **The estimated effect of oral contraceptive use on the cumulative risk of epithelial ovarian cancer.** Obstet Gynecl 1994; 83:419.

43. Risch HA, Marrett LD, and Howe GR. **Parity, contraception, infertility and risk of epithelial ovarian cancer. Am.** J Epidemiol 1994; 140: 585-97.

44. Daniel L, Clarke-Pearson M, and Yousif D. **Green's Gynecology: Essentials of Clinical Practice**; 4th ed., Little, Brown Company; 1990; pp. 531-541.

45. Wong C, Hempling RE, Piver MS, et al. **Perineal Talc exposure and subsequent epithelial ovarian cancer: A case control study.** Obstet Gynecol 1999; 93:372.

46. Bristow RE and karlan BY. **Ovulation induction, infertility, and ovarian**

cancer risk. Fertil steril 1996; 66:499.

47. Rodrigue ZC, Tatham LM, Calle EE, et al. **Infertility and risk of fetal ovarien cancer in a prospective cohort of U.S. women Cancer control** .Cancer Causes Control ; 1998 ;9 :645.

48. Rossing MA, Daling JR, Weiss NS, et al .**Ovarian tumor in a cohort of inferite women.** N Engl J Med. 1994; 331: 771.

49. **"General Information about Ovarian Epithelial Cancer" NCl Cancer.** Gov. web site (Http://www.cancer.gov.).

50. Smith LH and Oi RH. **Detection of malignant ovarian neoplasm's: A review of the literature I. Detection of the patient at risk, clinical, radiological and cytological detection.** Obstet Gynecol Surv.; 1984; 39:313.

51. Pollock RE. **Manual of Clinical Oncology**; 7th ed.; Wiley. Liss, Inc.; 1999; p.542.

52. Campbell S, Bhan V, Royston P, et al. **Transabdominal ultrasound screening for early ovarian cancer.** BNJ 1989; 299:1363.

53. Bast RC, Klug TL, St John E, Jenison E, Niloff JM, Lazarus H, Berkowitz RS, Leavitt T, Griffiths CT, parker L, zurawski VR, and knapp RC . **A radioimmunoassay using a monoclonal antibody to monitor the course of epithelial ovarian cancer.** N Eng J Med 1983; 309:883-887.

54. Schwartz PE, and Taylor Kjw. **Ovarian Cancer: Epidemiological perspectives with Developments in Early Diagnosis**; the Parthenon publishing group New York; 1994, p. 257.

55. James B, Wyngaarden Lloyd H, and smith JR, **Claude Bennett Cecil: textbook of Medicine.** 20th ed.; W.B. Saunders Company; 1996; pp. 1021-1022.

56. Celluzzi CM, Mayordomo CI, Storkns WJ, Lotze MT, and Falo LD. **Peptide-pulsed dentritic cells induce antigen-specific CTL-mediated protective tumor immunity.** J Exp Med 1996; 183:283.

57. Kawashima I, Hudson SJ, Tsai V, Southwood S, Takesako K, Appella E, Sette A, and Celis E. **The multiepitope approach for immunotherapy for cancer: identification of several ETL epitopes from various tumor associated antigens expressed on solid epithelial tumors.** Hum Immunol 1998; 59:1.

58. Vogle FD, Strickeler E, Weyermann M, Kohler T, Gill H, Negri G, kreienberg R, and Runnebaum IB. **p53 auto antibodies in patients with primary ovarian cancer are associated with higher age, advanced stage and higher proportion of a p53-posative tumor cell.** Oncology; 1999; 57:324.

59. Vikhanskaya F, D'Incalci, and Broggini M. **p73 competes with p53 and attenuates its response in a human ovarian cancer cell line.** Nucleic Acid Res 2000; 28: 513.

60. Werness BA, Freedman A, Piver MS, Romero-Gutierrez M, and petrow E. **Prognostic significance of p53 and p21 (waf1/cip1) immunoreactivity in epithelial cancer of the ovary.** Gynecol Oncol 1999; 75:413.

61. Presneau N, Laplace-Marieze V, sylvain V, Lortholary A, Hardouin A, Bernard- Gallon D, and Bignon Y. **New mechanism of BRAC1 mutation by deletion / insertion at the same nucleotide position in three unrelated fresh breast cancer.** Hum. Genet 1998; 103:334.

62. Lancaster JM, Garney M, and Futreal PA. **BRAC1 and 2: A genetic like to familial beast and ovarian cancer.** Medscape women's Health 1997; 2:7.

63. Woolas RP, xu FG, Jacobs IJ, Yu YH, Daly L, Berchuck A, Soper JT, Clarke- pearson DL Oram DH, and Bast RC. **Elevation of multiple serum markers in patients with stage I ovarian cancer.** J Natl Cancer Inst 1993; 85:1748.

64. kufe D, Inghirami G, Abe M, Hayes D, Justi-wheeler H, and schlom J. **Differential reactivity of a novel monoclonal antibody (DF3) with human malignant versus benign breast tumors.** Hybridoma 1984; 3:223.

65. Mckenzie SJ, Desombre KA, Bast BS, Hollis DR, Whitaker RS, Berchuck A, Boyer C M, and Bast RC. **Serum levels of HER-2 neu(C-erbB-2) correlate with over expression of p158 neu in human ovarian cancer.** Cancer 1993; 71:3942.

66. Hancock MC, langton BC, Chan T, Toy P Monahan JJ, Mischak RP, and Shawver L K. **A monoclonal antibody against the c-erbB-2 portion enhances the cytotoxicity of cis-diaminedichloro-platinum against human breast and ovarian tumor cell lines.** Cancer Res 1991; 51:4575.

67. Alexander WK and William RH. **Ovarian papillary serous tumors of low malignant potential (serous borderline tumors). A long term follow-up study, including patients with micro invasion, lymph node metastasis, and transformation to invasive serous carcinoma.** Cancer 1996; 78:278.

68. Thigpen JT, Lambuth BW, and Vance RB. **Management of stage I and II ovarian cancer.** Semin Oncol 1991; 18:596.

69. Kristensen GB and Trope C. **Epithelial ovarian carcinoma.** Lancet 1997; 349:113-117.

70. Kumar P, Rehani MM, Kumar L, Sharma R, Bhatla N, Chaudharg R, Thulkar S, Sunderam KR, and Kumar N. **Tumor marker CA125 as an evaluator and response indicator in ovarian cancer : its quantitative correlation with tumor volume.** Med Sci Monit 2005; 11: CR 84.

71. Colakovic S, Lukic V, Mitrovic L, Jelic S, Susnjer S, ,and Marinkovic J. **Prognostic value of CA125 kinetics and half time in advanced ovarian cancer.** Int J Biol. Marker 2000; 15:147-152.

72. Hempling RE, Piver MS, Natarajan N, Baker TR, Thompson JM, Hicks ML, and Metlin CJ. **Predictive value of serum CA125 following optimal cytoreductive surgery during weekly cisplatin induction therapy for advanced ovarian cancer.** J of Surg Onco 1993; 54:38-44.

73. Jacobs IJ and Bast RC. **The CA125 tumor –associated antigen: a review**

of the literature. Human Reproduction; 1989; 4:pp.1-12.

74. Backston T, Mahlck CA, and Kjellgrea O. **Progesterone as a possible tumor marker for nonendocrine ovarian malignant tumors.** Gynecol Oncol 1983; 16:129.

75. Heinnon PK, Tuimala R, Pyy KK, and Pystyam P. **Human placental alkaline phosphatase in benign and malignant ovarian neoplasia.** Br J Obstst & Gynecol 1982; 89:84.

76. Tholander B, Taube A, Lingew A, sjoberg O, Stendahi U, and Tamsen L. **Pretreatment serum level of CA125, CEA, tissue polypeptide antigen and placental alkaline phosphatase in patient with ovarian carcinoma.** Gynecol Oncol 190; 39:26-33.

77. Shabana A, Onsrud M. **Tissue polypeptide-specific antigen and CA125 as serum tumor markers in ovarian carcinoma.** Tumor Biol 1994; 15:361.

78. John R, Van Nagell JR, Pletsch A, and Goldenberg M. **A study of cyst fluid and plasma carcinoembrionic antigen in patients with cystic ovarian neoplasm's.** Cancer Res 1975; 35:1433-1437.

79. Negishi Y, Iwabuchi H, Sakunaga H, et al. **Serum and tissue measurement of CA72-4 in ovarian cancer patients.** Gyncol Oncol 1993; 48:149-54.

80. Berek JS and Martinez-Maza O. **Molecular and biological factors in the pathogenesis of ovarian cancer.** J Reprod Med 1994; 39:241-248.

81. Schwartz FE, Chambers SK, Chambers JT, Gutman J, Katopodis N, and Foemmel R. **Circulating tumor markers in the monitoring of gynecological malignancies** Cancer 1987; 60:353-61.

82. Berek JS, and Bust RC. **Ovarian cancer screening "the use of serial complementary tumor markers to improve sensitivity and specificity for early detection"** Cancer 1995; 76:2092-96.

83. Hanisch FG, and Dienst C. **CA125 and CA19-9: two cancer associated sialylsaccharide antigens on a mucus glycoprotein from human milk.** Eur J Biochem 1985; 149:323-330.
84. Sekine H, Ohno Tand Kufe DW. **Purification and characterization of a high molecular weight glycoprotein detected in human milk and breast carcinomas.** J Immunol 1985; 135:3610-3615.
85. Shimizu M, and Yamauchi K. **Isolation and characterization of mucn like glycoprotein in human milk fat globule membrane**. J Biochem 1982; 91: 515-524.
86. Tsubura A, Morii S, Vdea S, Sasaki M, Zother S , Waltzing V, Mooi W, Hageman PC, Hilkens J, and Tweel JV. **Immunohistochemical demonstration of MAM-3 and MAM-6 antigen in normal human skin and their tumors.** Arch Dermatol Res. 1987; 279:550-557.
87. Sekin H, Hayes DF, Ohno T, et al. **Circulating DF3 and CA125 antigen levels from patients with epithelial ovarian carcinoma.** J Clin Oncol 1985; 3:1355-63.
88. Harbest AL. **The epidemiology of ovarian carcinoma and the current status of tumor markers to detect disease.** J Obstet Gynecol 1994; 170:1099-107.

89. Berek JS, Chung C, kaldi K, Watson JM, Knox RM, and Martinez Maza O. **Serum interleukin-6 levels correlate with disease status in patients with epithelial ovarian cancer**. J Obstet Gynecol 1991; 164:1038-43.
90. Gotlib WH, Abrams JS, Watson JM, Velu T, Martine Z, Mazo O, and Berek JS. **Presence of interleukin 10 (IL 10) in the ascites of patients with ovarian and other intra abdominal cancer.** Cytokine 1992; 4:385-90.
91. Ramakrishhan S, Xu FJ, Brandt SJ, Niedel JF, Bast RC, and Brown EL .**Constitutive production of macrophage colony-stimulating factor by human ovarian and breast cancer cell lines.** J Clin invest 1989;83:921-

926.

92. Xu FJ, Ramakrishhan S, Daly L, Soper JT, Berchuck A, Clarke PD, et al. **Increased serum levels of macrophage colony stimulating factor in ovarian cancer.** Is J Obstet Gynecol 1991; 165:1356-62?

93. Xu FJ, Yu YH, Daly L, Desombre K, Anselmino L, Hass GM, et al. **The OVX1 radioimmunoassay complements CA125 for predicting the presence of residual carcinoma at second-look surgical surveillance procedures.** J Clin Oncol 1993; 11:1506-11.

94. Knauf S, Anderson DJ, Knapp RC, and Bast RC. **A study of NB/70K and CA125 monoclonal antibody radioimmunoassay for measuring serum.** Am J Obstet Gynecol 1985; 152(7):911-913.

95. Schwartz PE, Chaambers JT, Taylor KJ, et al. **Early detection of ovarian cancer: preliminary results of the Yale Early Detection Program Yale.** J Biol Med 1991; 64:573-82.

96. Soper JT, Hunter VJ. Daly L, Tanner M, Creasman W, and Bast RC. **Preoperative serum tumor-associated antigen levels in women with pelvic masses.** Obstet Gynecol 1990; 75:249.

97. Davis HM, Zurawski VR, Bast RC, and Klug TE. **Characterization of the CA125 antigen associated with human epithelial ovarian carcinomas.** Cancer Res 1986; 46:6143-6148.

98. Nagata A, Hirota N, Sakai T, Fujimoto M, and Komoda T. **Molecular nature and possible presence of a membranous glycophosphatidylinositol anchor of CA125 antigen.** Tumor Biol 1991; 12:279.

99. Bast RC, Boyer JI, Xuf J, Wiener J, Kohler M, and Berckuck A. **Cell growth regulation in epithelial ovarian cancer.** Cancer 1993; 71:1597-1601.

100. O'Brien TJ, Beard JB, Underwood LJ, and Shigemasa K. **The CA125 gene: A new discovered extension of the glycosylated N-terminal domine**

doubles to size of this extracellular superstructure. Tumor Biol 2002; 23: 154-169.

101. O'Brien TJ, Beard JB, Underwood LJ, Dennis RA, Santin AD, and York L. **The CA125 gene: an extacllular superstructure dominated by erepear sequences.** Tumor Biol 2001; 22:348-366.

102. Kui Wong N, Easton RL, Panico M, Sutton Smith M, Morrison JC, Lattanzio FA, Morris HR, Clark GF, Dell A, and Patankar MS. **Characterization of the oligosaccharides associated with the human ovarian tumor marker CA125.** J Biol Chem 2003; 278: 28619-28634.

103. Yin BW and Lloyd KO. **Molecular cloning of the CA125 ovarian cancer antigen identification as a new mucin, MUC16.** J Biol Chem 2001; 276, 27371-27375.

104. Wreschner DH, McGuckin MA, Williams SJ, Baruch A, Yoeli M, Ziv R, Okun L, ZareTsky J, Smorodinsky N, Keydar I, Neophytou P, Stacey M, Lin HH, and Gordon S. **Generation of ligand-receptor alliances by "SEA" model-mediated cleavage of membrane-associated mucin proteins.** Protein Sci 2002; 11:698-706.

105. Hardardottir H, Parmely TH, Quirk JG, Sanders MM, Miller FC, and O' Brien TJ. **Distribution of CA125 in embryonic tissue and adult derivation of the fetal periderm.** J Obstet Gynecol 1990; 163:1925-1931.

106. Fukuda M, **Roles of mucin-type O-glycans in cell adhesion.** Biochim Biophys Acta 2002; 1573:394-405.

107. Bresalier RS, Byrd J, Wang L, and Raz A. **Colon cancer mucin: A new ligand for the beta-galactoside binding protein galactin-3.** Cancer Res 1996; 56: 4354-4357.

108. Seelenmeyer C, Wegehingel S, Lechner J, and Nickel W. **The cancer antigen CA125 represents a novel counter receptor for galactine-1.** J Cell Science 2003; 116:1305-1318.

109. Perillo NL, Marcus ME and Baum LG. **Galectins: versatile modulators**

of cell adhesion, cell proliferation, and cell death. J Mol Med 1998; 76: 402-412.

110. Gaetje R, Winnekendonk DW, Scharl A, and Kaufmann M. **Ovarian cancer antigen CA125 enhances the invasiveness of the endometriotic cell line EEC145**. J Soc Gynecol Investig 1999; 6: 278-281.

111. Rump A, Morikawa Y, Tanaka M, Minami S, Umesaki N, Takeuchi M, and Miyajima A. **Binding of ovarian cancer antigen CA125/MUC16 to mesothelin mediates cell adhesion.** J Biol Chem 2004; 279(10): 9190-9198.

112. Hassan R, Bera T, and Pastan I. **Mesothelin: A new target for immunotherapy.** Clin cancer Res 2004; 3937-3942.

113. Bast RC, Siegal FP, Runowiecz C, Klug TL, and Knapp RC. **Elevation of serum CA125 prior to diagnosing of an epithelial ovarian carcinoma.** Gynecol Oncol 1985; 22:115-120.

114. Bon GG, Kenemans P, Verstraeten R, Van kamp GJ and Hilgers J. **Serum tumor marker immunoassay in gynecologic oncology : establishment of reference values.** J Obstet Gynecol 1996 174:107-114.

115. Lloyd KO and Yin BW. **Synthesis and secretion of the ovarian cancer antigen CA125 by the human cancer cell line NIH: OVCAR-3.** Tumor Biol 2001; 22: 77-82

116. Meyer T, and Rustin GJ. **Role of tumor markers in monitoring epithelial ovarian cancer.** Br J Cancer 2000; 82:1535-1538.

117. Bast RC, Feeney M, Lazarus H, Nadler LM, Colvin RB, and Knapp RC. **Reactivity of monoclonal antibody with human ovarian carcinoma.** J Clin Invest 1981; 68: 1331-1337.

118. Nustad, et al. **Specificity and affinity of 26 monoclonal antibodies against the CA125 antigen: first report from the ISOBM TD-1 workshop.** Tumer Biol 1996; 17:196-219.

119. Lehtovirta P, Apter D, and Stenman VH. **Serum CA125 levels during the**

menstrual cycle. Br J Obstet Gynecol. 1999; 97: 930-933.

120. Bonfrer JMG, Korse CM, Verstraeten RA, Van Kamp GJ, Hart AAM, and Kenemans. **Clinical evaluation of the BYK LIA-mat CA125 II assay: Discussion of a reference value.** Clin Chem 1997; 43: 491-497.

121. Guadagni F, Marth CH, Zeimet AG, Ferroni F, Spila A, Abbolito R, Roselli M, Greiner JW, and Schlom J. **Evaluation of markers in patients with gynecologic diseases.** AMJ Obstet Gynecol 1994; 171:1183-91.

122. Austoker J. **Screening for ovarian, prostatic and testicular cancer.** Br Med J 1994; 309:315-320.

123. Monagham JM. Malignant diseases of ovary. Dewhursts text book of Obstetrics and Gynecology for postgraduates, 6 editions; Blackwell science Ltd. 1999; PP.590-592.

124. Zurawski VR, Orjaseter H, Andersen A, et al. **Elevated serum CA125 levels prior to diagnosis of ovarian neoplasia: relevance for early detection ovarian cancer** Int J Cancer 1988; 42:677.

125. Roupaz FE, Raftopoulos V, Tzavelas G, Kotrotsiou E, Sotiropoulou P, Karanikola E, Skifla, and Ardavanis A. **Serum CA125 combined with transvaginal (TSV) ultrasonography for ovarian cancer screening.** Invivo 2004;18(6):831-836

126. Bast RC, Xu F, Woolas RF, Yu Y, Conaway M., O' Briant K, et al. **complementary and coordinate markers for detection of epithelial ovarian cancers,** In: sharp F., Mason P, Blackett T, and Berek JS, editors. Covarian Cancers 3; Chapman and Hill; London; 1995; P.P. 189-192.

127. Schutter EMJ, Kenemans P, Sohn C, Kristen P, Crombach G, Westermann R et al. **Diagnostic value of pelvic examination, ultrasound and serum CA125 in post-menopausal women with pelvic mass.** Cancer 1994; 74:1398-1406.

128. Rustin GJS. **The clinical value of tumer markers in the malignant of ovarian cancer.** Ann Clin Biochem 1996;33:284-289.

129. Wagner U, Kohler S, Prietl G, Giffels P, Schmidt-Nicolai S, Schlebusch H, et al. **Monoclonal antiidiotypic antibodies in immunotherapy of ovarian carcinoma (MAB CA125) and breast carcinoma** .Zentrabl Gynakol 1999; 121:190.

130. Wagner U, Schlebusch H, Kohler S, Schmolling J, Grunn U, and Krebs D. **Immunological responses to the tumor associated antigen CA125 in patient with advanced ovarian cancer induced by the murin monoclonal anti-idiotypic vaccine A CA125.** Hybridoma 1997; 16:33-40.

131. Nusted K, Lloyd KO, Nilsson O, and O'Brient TJ. **Epitopes on CA125 from cervical mucus and ascites fluid and characterization** Tumer Biol 2002; 23:303-314.

132. Einhorn N, Sjovall K, Knapp RC, Hall P, Scully RE, Bast RC, and Zurawski VR. **Prospective evaluation of serum CA125 levels for the early detection of ovarian cancer.** Obstet Gynecol 1992; 80: 14-18.

133. Boerman OC, Thomas GMG, Segers MFG, Kenemans P, Lovgren, Zurawski VR, Haisma HJ, and Poels LG. **Time-resolved immunoflurometric assay for the ovarian carcinoma-associated antigenic determinant CA125 in serum.** Clin Chem 1987; 33(12): 2191-

134. Schollerr N, Crawford M, Sato A, Drasche CW, O'Biant KC, Kiviat N, Andrson GL, and Urban N. **Bead-based ELISA for valedation of ovarian cancer : Erley detection markers .** Clin Cancer Res 2006 ;12:2117-2124.ancer

135. **Bast RC and Knapp CC. CA125: History, current status, and future prospects. MJM**, 1997; 3:67-71.

136. Lowry OH, Rosenrough NJ, Farr AL, and Randel RJ. **Protein measurement with folin phenol reagent.** J Biol Chem 1951; 193: 365-375.

137. Fleuren GJ, NAP M, Aalders JG, Trimbos JB, and DE Bruijn NWA.

Explanation of the limited correlation between tumor CA125 content and serum CA125 antigen levels in patients with ovarian tumors. Cancer 1987; 60: 2437-2442.

138. Al-Barazanji AK. (2002) **"The accuracy of malignant risk index based onCa125, ultrasound and menopausal state"**. Thesis, supervised by Kais Kubba and Suhail Najim Al-Salam, submitted for the degree of fellowship of Arab Board of Obstetrics and Gynecology.

139. Malkasion G.D. Jr., Knapp R.C., Lavin ph. T., Zurawski V.R. Jr., Podratz K.C., Stonhope CR, Mortel R, Berck JS, Bast RC, and Ritts RE. **Preoperative evaluation of serum CA125 levels in pre-menopausal and post-menopausal patients with pelvic masses: Discrimination of benign form malignant disease. J Obestet Gynecol** 1988; 159:341-6.

140. James T Wu, Terry M, Joseph AK, and David PK. **Improved specificity of the CA125 Enzymeimmunoassay for ovarian carcinomas by use of the ratio of CA125 to carcinoembryonic antigen.** Clin Chem 1988; 34/9: 1853-1857.

141. Nagell JR, Meeker WR, Parker J., and Harraison JD. **Carcinoembryonic antigen in patients with gynecologic malignancy.** Cancer 1975; 35: 1372-1376.

142. Nagell JR, Donaldson ES, Gay EC, Sharkey RM, Rayburn P, and Goldenberg DM. **carcinoembryonic antigen in ovarian epithelial cystadenocarcinomas. Cancer** 1978; 41: 2335-2340.

143. Donaldson ES, Nagell JR, Pursell S, Gay EC, Meeker WR, Kashmiri R, and Voorde J. **Multiple biochemical marker in patients with gynecologic malignancies.** Cancer 1980; 45: 948-953.

144. Freifrlder D. **"Physical Biochemistry: Application to Biochemistry and Molecular Biology"**; 2nd ed.; San Francisco: W.H. Freeman & Company. 1982; Chapter 14; pp. 494-591.

145. Changux JP. **Responses of actylcholinesterase from torepedo marmorata to salts and curarizing drugs**. Mol. Pharmacol 1966, 2:369.

146. Helen CH, Mansel H, Siraj M, and Niel S. **Essential of Clinical Immunology**; 4th ed.; London Blackwell Science Ltd; 1999; Chapter 19:pp.314-321.

147. Clackson T, Hoogenboon HR, Griffiths AD, and Winter G. **Marking antibody fragments using phage display libraries.** Nature 1991; 352:624-628.

148. Dixon M, and Webb E, **Enzymes**; 3rd ed.; London; Longman Group Limited; 1979; pp.273.

149. Devlin TM. **Text Book of Biochemistry with Clinical Correlation**; 2nd Ed; John Wiley and Sons Inc.; New York; 1986; pp.125-66.

150. Melander W and Horvath C. **Salt effect on hydrophobic interactions in precipitation and chromatography of proteins: an interpretation of the lyotropic series.** Arch Biochem Biophys 1977; 183: 200-215.

151. Collins KD. **Charge density-dependent strength of hydration and biological structure**. Biophys J.; 1997; 72: 65-76.

152. Evans JS and Levine BA. **Protein–protein interaction sites in the calcium modulated skeletal muscle troponin complex.** J Inorg Biochem 1980; 12:695.

153. Jones S, and Thornton JM. **Principles of protein –protein interactions.** Proc Natl Acad Sci 1996; 93:13-20.

154. O'Brien TJ, Hardin JW, Bannon GA, Norris JS, and Quirk JG. **CA125 antigen in human amniotic fluid and fetal membranes.** Am J Obstet Gynecol 1986; 155(1): 50-55.

155. Scopes RK, **Protein Purification Principles and Practice**; New York; Springer Verlag. 1982; pp. 162-197.

156. Price NC, and Stevens L. **Fundamentals of Enzymology**; 2nd ed.;

Newyork, Oxford University Press; 1986; pp. 125.

157. Ormerod MG, Steel K, Westwood JH, and Mazzini MN. **Epithelial membrane antigen: partial purification, assay and properties.** Br J Cancer 1983; 48:533-541.

158. Segal I.H.; **Biochemical Calculations**; 2nd ed.; John Wiley and Sons; 1976; pp. 278-373.

159. Haisma HJ, Battaile A, Stradtman EW, Knapp RC, and Zurawski VR. **Antibody antigen complex formation following injection of CA125 monoclonal antibody in patients with ovarian cancer.** Int J Cancer 1987; 40: 758-762.

160. Wiseman T, Williston S, Randts J, and Lnng-Nam Lin. **Rapid measurement of binding constants and heats of binding using a new titration calorimeter.** Anal Biochem 1989; 179:131-137.

161. Rosier JS, Gokulrangan G, Girault H, Sovojanovsky S, and Wilson GS. **Characterization of protein adsorption and immunosorption kinetic in photoabelated polymer microchanals**. Langmuir 2000; 16: 8489-8494.

162. Weiland GA, Minneman KP, and Molinoff PB. **Thermodynamic of agonist and antagonist interactions with mammalian β adrenergic receptors.** Mol. Pharmacol 1980; 18: 341.

163. Camacho Cj, Weng Z, Vajda S, and Delisi C. Free energy landscapes of encounter complexes in protein-protein association. Biophys J 1999; 76:1166-1178.

164. Seeley DH, Wang WY, and Salhanick HA. Temperature dependence of kinetic interactions between progesterone and uterine cytoplasmic receptor. **Biochem Biophy Acta** 1980; 632: 536-543.

165. Forde A, and Coley J. Choosing and characterizing antibodies. In: Goaling JP. Editor. Immunoassays A practical approach ; Oxford university press London; p.p.62-63

166. Weiland GA and Molinoff PB. **Qutitative analysis of drug-receptor**

interaction I. Determination of kinetic and equilibrium properties. Life Science; 1981; 29: 314.

167. Nemethy G and Scherag AJ. **The structure of water and hydrophobic bonding in proteins: III the thermodynamic properties of hydrophobic bond in protein.** Phys Chem 1962; 66:1775.

168. Waelbroeck M, Van Obberghen E, and De Meyts p. **Thermodynamics of the interaction of insulin with its receptor.** J Biol Chem 1979; 259:7736.

169. Haro LS, and Talamantes FJ. **Thermodynamics and kinetics of mouse prolactin-hepatic receptor interaction.** Mol Cell Endocrinol 1985; 43:199

170. Ross PD and Subramanian S. **Thermodynamics of protein association reaction: Forces contributing to stability.** Biochemistry 1981; 20:3096.

171. Blumenthal DK and Stull JT. **Effect of pH, ionic strength, and temperature on activation by calmodulin and catalytic activity of myosin light chain kinase.** Biochemistry 1982; 21:2386-2391.

172. Laport DC, Wireman EM, and Storm DI. **Calcium-induced exposure of a hydrophobic surface on calmodulin.** Biochemistry 1980; 19: 3814.

173. Johnstone A and Thorpe R. **Immunochemistry in Practice**; 3rd ed.; Blackwell Science Ltd.; 1996; p.p. 1-4, 292-311.

174. Bujalowski W and Jezewska MJ. Quantitative determination of equilibrium binding isotherms for multiple ligand-macromolecule interactions using spectroscopic methods. In: Michael G. Spectrophotometry and spectrofluorimetry: a practical approach .New York: Oxford; 2000; pp. 141.

175. Nolta K and Steck. **Isolation and initial characterization of the bipartite contractile vacuole complex from dictyostelium discoideum.** J Biol Chem 1994; 269:2225.

176. Scheraga HA. **Protein Structure**; New York: Academic Press; 1961; pp. 365-571.

177. Kiernan JA. **Histological and Histochemical Methods Theory and Practice**; 3rd ed., Reed Educational and Professional Publishing Ltd.; 1999;

Chapter 19: pp. 391-398.

178. Williams CA and Chanse MW. **Methods in immunology and immunochemistry**; New York., Academic Press; 1968; vol II; Chapter10: pp 163-174.

179. Haider TM. (2004) **"Development of Radio Receptor Technique for Measurement of CA125 in Malignant and Benign Breast Tumors"**. Thesis, supervised by Al-Mudhaffar S.A., College of Science, Baghdad University.

180. Al-Jobory E. (2004) **"Biochemical Characterization of CA125 in Sera and Tissue of Some Colorectal Tumors"**. Thesis, supervised by Al-Mudhaffar S.A., College of Science, Baghdad University.

181. Mathews Ch k, and Holde KE. **"Biochemistry"** California the Benjamin /Cummings Publishing Co.; 1990; Chapter 6: pp. 191.

182. Sheinerman FB, Norel L, and Honig B. **Electrostatic aspects of protein-protein interaction.** Curr Opin Struct Biol 2000; 10:153-159.

183. Nils H Axelsen. **"Hand book of immuno precipitation"-in Gel Techniques**; 3rd ed.; WA. Benjamin Inc. London; 1983.

184. Nagacura S, and Baba H. **Dipole moment and near ultraviolet absorption of some monosubstituted benzenes: The effect of solvent and hydrogen bonding.** Am Chem. Soc 1952; 74:5693.

185. Pimentel GC. **Hydrogen bonding and electronic transitions: The role of the Franck-Condon principle. J Am Chem Soc** 1957; 79:3323.

186. Silvestien. RM, Bassalar GC, and Marril. TC. **"Spectrophotometric identification of organic compounds"**; New York: John Wiley and Sons; 1981; pp.181.

Leach SJ. **physical principles and techniques of protein chemistry**; New

Third
Molecular Characterization of Prolactin in Ovarian Tumors

Sami A. AlMudhaffar

Hiba Itemad Yousif Nahab

Chapter one

The Ovaries

Anatomy

The female reproductive system (Figure 1-1) consists of **two ovaries, two oviducts (uterinetubes), the uterus, the vagina, and the external genitalia**. Between menarche and menopause, the system undergoes cyclic changes in structure and functional activity [1]. The ovary is essentially intraperitoneal organ as indicated by its peritoneal doubling known as the mesovarium, which is found on the posterior aspect of the broad ligament of the uterus. The paired ovaries are found close to the lateral wall of the lesser pelvis at the angle formed by external and internal iliac arteries and in close association with the ureter separated from these structures by the parietal peritoneum [2,3].

The mesovarium, ovarian ligament and infundibular pelvic (suspensory ligament of the ovary) ligaments determine the anatomic mobility of the ovary, the suspensory ligament attaches the ovary to the lateral pelvic walls and contains the ovarian artery, veins and accompanying nerves [4,5]

During the reproductive years, the ovary weighs 4 to 8 g and measures approximately 3 cm long, 1.5 cm wide, and 1cm thick. However, the weight varies during the menstrual cycle [4,6].

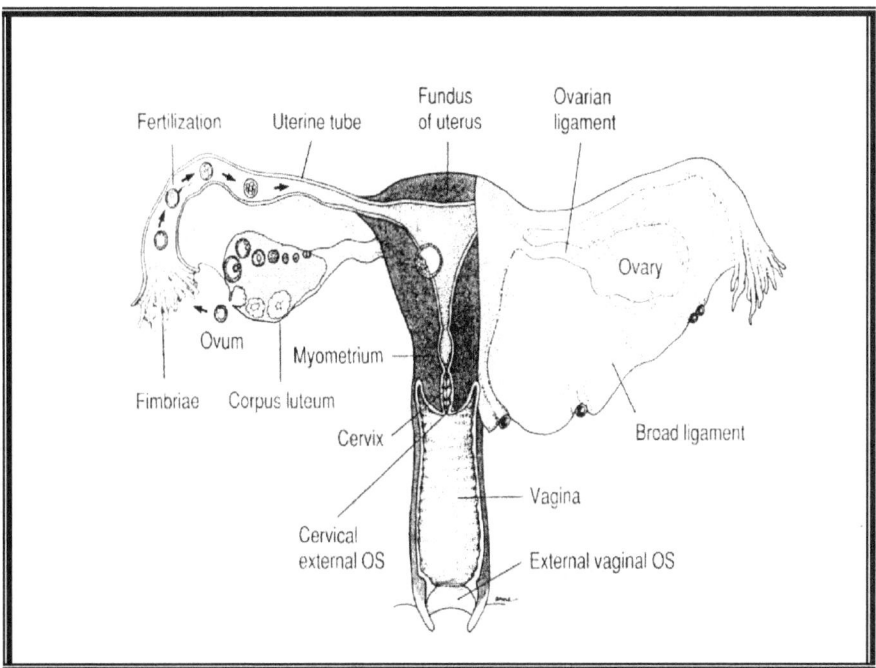

Figure (1-1): Internal organs of the female reproductive system. [1]

Histology

The ovary consists of following parts [1,7,8]. (Figure 1-2)

- **Medullary region**: containing a rich vascular bed within a cellular loose connective tissue and contains blood vessels, nerves, lymphatics and smooth muscle fibers.
- **Cortical region**: contains the ovarian follicles in all stages of development, surrounded by the connective tissue elements of the stroma and the hilar cells.
- **The germinal epithelium**: is a layer of simple squamous or cuboidal epithelium that covers the surface of the ovary.
- **The tunica albuginea**: is a dense layer of connective tissue under the epithelium.
- **The ovarian follicles**: are embedded in the stroma of the cortex, and consists of an oocyte, surrounded by one or more layers of cells. When the surrounding cells form a single layer, they are called **follicular cells**;

later in development, when they form several layers, they are called **granulosa cells**.

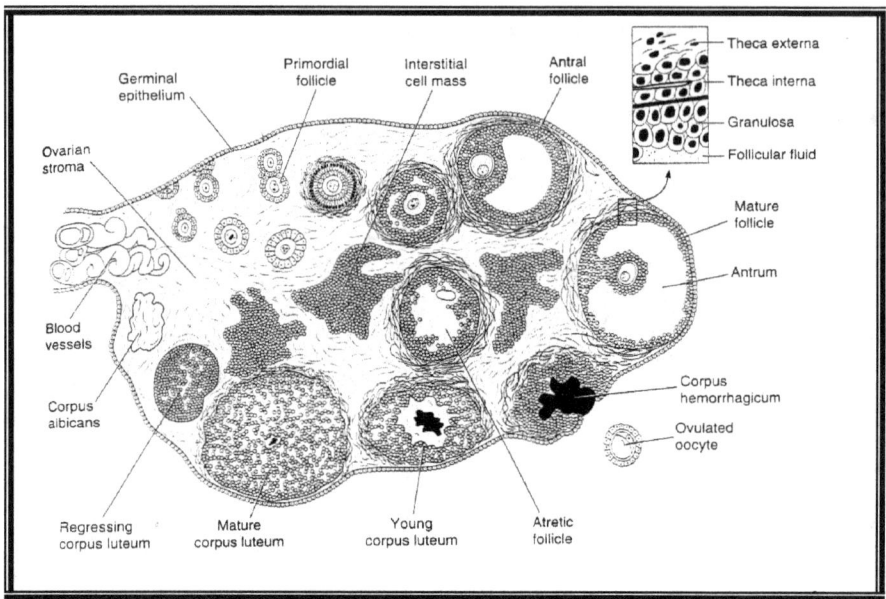

Figure (1-2): Histology of the ovary [7]

- **A corpus luteum**: is a transient endocrine organ that secretes principally progesterone for about 14 day. After ovulation, the granulosa cells and those of the theca interna that remain in the ovary called corpus luteum (yellow body).

Ovarian Physiology

Ovarian Function

The ovaries perform two important physiological functions, **reproduction and control of secondary sex characteristics** [9,10]. The hypothalamus plays an important role in the hormonal regulation of female reproductive function (Figure 1-3). The hormonal control of reproduction has progressed from the identification of ovarian steroids and pituitary gonadotropins to the discovery of hypothalamic releasing factors [3].

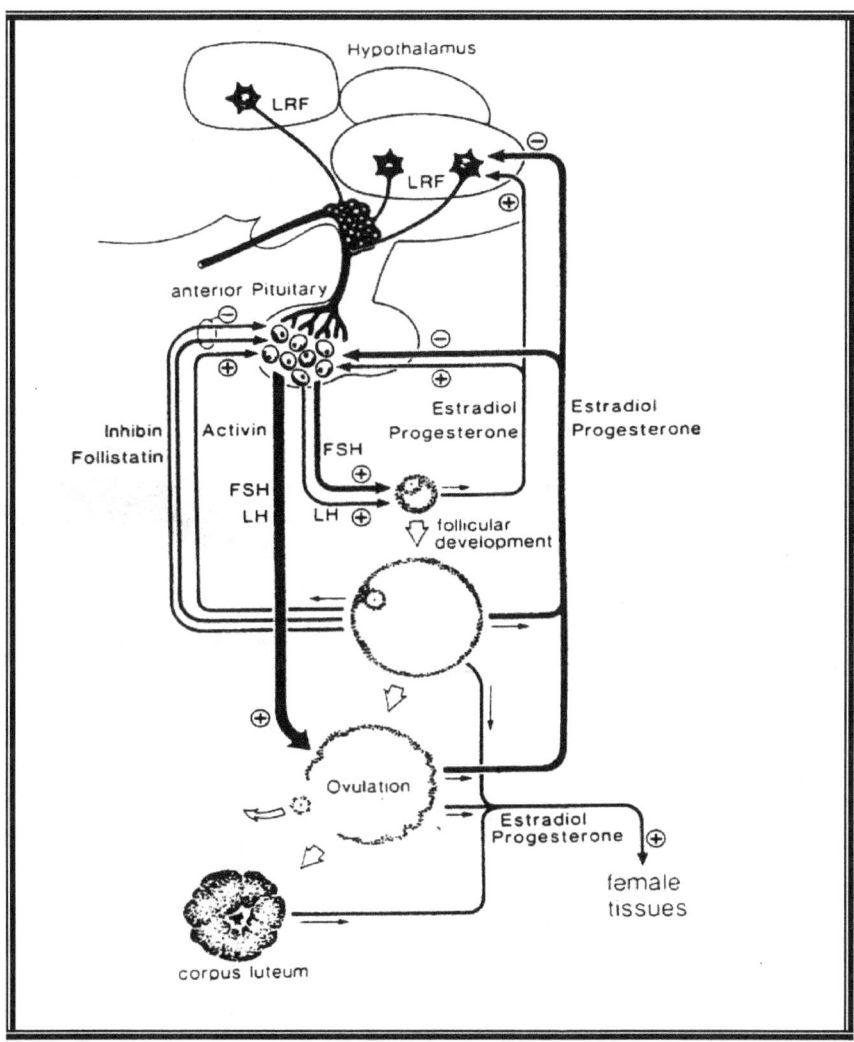

Figure (1-3): A diagrammatic representation of the hypothalamic – **pituitary – ovarian axis** [3].

The hormonal functions, which makes fertility possible by releasing the ovum and regulating the menstrual cycle through the secretion of progesterone and estrogen, which stimulate the development of female secondary sex characteristics [10].

The other ovarian function during embryonic life because of the stimulation by another gonadotrophic hormone, **human chorionic gonadotrophin (HCG)** secreted by the placenta, after birth the stimulation is lost and the ovaries become almost dormant until the prepubertal period [11].

Menstrual Cycle.

The female reproductive system undergoes a series of regular cyclic changes termed the menstrual cycle, the most obvious of these changes is periodic vaginal bleeding, resulting from shedding of the endometrial lining of the uterus. The ovary plays a central role in this process, since it appears to be responsible for regulating both the cyclic changes and the length of the menstrual cycle [7,12].

The length of the menstrual cycle is defined as the period from onset of one menstrual bleeding until onset of the next, the median length of the normal cycle in women of reproductive age is 28 day.

The menstrual cycle is usually divided into two phases: follicular or proliferative phase and luteal or secretary phase [13] (Figure 1-4). The interval from the onset of menses to ovulation (follicular phase) is variable in duration and accounts for the range of cycle lengths observed in ovulating women [3,14].

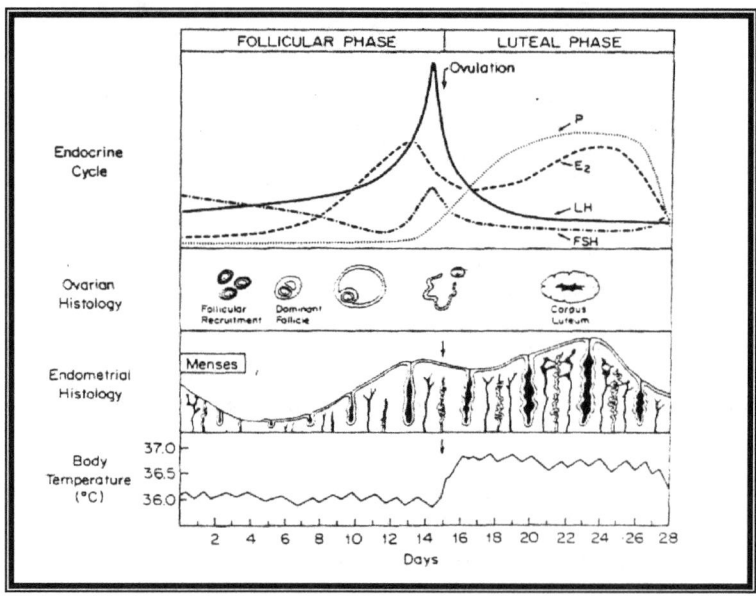

Figure (1-4): Menstrual Cycle [3]

At follicular phase, a particular follicle begins to enlarge under the general influence of follicle stimulating Hormone (FSH). Estradiol (E2) levels are low during the first week of the follicular phase, but they begin to rise progressively as the follicle enlarges, luteinizing Hormone (LH) is released either in response to high level of E2 in a "positive feedback". Progesterone levels are very low during the follicular phase[15]. After ovulation, the residual follicle undergoes dramatic changes in structure and function that convert into the corpus luteum. During the last few days of the previous luteal phase, progesterone and estrogen levels decline because of demise of the corpus luteum, and FSH level rise. This rise in FSH initiates the development of follicles and the beginning of the next menstrual cycle. The luteal phase is relatively constant and approximately 14 day in most women[3,15,16].

Ovarian Hormones

The ovarian hormones are classified on the basis of chemical structure and principal biologic function and consist of three major types: **estrogen, progesterone** and **androgens**[3,17]. (Figure 1-5).

Estrogens **are required for the normal maturation of the female, they stimulate growth of uterus, fallopian tubes, thickening of the vaginal mucosa, promotion of breast development, maturation of external genitalia, and they promote development of the secondary sexual characteristics of women**[18].

Estradiol — Progesterone — Testosterone

Figure (1-5): Chemical formulas of the female sex hormones [3,7]

Progesterone is the principal secretary product of the corpus luteum and is responsible for the progestational effects. This hormone supports follicular growth and function as well as primes the cells of the uterine wall for proper future implantation of the embryo. It is also inhibits uterine contractions, increases the viscosity of cervical mucus, and promotes glandular development of the breast[19,20].

Androgens are produced by the theca cells and to a lesser degree by the ovarian stroma. The normal ovary secretes potent androgens, including testosterone, dihydrotestosterone, androstenedione and dehydroepiandrosterone (DHEA)[7,19]. Some studies suggest that androgens may have important anabolic effect on protein metabolism[21].

Ovarian Tumors

Ovarian tumors are common, most are benign, but malignant ovarian tumors are the leading cause of death from reproductive tract cancer [22]. According to the bases of distinct clinical and pathologic features, ovarian tumors can be separated into three major entities: **epithelial tumors, germ cell tumors,** and **sex cord-stromal tumors** [23,24].

The vast majority of ovarian cancer is epithelial tumors, these account 90% of malignant ovarian tumors [23,25]. The classification of common epithelial tumors has been developed by the **World Health Organization (WHO)** and the **International Federation of Gynecology Obstetrics (FIGO)** [23,26]. (Table 1-1).

Epithelial ovarian tumors are classified as benign, borderline and malignant [27,28,29]. Approximately 10-20% of the common epithelial tumors are borderline malignancy (low malignant potential), these tumors are neither benign nor clearly malignant [30]. Epithelial tumors of the ovary metastasize primarily by direct extension, implantation of tumor cells on the peritoneal surface and lymphatic spread [31].

Serous epithelial ovarian tumors are the most common form of epithelial neoplasms and account for 46% of all epithelial tumors. Approximately 20% of serous tumors are adenofibroma consisting of a firm, white fibroma component containing multiple neoplastic cysts [32,33].

Table (1-1): World Health Organization (WHO) classification of Ovarian Tumors [23,26]

Epithelial tumors	Malignant serous tumors	Adenocarcinoma, papillary adenocarcinoma, papillary cystadenocarcinoma	
		Surface papillary carcinoma	
		Malignant adenofibroma, cystadenofibroma	
	Malignant mucinous tumors	Adenocarcinoma, cystadenocarcinoma	
		Malignant adenofibroma, cystadenofibroma	
	Malignant endometrioid tumors	Carcinoma	Adenocarcinoma
			Adenocanthoma
			Malignant adenofibroma, cystadenofibroma
		Endometrioid stromal sarcomas	
		Clear cell (mesonephroid) tumors, malignant	
		Brenner tumors, malignant	
		Mixed epithelial tumors, malignant	
		Undifferentiated carcinoma	
Sex cord-stromal tumors	Granulosa-stromal cell tumors	Granulosa cell tumor	
		Tumors in the thecoma-fibroma group	
		Fibroma	
	Androblastomas: sertoli-leyding cell tumors	Tubular Androblastomas, sertoli cell tumor	
		Sertoli-leyding cell (tubular adenoma with leyding cells)	

Germ cell tumors	Dysgerminoma.		
	Endodermal sinus tumor.		
	Polyembryoma.		
	Teratomas.		

Incidence

Epithelial ovarian cancer (EOC) is the fifth most common cause of death from cancer in women and accounts for about 4% of incident cancer in most cancer registries. It is leading cause of death from gynecologic malignancies [34,35,36]. The incidence of epithelial ovarian cancer occurs infrequently in women under age 40 [37]. The vast majority of (EOC) is diagnosed in postmenopausal women. However, the median age diagnosis is 63 years, with 38% of all cases diagnosed at age 65 or older [23,38].

Etiology

The etiology of ovarian cancer due to, reproductive factor, genetic, environmental all have been identified as playing an important role in the development of ovarian cancer [33,39,40].

Reproductive risk factor associated with an elevated risk for the development of ovarian cancer include those associated with an increased number of ovulation in a woman's lifetime [33]. Conversely factors that decrease the number of ovulatory cycles, such as oral contraceptive use and pregnancy, are associated with a decreased risk for the development of ovarian cancer [41].

The genetic etiology of hereditary ovarian cancer is well understood, approximately 5% to 10% of all ovarian cancers are thought to be hereditary in etiology [42]. They found if a woman is a member of a hereditary breast and ovarian cancer family or a hereditary ovarian cancer family, has risk of 50% to develop ovarian cancer [33]. The majority of hereditary ovarian cancer results from inherited mutation in two genes BRCA1 and BRCA2 [43]. However, it is known that mutation of BRCA1 and BRCA2 genes are responsible for most cases of familial ovarian cancer [44,45].

The environmental risk factor that has been consistently associated with an increased risk for the disease is the exposure to talc powder on the perineal area [33].

Staging of Ovarian Tumors

Staging of ovarian cancer is based on the extent and location of disease found at surgical exploration [29]. The staging classification is based on findings after opening the abdomen but not after surgical debulking. The surgeon must define the amount of disease after opening the abdomen [26].

The majority of studies on staging of ovarian cancer is based on the **International Federation of Gynecology Obstetrics (FIGO)**[23,26,46], as it is shown in Table (1-2). Several studies suggest that 70% of ovarian cancer are (FIGO) stage III/IV at presentation. Although survival rates for women with early stage ovarian cancer are 70-90%, but for advanced disease, the survival rate is only 20-30% thus, it seems likely that early detection of disease, perhaps by screening, would be beneficial [47].

Clinical Presentation (Symptoms)

Ovarian cancer has no specific signs or symptoms, particularly in early-stage disease. The most common symptoms of epithelial ovarian cancer include abdominal distension due to ascites, pleural effusions may also be present with ascites. Other symptoms include nausea, dyspepsia, lower abdominal discomfort, early satiety and abnormal vaginal bleeding. It is important to note that most of these symptoms may be associated with a variety of other intra-abdominal and gastrointestinal conditions [26,33,48].

As the disease progress, symptoms become more specific and constant, related to pain and pressure caused by enlarging tumor or ascites that is not uncommon [49].

Table (1-2): (FIGO) staging of Ovarian Tumors [23].

Stage I	Growth limited to the ovaries
Stage 1 a	Growth limited to one ovary, no ascites, no tumor on external surface, capsule intact.
Stage1 b	Growth limited to both ovaries, no ascites, no tumor on the external surface, capsules intact
Stage 1 c	Tumor either stage 1a or 1b but with tumor on the surface of one or both ovaries, with capsules ruptured, with ascites present containing malignant cells, or with positive peritoneal washings.
Stage II	Growth involving one or both ovaries with pelvic extension.
Stage II a	Extension or metastases to the uterus or the tubes.
Stage II b	Extension to other pelvic tissues.
Stage II c	Tumor either stage IIa or IIb but with tumor on the surface of one or both ovaries, with capsules ruptured, both ascites present containing malignant cells or with positive peritoneal washings.
Stage III	Tumor involving one or both ovaries with peritoneal implants outside the pelvis or positive retroperitoneal or inguinal nodes, superficial liver metastases equal stage III. Tumor limited to the true pelvis but with histologically proved malignant extension to small bowel or omentum.
Stage III a	Tumor grossly limited to the true pelvis with negative nodes but with histologically confirmed microscopic seeding of abdominal peritoneal surfaces.
Stage III b	Tumor of one or both ovaries with histologically confirmed implants of abdominal peritoneal surfaces, none exceeding 2cm in diameter. Nodes are negative.
Stage III c	Abdominal implants greater than 2cm in diameter, or positive retroperitoneal or inguinal nodes.
Stage IV	Growth involving one or both ovaries with distant metastases. If pleural effusion is present, there must be positive cytology to allot a case to stage IV.

Parenchymal liver metastases equal stage IV

Diagnosis

Ovarian malignant tumors are often diagnosed in women who are in their fifth or sixth decade of life [50]. The stage of epithelial ovarian tumor, is the greatest prognostic factor [33]. Approximately 70% of patients are diagnosed as having stage III or IV disease [51]. Other diagnostic factor that may be important to include, grade of the tumor, histopathologic subtype, performance status and age of patient, volume of disease prior to surgery, volume of disease remaining after primary surgery and presence of ascites [33,52,53].

Studies have shown that **Color Doppler Ultrasound (CDU)** may be able to detect neovascularization in some solid tumors of the ovary, endometrium, breast, and kidney [54]. Although small ovarian cysts are often identified with use of **ultrasound examination** of postmenopausal ovaries. Approximately 8% to 9% of postmenopausal women who do not have clinically palpable ovaries are found by ultrasound examination to have ovarian cysts between 1.5 and 3 cm in size [23].

The combined use of **serum CA125, physical and pelvic examination** and **transvaginal ultrasound (TVS)** detects the disease progression [55,56,57]. Although **computer tomography (CT)** scanning is useful in preoperative evaluation of the extent of disease [23]. Several studies show comparison between the diagnostic value of CA-125 with that of computer tomography (CT) and nuclear magnetic resonance imaging(MRI) in the tumor progression of patients with ovarian tumors[58].

Ovarian Tumor Markers

A tumor marker is a substance present in or produced by a tumor itself or produced by the host in response to a tumor that can determine the presence of a tumor based on measurement in the blood or secretions [59].

Tumor marker capable of detecting early ovarian cancer would be valuable because most patients are not diagnosed until the disease is advanced. Although markers are helpful in detecting and monitoring germ cell and some epithelial malignant[26].

A carbohydrate antigen (CA-125) is a marker for ovarian and endometrial carcinomas [60]. Several studies explored the use of serum CA-125 level in the early detection of ovarian carcinoma [26] CA-125 is elevated in 80-90% of women with epithelial ovarian cancer, decrease of level have been shown to be associated with response to therapy [22,61]. CA-125 is elevated in 50% of patients with stage I disease, 90% with stage II, and more than 90% with stages III and IV, it is also elevated in women in the follicular phase of the menstrual cycle and in benign conditions such as cirrhosis, hepatitis, endometriosis, pericarditis and early pregnancy. CA-125 is also useful in differentiating benign from malignant disease in patients with palpable ovarian masses, but it cannot be used to differentiate ovarian tumor from other malignancies [59]. Carcinoembryonic Antigen (CEA) levels are elevated in approximately 58% of patients with stage II epithelial ovarian tumor. The frequency of elevated CEA levels progressively increases with advancing stage and bulk tumor [26].

Treatment

The treatment of ovarian cancer remains combination of surgery and chemotherapy [62] the treatment of early- stage ovarian cancer consists of thorough surgical staging and in selected cases, no treatment with chemotherapy. In patients with high-grade or clear–cell tumors of ovary, treatment with chemotherapy is recommended. In advanced-stage ovarian cancer, the treatment consists of tumor cytoreductive surgery and chemotherapy [32,33].

Surgical management of early-stage ovarian cancer

Approximately 10% to 15% of patient will present with early- stage ovarian cancer. However, in this stage treatment with chemotherapy will not be necessary. The surgical staging procedure is based on the patterns of spread of ovarian cancer and includes a thorough visual inspection of all peritoneal surfaces alone with biopsies and through evaluation of pelvic and para-aortic lymph nodes[33]. Patients with apparent early-stage disease often require different therapy from these with microscopic metastases and proper evaluation of the upper abdomen is rarely possible through a lower abdominal incision. If there is gross disease in the upper abdomen, proper resection requires adequate exposure [26,63].

Surgical management of advanced-stage ovarian cancer

The primary aim for surgical management of advanced-stage epithelial ovarian cancer is the removal of as much tumor as possible at the time of initial surgery. The generally accepted treatment for patients with advance-stage (stage III, IV) ovarian cancer was similar to cytoreductive surgery followed by chemotherapy. The theory supporting the principle of maximal surgical cytoreduction is that epithelial ovarian cancer is a chemosensitive tumor and that, by removing a large proportion of the tumor, the remaining cells will be thrown into active division and will therefore be more sensitive to chemotherapy [23,33,64].

The Prolactin (PRL):

Prolactin (PRL) is a poly peptide hormone with a molecular weight of 22000 Dalton and an amino acid sequence of 199 amino acids, it is synthesized and secreted by the lactotrophs of the pituitary [65,66]. The lactotrophs can be identified by immunoperoxidase staining by using specific antisera and believed to arise directly from the acidophil stem cell line [67]. The relative number and PRL content of lactotropic cells is increased in fetal pituitary glands and during pregnancy. The increase in the number of lactotropic cells is the result of elevated concentration of estrogens during pregnancy [68].

Regulation of Prolactin Secretion :

The normal plasma prolactin concentration is approximately 8ng /ml in women and 5ng/ml in men [12]. Secretion of PRL, as for other hormones released by the anterior lobe of the pituitary gland falls under hypothalamic control Figure (1-6) [3]. However, PRL is unique among adenohypophyseal hormones in that the primary control of its secretion is Inhibitory (prolactin inhibitory factor, PIF) rather than stimulatory (prolactin-releasing factor, PRF)[68].

Dopamine, the most important PIF, which is secreted by the tuberoinfundibular dopaminergic pathways and is present in hypophyseal portal vessel blood in sufficient concentration to inhibit PRL release [69]. Although dopamine suppresses virtually all aspects of PRL synthesis and secretion [70].

Although the most important of the PRFs are **thyrotropin releasing hormone (TRH)**, this factor is secreted into the hypophyseal-portal blood and stimulates PRL secretion within minutes when injected intravenously into human subjects [68,71,72]. TRH, however, is not the only PRF. Factors such as **vasoactive intestinal peptide (VIP)** has also been shown to stimulate PRL release [68]. Another candidate PRF is **vasopressin**, this factor also stimulates

PRL release and can not be excluded as a physiological PRF. It is present in hypophyseal-portal blood and is released during stress and shock [3].

In humans, exercise, surgical and psychological stresses, and stimulation of the nipple increase PRL secretion. The PRL level rises during sleep, the rise starting after the onset of sleep and persisting throughout the sleep period. Also PRL secretion is increased during pregnancy, reaching a peak at the time of parturition [12]. Finally, an important influence on PRL regulation appears to be exerted by PRL itself by short feedback loop between the pituitary and hypothalamus. Short feedback-loop inhibition of gonadotrophin releasing hormone (GnRH) secretion by PRL has also been suggested as the cause for inhibition of gonadotrophin (Gn) secretion that occurs in women who are nursing and in patients with PRL- secreting adenomas of the pituitary gland [68].

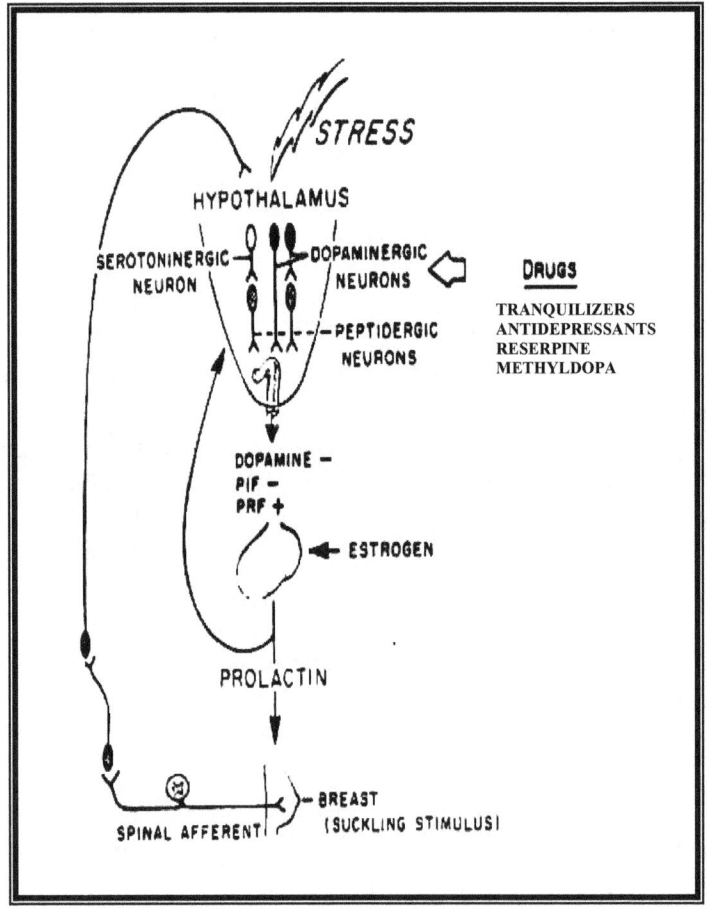

Figure (1-6): Hypothalamic regulation of PRL secretion [3]

The Structure of Prolactin

The structure of human pituitary prolactin contains 199 amino acids residues and has three intramolecular disulfide bridges with a molecular weight of 22000-25000 D [12,73](Figure 1-7). Most of studies concerning PRL chemistry were performed on ovine prolactin [74].

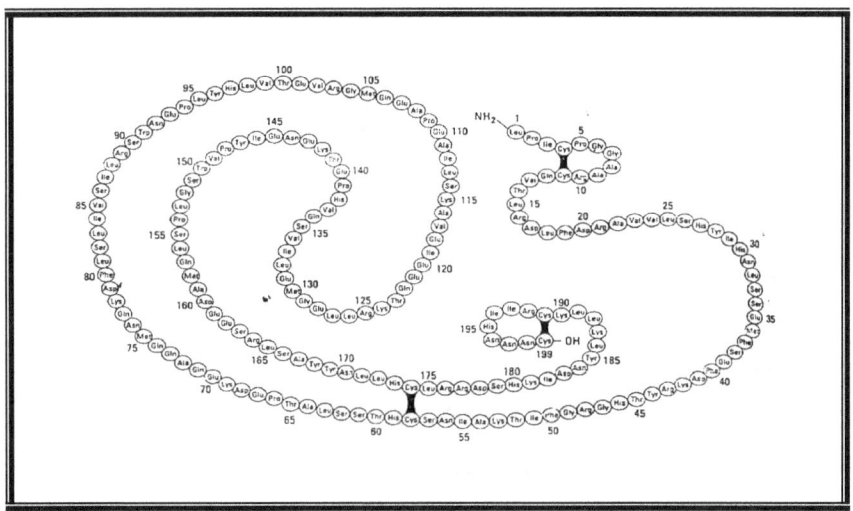

Figure (1-7): Structure of human prolactin [12].

The structure of 0-PRL is similar to that of human growth hormone (hGH) and human chorionic somatomamotropin (hCS). The half-life of PRL, like that of GH, is about 20 minutes. Each of PRL, GH has a single tryptophan residue, and each has two homologous disulfide bonds, GH has disulfide bond between residues 53-165 and 182-189 while PRL has disulfide bonds between residues 4-11, 58-173 and 190-198 [15]. Figure (1-8).

The secondary structure of 0-PRL was determined by using **Circular Dichroism Technique (CD)**, which gave a strong negative band at 233 nm and a second weak band at 209nm. Because of many properties of 0-PRL are similar to those of hGH, therefore spectra of 0-PRL is similar to those of hGH [75].

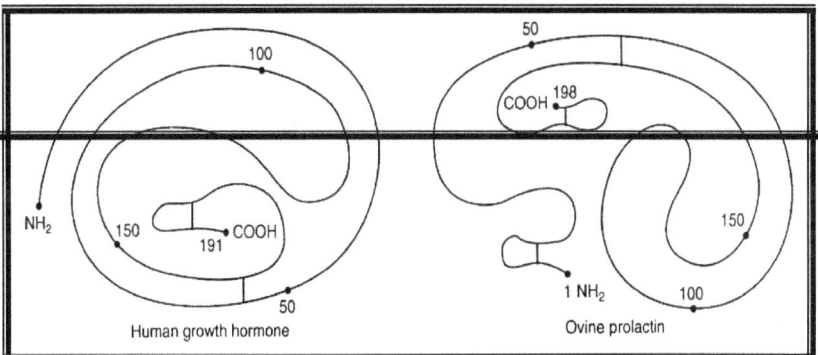

Figure (1-8): The structures of human growth hormone and ovine prolactin [15]

Function of Prolactin:

PRL function can be classified into two main types:

Non –Reproductive Function

These functions of PRL have been demonstrated in different organs such as adrenal gland and liver

Adrenal Gland

Adrenal cortical tissue has the highest concentration of PRL receptor in the body, the adrenal cortex responds to PRL with activation of both ornithine decarboxylase and adenyl cyclase [76]. There is some evidence that PRL may regulate aldosterone levels and good evidence that it regulates plasma levels of dehydroepiandrosterone (DHEA) and (DHEA) sulphate [77].

Liver

Hepatic PRL receptors have been studied in greater detail than any others [78]. Several studies suggested that hepatic PRL receptors are regulated by sex steroids [79]. There is evidence that female rat liver contains much greater hepatic PRL than in male [80].

Reproductive Functions
Prolactin and Male Reproductive System

PRL is widely expressed in different tissues, and it is presumed to have both local and systemic actions. In males it is known to influence reproductive functions but the significance and mechanisms of PRL action in male accessory reproductive tissues are poorly understood [81].

In reproduction PRL has been shown to have luteotropic actions and to regulate testicular function by increasing the binding of luteinizing hormone (LH) to leyding cells [82]. PRL has also been suggested to be involved in the regulation of abnormal prostatic function [83,84,85,86]. However, about the specific and direct effect of PRL on human prostate, the source of PRL and the mechanisms underlying the responses of prostatic cells to PRL have remained unclear [87,88,89]. The increasing evidence that PRL is involved in the regulation of male reproductive function has led to several studies of receptors in male reproductive organ [76].

Prolactin and Female Reproductive System: (PRL and Ovary)

PRL levels in women are slightly but consistently higher than in men. Several studies suggested that PRL level may fall after the menopause due to the loss of estrogen stimulation. Some PRL is necessary for normal luteal phase progesterone production but too much inhibits progesterone secretion. In vivo and vitro studies indicate that part of the PRL effect is at the ovary with both estrogen and progesterone production less than are appropriate for the LH and FSH levels [76]. However part of the PRL effect is at the hypothalamic-pituitary level with FSH and LH levels inappropriately low in relation to the low ovarian steroid levels [90]. (Figure 1-9) shows the interactions of the hypothalamic control of gonadotrophins (LH, FSH) and PRL secretion during the follicular and luteal phase [91].

PRL concentrations are lowest in the early follicular phase, rise in the late follicular phase to an ovulatory peak and then fall back in the luteal phase to levels which are still higher than in the follicular phase [77]. In addition PRL concentrations seem to be positively correlated with those of estrogen but not with those of progesterone, FSH or LH [92].

Ovarian dysfunction has reported to primarily result from the lack ormone (FSH), as well as the direct effect of PRL on the ovary [93]

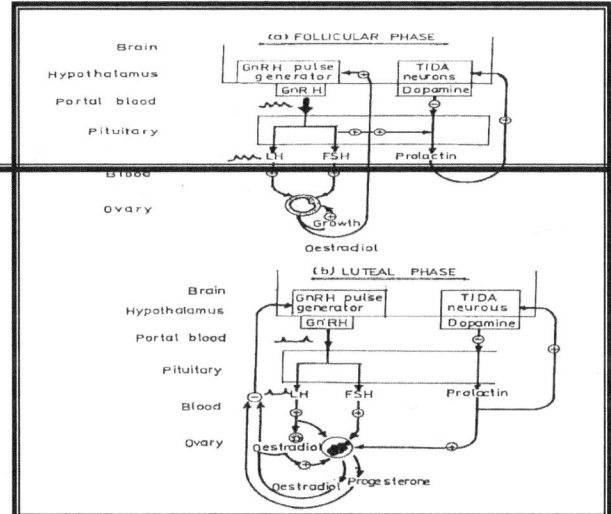

Figure (1-9): Interaction between the hypothalamic control of gonadotrophins (LH&FSH) and Prolactin [91].

Disorders of Prolactin Secretion

PRL exists as three mains molecular, the 23-KDa monomer is the predominant form in general population, but other circulating species include the 50-KDa form (big PRL) and the 150 to 170 KDa macroprolactin (big-big PRL) [94,95,96].

The presence of macroprolactin, which is physiologically inactive, may contribute to the apparent hyperprolactinemia, therefore it becomes important to determine whether the patient is hyperprolactinemic due an increase in monomeric PRL or due to the non-clearance of the macroprolactin [97].

Hyperprolactinemia is common and the cause is usually apparent [98]. In women it is often present with galactorrhea, amenorrhea, oligomenorrhea, and anovulation with infertility [99,100]. A cause of increasing PRL production is PRL-secreting pituitary adenomas **prolactinoma**, the most common secretary pituitary tumor, the natural history of prolactinoma is not known precisely, but most of these tumors grow slowly over years [3].

Several studies make some important points about hyperprolactinemia in women with the polycystic ovary syndrome (PCOS)[101]. The prevalence of hyperprolactinemia in women with (PCOS) may have been overestimated. The level of PRL in the patients with PCO was significantly higher than in normal women [93,102,103]. Women who have infertility due to anovulation in association with (PCOS) are particularly difficult to treat [104]. Although polycystic ovaries (PCO) are found in at least 20% of women of reproductive age and up to half of these will have symptoms of (PCOS)[105].

Basal PRL level are used in the assessment of hyperprolactinemia. The normal level of PRL in the serum of the nonpregnant, nonlactating female is 5 to 20 ng/ml .In Patients with drug-induced hyperprolactinemia and in functional variety, the level range between 50 to 100ng/ml. The PRL level in patients with pituitary microadenoma range between 100 and 250ng/ml, levels in excess of 300ng/ml usually are encountered with larger tumors. Highest levels of PRL are encountered in patients harboring PRL- secreting macroadenomas that have invaded above and sectioned the stalk [67]. Therefore, an increased serum PRL level must be interpreted in conjunction with anatomic findings (MRI and CT) to determine whether the hyperprolactinemia is due to a prolactinoma or to some other process [3].

Methods For The Determination Of Prolactin

Different methods are used to detect PRL effect on different target organs, the assay methods for determination of PRL can be classified as follows:

Bioassays

The levels of PRL were estimated by using inconvenient bioassays, the classical of bioassays were based on the growth-promoting action of PRL using the pigeon crop sac or the rat mammary gland [68]. There is fast proliferation of the epithelial lining of the crop sac, which contact with basophilic changes in the cytoplasm and they are sensitive to PRL, these changes were used as an indicated to the effect of the hormone [106].

Radioimmunoassay (RIA)

Radioimmunoassay (RIA) has been a popular method for clinical endocrine determination [107,108]. RIA is a competitive protein binding (CPB) technique that uses radio-labeled hormone as the tagged hormone and antisera prepared against the specific hormone as a binding site. Competition between unlabeled hormone in the patient sample and the added-labeled hormone for a limited number of antibody–binding sites forms the basis of the assay. Although RIA is a good technique when high sensitivity is required [18,109].

Immunoradiometric assay (IRMA) [18,68,110]

These methods are similar to (RIA) in that a radio labeled substance is used in an antibody-antigen reaction. However, the radioactive label is attached to the antibody instead of the hormone (Antigen). In addition, an excess of antibody is present in the assay, rather than a limited quantity, is present in the assay. Because the entire unknown antigen becomes bound in IRMA rather than just a portion as in RIA, so that IRMA assays are more sensitive.

Both one-site and two-site IRMAs exist. In the **one site assay**, the excess antibody that is not bound to the patient sample is removed by addition of a precipitating binder, this binder is antigen bound to some solid support. In the **two-site assay (Sandwich technique)**, a hormone with at least two antibody-binding sites is adsorbed into a solid phase to which one of the antibodies is firmly attached to the walls of the assay tube. After binding to this antibody is completed, a second antibody labeled with ^{125}I is added to the assay. This antibody reacts with the second antibody-binding site to form the Sandwich comprising antibody-hormone-labeled antibody.

Mechanism of Action of Prolactin

Most experimental information regarding the mechanism of action of PRL. Since PRL is a relatively large polypeptide hormone. PRL, like other pituitary hormones, binds to a specific receptor on the cell membrane of its target organs (breast, adrenal, ovaries, testes, prostate, kidney, and liver). However the exact intracellular mechanism of PRL action is not known [68].

Several studies proposed a mechanism for the PRL action on the mammary gland [111]. Figure (1-10).

- PRL molecule interacts initially with the receptor sites located on the outer surface of the plasma membrane.
- The receptor-hormone complex leads to activation of phospholipase (PLA) and this activation leads to the release of poly unsaturated fatty acids (PUFA), including Arachidonic acid (AA), from membrane phospholipids.
- Arachidonic acid is converted to prostaglandin (PG) via prostaglandin synthetase complex (PGS).
- Prostglandin (PG) stimulate guanylate cyclase to increase cyclic guanycine monophosphate (cGMP) synthesis.
- The newly-synthesized cGMP may stimulate cyclic adenosine mono phosphate phosphodiesterase (cAMP PD) and reduce the rate of cAMP synthesis.
- The altered (cAMP) levels may stimulate casein synthesis, then stimulate RNA synthesis.

Studies on the mechanism of PRL action have demonstrated the existence of a low-molecular-weight soluble factor (second messenger) which transfers the hormonal information from the receptor to the nuclei [112].

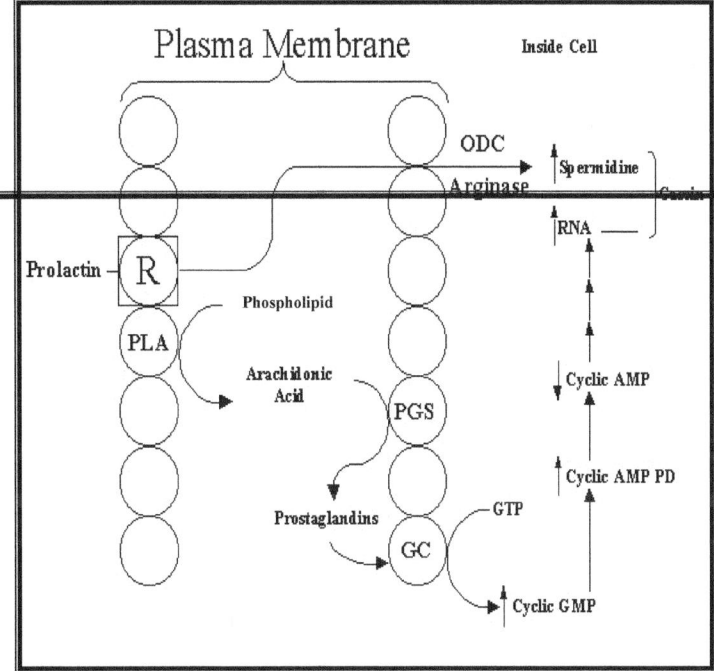

Figure (1-10): The mechanism for Prolactin actions on mammary tissues [111].

Chapter Two

Patients

Two groups of premenopausal patients, and one group postmenopausal patients were included in this study, group I consisted of 10 premenopausal patients with benign serous ovarian tumor, cystadenoma, (Age = 17- 38 years), group II consisted of 6 postmenopausal patients with benign serous ovarian tumor, cystadenoma, (Age = 51- 60 years), group III consisted of 4 premenopausal patients with malignant serous ovarian tumor, cystadenocarcinoma, (Age = 27- 33 years).

Blood Sampling

Blood samples (5-10 ml) were obtained from premenopausal and postmenopausal patients immediately before surgery and by veinpuncture. Age matched sera were obtained from (10) healthy female volunteers (Age=26-35 years) Group (IV) represented premenopausal patients.

Blood samples were centrifuged at 1500xg for 10min after allowing the blood to clot at room temperature and kept at -20 °C until assaying.

Collection of Specimens

The tumor tissues were surgically removed from ovarian tumor patients by hysterectomy. The specimens were cut off and immediately rinsed with ice-cold isotonic saline solution. They were collected individually in plastic receptacles and stored at -20 °C until homogenization.

Preparation Of Ovarian Tumors Tissue Homogenate

The frozen tissue was thawed, sliced finely with a scalped in petridish standing on ice bath. The slices were further minced with scissors, then homogenized at 4 °C in (ST) buffer solution (0.01M) with ratio of 1:5 (weight:volume), using manual homogenizer. The homogenate was filtered through several layers of nylon gauze, then centrifuged at 1500xg for 15 min in a cooling centrifuge at 4 °C. The supernatants were used through out our study.

Determination Of Total Protein Content In Benign and Malignant Serous

The total protein of ovarian tumors was determined by **Lowry et al** [114] method using bovine serum albumin (BSA) as a standard protein. The details of the methods described according to the following steps:

1- One milliliter of each of standard BSA (0,20,40,80,120,160) µg/ml was pipette in a set of test tubes. The experiment was carried out in duplicate.

2- One hundred microliters of ovarian tumors homogenate was also pipetted in test tubes and the, volumes were made up to 1ml with distilled water.

3- Five milliliters of reagent C was added to all assay tubes. Then the contents were mixed by vortexing and allowed to stand for 10min at room temperature.

4- Half milliliters of reagent D was added drop by drop with vigorous mixing to all assay tubes. The mixture was left to stand for 30min at room temperature.

5- The absorbency of the developing color was read at 600nm against the appropriate blank.

6- The standard curve was obtained by plotting the absorbency against the corresponding concentration of standard protein and used to determine the unknown protein concentration of the sample (ovarian tumors homogenate). Figure (2-1).

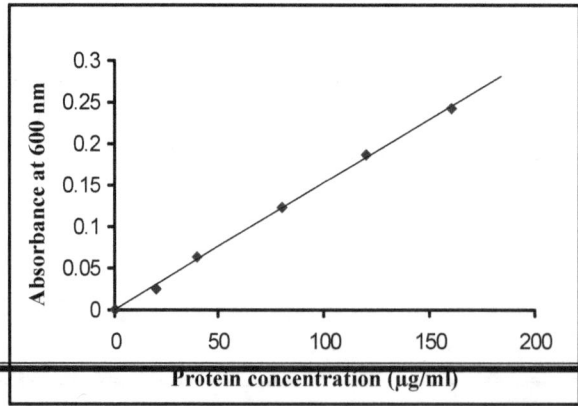

Figure (2-1): Standard curve of protein determination

Determination of hPRL Levels in Sera of Benign and Malignant Serous Ovarian Tumors Patient and Controls

Serum levels of human PRL were determined by an Immunoradiometric assay (IRMA). The method is based on the use of antibody-coated tubes, employing to mouse monoclonal antibodies directed against different epitopes on the hPRL molecule. The assay protocol is described in Table (2-1).

Table (2-1): IRMA assay protocol of serum hPRL (ng/ml).

	hPRL standard (ng/ml)						Control	Unknown samples		
	0	1	2	3	4	5	—	1	2	3
Coated tube no.	1,2	3,4	5,6	7,8	9,10	11,12	13,14	15,16	17,18	19,20
Standard (µl)	50	50	50	50	50	50	—	—	—	—
Control serum or sample (µl)	—	—	—	—	—	—	50	50	50	50
Tracer (µl)	500	500	500	500	500	500	500	500	500	500

- Dispense reagents in the bottom of coated tubes according to the scheme above.
- Dispense 500μl tracer into all tubes. Prepare two additional non-coated tubes for total activity computation containing only 500μl tracer and set them aside until counting.
- Mix the contents of tubes with a Vortex and incubate for one hour at room temperature while continuously shaking (300- 350 rpm).
- Carefully aspirate the incubation mixture and wash twice with 2ml wash solution.
- Measure the radioactivity of tubes.

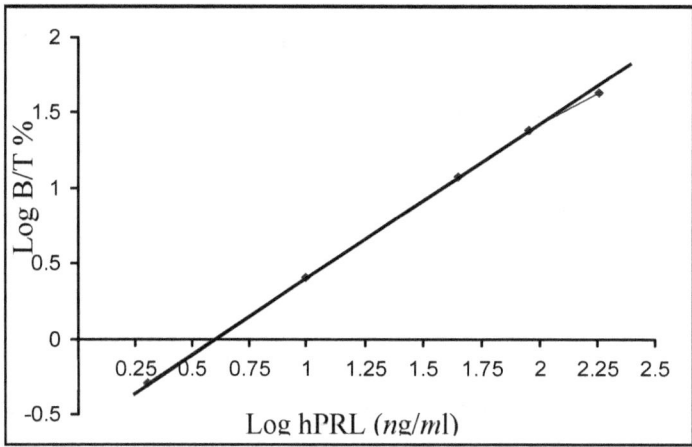

Figure (2-2): Standard curve of hPRL in human serum samples

Calculations

1- The mean net count for each group of tubes was counted in a gamma counter for 1min.

2- The B/T ratio was computed for each standard and unknown sample as follows:

$$\text{B/T \%} = \frac{\text{Standard or samples mean counts}}{\text{Total activity mean counts}} * 100$$

3- A standard curve was drawn by plotting the percent value for each standard against the corresponding hPRL standard concentration (in log-log coordinates), Figure (2-2).

4- hPRL concentrations of the unknown were calculated from the standard curve by using the mean of their duplicate counts.

Determination Of hPRL Concentration in Benign and Malignant Serous Ovarian Tumors Tissue by IRMA.

The concentration of hPRL Benign and malignant ovarian tissue homogenate was determined by the same Immunoradiometric assay used for serum hPRL determination that is mentioned in section (2.3) and following the assay protocol described in table (2-1).

Calculations

The hPRL concentration in (ng/ml) of the benign and malignant ovarian tissue homogenate was estimated according to section (2.3).

Binding studies of hPRL in Benign and Malignant Serous Ovarian Tumors Homogenate with ^{125}I – Anti hPRL Antibody.

Preliminary Test of the Binding of hPRL in Benign and Malignant Serous Ovarian Tumors Homogenate with ^{125}I – Anti hPRL Antibody.

1- Fifty microliters which contain (100µg protein) of premenopausal benign tumor homogenate were incubated with 50µl (91.6µg/ml protein) of ^{125}I –anti hPRL antibody (mouse monoclonal IgG) in duplicate tubes and the volume was completed to 500µl with ST buffer pH(7.4) at room temperature (25 ºC) for one hour with continuously shaking.

2- Two additional tubes containing 50µl of ^{125}I – anti hPRL antibody only (for total activity computation) were set a side until counting.

3- After incubation, the tubes were centrifuged at 1500 xg and 4 ºC for 20min in order to separate the complex formed.

4- The supernatant was discarded by decanting the assay tubes. Then, the tubes were inverted on a filer paper for 10min.

5- The rims of the tubes were swabbed with cotton piece.

6- The amount of bound radioactivity (C.P.M) was counted in a gamma counter for one min.

7- The steps 1 to 6 above were repeated for other patient groups postmenopausal benign tumor homogenate and premenopausal malignant tumor homogenate.

Calculation

1- The counted radioactivity in each tube (expressed in C.P.M) represents the bound fraction (B), (^{125}I- anti hPRL antibody/hPRL) complex.

2- The counted radioactivity in the tubes containing ^{125}I – anti hPRL antibody only represents the total activity (T).

3- The B/T ratio for each tube was counted as follows :

$$(B/T)\% = \frac{\text{Sample mean counts (B)}}{\text{Total activity mean count (T)}} *100$$

Most Appropriate Conditions of the Binding of hPRL in Benign and Malignant Serous Ovarian Tumors Homogenate with ^{125}I–Anti hPRL Antibody.

The Effect of Different Protein Concentration of Benign and Malignant Serous Ovarian Tumors Homogenate on the Binding of hPRL with ^{125}I – Anti hPRL Antibody.

1- Fifty microliters of increasing amounts (25,50,75,100,150,and 200µg protein) of premenopausal benign tumor homogenate was added to 50µl (91.0µg protein) of ^{125}I –anti hPRL antibody (mouse monoclonal IgG) in duplicate tubes. The volume was completed to 500μl with ST buffer pH (7.4), the assay tubes were incubated at 25 °C for one hour.

2- The steps 2 to 6 of the experiment (2.5.1) were repeated.

3- The steps above were repeated for other patient groups postmenopausal benign tumor homogenate and premenopausal malignant tumor homogenate.

Calculations

1- The B/T percent values were determined according to section (2.5.1).

2- The percent of binding values B/T % were plotted against the increasing amounts of protein of the benign and malignant serous ovarian tumor tissue homogenate.

The Effect of Different Concentrations of ^{125}I –Anti hPRL Antibody on the Binding with hPRL in Benign and Malignant Serous Ovarian Tumors Homogenate

1- Increasing volumes (10,15,20,25,50,and 75μl) of ^{125}I anti hPRL anti hPRL antibody (mouse monoclonal IgG) containing (18.32, 27.48, 36.64, 45.8, 91.6, 137.4 μg protein) respectively were each added to 50μl (100μg protein) of premenopausal benign tumor homogenate in duplicate tubes. The volume was completed to 500μl with ST buffer pH (7.4). The assay tubes were incubated at 25°C for one hour.

2- A set of tubes containing the same increasing volumes of ^{125}I –anti hPRL antibody (10, 15, 20, 25, 50 and 75μl) only, for total activity computation, were set a side until counting.

3- The steps 3 to 6 of the experiment (2.5.1) were repeated.

4- The steps above were repeated for other patient groups postmenopausal benign tumor homogenate (50μg protein), and malignant tumor homogenate (100μg protein).

Calculation

1- The B/T percent values were determined according to section (2.5.1).

2- The percent of binding values B/T % were plotted against the increasing volume of ^{125}I –anti hPRL antibody.

The Effect of Different pH on The Binding of hPRL in Benign and Malignant Serous Ovarian Tumors Homogenate with ^{125}I –Anti hPRL Antibody

1- Fifty microliters (100μg protein) of premenopausal benign tumor homogenate was added to 25μl (45.8μg protein) of ^{125}I-anti hPRL antibody in duplicate tubes and the volume was completed to 500 μl with ST buffer of different pH (6.8, 7, 7.4, 7.8, 8, 8.2, 8.6 and 9), the assay tubes were incubated at 25 °C for one hour.

2- The steps 3 to 6 of the experiment (2.5.1) were repeated.

3- The steps above were repeated for other patient groups, postmenopausal benign tumor homogenate (50μg protein) with 25μl (45.8μg protein) of ^{125}I –anti hPRL antibody, and malignant tumor homogenate(100μg protein) with 25μl (45.8μg protein) of ^{125}I –anti hPRL antibody.

Calculations:

1- The B/T percent values were determined according to section (2.5.1).

The percent of binding values B/T % were plotted against their corresponding pH value.

Effect of Temperature on The Binding of hPRL in Benign and Malignant Serous Ovarian Tumors Homogenate with ^{125}I – Anti hPRL antibody

1- Fifty microliters (100μg protein) of premenopausal benign tumor homogenate was added to 25μl (45.8μg protein) of ^{125}I –anti hPRL antibody in duplicate tubes, and the volume was completed to 500μl with ST buffer pH (7.4). The assay tubes were incubated at 4°C for one hour.

2- The steps 3to 6 of the experiment (2.5.1) were repeated.

3- The experiment was repeated at different temperatures (10, 25, 37, 45 and 55°C).

4- The steps above were repeated for other groups, postmenopausal benign tumor homogenate (50µg protein) with 25µl (45.8µg protein) of ^{125}I –anti hPRL antibody, buffer pH (7.8) and malignant tumor homogenate (100µg protein) with 25µl (45.8µg protein) of ^{125}I- anti hPRL antibody, and ST buffer pH(7.4).

Calculations

1- The B/T % values were determined according to section (2.5.1).

2- The percent of binding values were plotted against the different temperature of incubation.

The Choice of The Most Appropriate Incubation Time for the Binding of hPRL in Benign and Malignant Serous Ovarian Tumors Homogenate with ^{125}I-Anti hPRL Antibody

1- Fifty microliters (100µg protein) of premenopausal benign tumor homogenate was added to 25µl (45.8µg protein) of ^{125}I-anti hPRL antibody in duplicate tubes and the volume was completed to 500µl with ST buffer pH (7.4).

2- The assay mixtures were incubated at 10 °C for different time intervals (30, 60, 90, 120, 150 and 180 min).

3- The steps 3 to 6 of the experiment (2.5.1) were repeated.

4- The steps above were repeated for other groups, postmenopausal benign tumor homogenate (50µg protein) with 25µl (45.8µg protein) of ^{125}I-anti hPRL antibody, ST buffer pH 7.8, temperature 4 °C and premenopausal malignant tumor homogenate (100µg protein) with 25µl (45.8µg protein) of ^{125}I-anti hPRL antibody, ST buffer pH 7.4, temperature 45°C for different time (30, 60, 90, 120, 150 and 180 min).

Calculations

1- The B/T % values were determined according to section (2.5.1).

2- The percent of binding values were plotted against the different times of incubation.

The Effect of Different Halides on The Binding of hPRL in Benign and Malignant Serous Ovarian Tumors Homogenate with ^{125}I-Anti hPRL Antibody

The experiment was carried out at the optimum conditions according to the following:

1- Fifty microliters (100μg protein) of premenopausal benign tumor homogenate was added to 25μl (45.8μg protein) of ^{125}I-anti hPRL antibody in duplicate tubes. The volume was made up to 500μl with ST buffer pH 7.4 containing (0.1M) of each of the following halides: NaF, NaCl, NaBr, NaI. (A sample without the addition of any salt was used as a control).

2- The assay tubes were incubated at 10°C for 60min.

3- The steps 3 to 6 of the experiment (2.5.1) were repeated.

4- The steps above were repeated by using: postmenopausal patients with benign tumor homogenate at it's optimum conditions of (50μg protein) with 25μl (45.8μg protein) of ^{125}I-anti hPRL antibody, ST buffer pH (7.8), temperature 4 °C and the time of incubation 30min. Other group, premenopausal malignant tumor homogenate (100μg protein) with 25μl (45.8μg protein) of ^{125}I –anti hPRL antibody, pH (7.4), temperature 45 °C and the time of incubation 180min.

Calculations

1- The B/T % values were determined according to section (2.5.1).

2- The percent of binding values were plotted against halide concentrations.

The Effect of Divalent Cations on the Binding of hPRL in Benign and Malignant Serous Ovarian Tumors Homogenate with ^{125}I-Anti hPRL Antibody.

The experiment in section (2.5.2.6) was repeated but instead of completing the volumes to 500µl with ST buffer containing halide, the volumes were completed to 500µl with ST buffer containing 25mM of each of the following salts: $CaCl_2$, $CuSO_4.5H_2O$, $MgCl_2.6H_2O$, $MnCl_2$, $ZnCl_2$, pH 7.4 for premenopausal benign and malignant ovarian tumors, pH 7.8 for postmenopausal benign ovarian tumors homogenate.

Calculations

1- The B/T % values were determined according to section (2.5.1).

2- The percent of binding values were plotted against the salt concentration.

2.5 The Kinetic and Thermodynamic Studies of hPRL Binding in Benign and Malignant Serous Ovarian Tumors Homogenate with ^{125}I-Anti hPRL Antibody

The Time Course of The Binding of hPRL in Benign and Malignant Serous Ovarian Tumors Homogenate to ^{125}I-Anti hPRL Antibody

1- Fifty microliters (100µg protein) of premenopausal benign tumor homogenate was added to 25µl (45.8µg protein) of ^{125}I-anti hPRL antibody in duplicate tubes. The volume was made up to 500µl with ST buffer pH 7.4

2- The reaction mixture was incubated at 10°C for several times intervals (10, 20, 30, 60, 90, 120, 150 and 180min).

3- The steps 3 to 6 of the experiment (2.5.1) were repeated.

4- The experiment above was repeated at different temperatures (4, 25, 37 and 45 °C) for several time intervals (10, 20, 30, 60, 90, 120, 150 and 180min).

5- To determine the time course for other groups, postmenopausal benign tumor homogenate (50µg protein) with 25µl (45.8µg protein) of ^{125}I-anti hPRL antibody and ST buffer pH 7.8, and different incubation time(10, 20, 30, 60, 90, 120, 150 and 180min). Other group premenopausal malignant tumor homogenate (100μg protein) 25μl (45.8μg protein) of ^{125}I-anti hPRL antibody and ST buffer, pH 7.4, the experiment was performed at five temperatures (4, 10, 25, 37 and 45 °C). Each temperature at different time intervals (10, 20, 30, 60, 90, 120, 150, 180 and 210min).

Calculations

1- The B/T % percent values were determined according to section (2.5.1).

2- The percent of binding values were plotted against the different times of incubation at each temperature.

Determination of The Affinity Constant (Ka) and The Maximal Binding Capacity (Bmax) of hPRL in Benign and Malignant Serous Ovarian Tumors Homogenate Associated with ^{125}I –Anti hPRL Antibody

1- Fifty microliters (100μg protein) of premenopausal benign tumor homogenate was incubated with increasing volumes (10, 15, 20, 25, and 30μl) of ^{125}I-anti hPRL antibody (18.32, 27.48, 36.64, 45.8 and 54.96 μg protein). The final volume was made up to 500μl with ST buffer pH (7.4). The incubation was carried out at 10 °C for 60min.

2- The steps 3 to 6 of the experiment (2.5.1) were repeated.

3- The previous steps were performed at different temperatures (4, 25, 37 and 45 °C). The times of incubation needed to get to the equilibrium state were as the following :

Temp(°C)	Time(min)
4	150
25	90

37	150
45	120

4- The steps 1 and 2 of this experiment were repeated by using postmenopausal patients with benign tumor homogenate (50µg protein), ST buffer pH (7.8). the times of incubation needed to get the equibrium state were 60 min at (25, 37, and 45 °C), 120 min at 10 °C and 30 min at 4 °C. Other groups, premenopausal malignant ovarian tumor homogenate (100µg protein) and ST buffer pH (7.4), the times of incubation needed to get the equibrium state were 60 min at (4 °C and 10 °C), 150 min at (25 and 37 °C) and 180 min at 45 °C.

Calculations

1- The B/T % ratio was computed for each tube, where:

B: is the bound radioactivity mean counts (c.p.m), which represents the (^{125}I-anti hPRL antibody/hPRL) complex.

F: is the free radioactivity mean counts (c.p.m), which represents the non-bound ^{125}I-anti hPRL antibody.

T: is the total radioactivity mean of the counts.

F = Total counts (T) – Bound radioactivity (B)

2- The concentration of the (^{125}I-anti hPRL antibody/hPRL) complex in mg/ml that formed after time (t) was calculated from the following equation:

$$B(mg/ml) = \frac{B(c.p.m)}{T(c.p.m)} * \text{Concentration of } ^{125}\text{I- anti hPRL antibody in the incubation medium (mg/ml)}.$$

3- The affinity constant and maximal binding capacity were determined according to scatchard equation[115].

$$B/F = 1/Kd\ (Bmax - B)$$

$$Ka = 1/Kd$$

Where:

Ka = Affinity constant.

Kd = Dissociation constant.

Bmax = Maximal binding capacity.

4- The values of the ratio B/F were plotted against the values of the (B) in (mg/ml), give a linear relationship. The values of the affinity constant of the binding (Ka) at each temperature can be calculated from the slope of the straight line, while the value of the total concentration of hPRL (Bmax) in Benign and malignant serous ovarian tumor tissue was calculated from the intercept with the x-axis.

The Thermodynamic Studies of hPRL Binding in Benign and Malignant Serous Ovarian Tumors Homogenate with ^{125}I-Anti hPRL Antibody

According to the steps of the explained in section (2.6.2). The thermodynamic parameters were calculated.

Calculations

1- The thermodynamic parameters of standard state (ΔH^o, ΔG^o, ΔS^o) were obtained from **Van't Hoff** plot, the values of the natural logarithm of equilibrium constant (affinity constant Ka) obtained at different temperatures were plotted against the reciprocal values of obsolute temperatures in Kelvin (1/T) was calculated according to the following equation:

$$LnKa = \Delta S°/R - \Delta H°/RT$$

Where: -

$\Delta H°$: the enthalpy change of the standard state.

$\Delta S°$: the entropy change of the standard state.

R   : the gas constant (8.31441 J.K^{-1}.mole^{-1}).

$\Delta H°$ value was obtained from the slope of the linear relationship of the plot. The change in Gibbs free energy of the standard state ($\Delta G°$) was obtained from the following equation:

$$\Delta G° = -RT\, LnKa$$

While the standard state entropy change was obtained from the following equation:

$$\Delta S° = (\Delta H° - \Delta G°) / T$$

2- The thermodynamic parameters of the transition state were obtained from **Arrhenius** plot of LnK_{+1} values against (1/T) values, that gives a linear relation ship according to the following equation:-

$$LnK_{+1} = LnA - (Ea/RT)$$

Where:

A: Arrhenius constant.

Ea: Apparent energy of activation.

T: Absolute temperature in Kelvin.

The value of Ea of the Binding reaction can be determined from the slope of the straight line.

The enthalpy of transition state (ΔH^*) was obtained from:

$$\Delta H^* = Ea - RT$$

The free energy change of the transition state (ΔG*) was calculated using the following equation: -

$$\Delta G^* = -RT Ln K_{+1} + RT\, Ln(KT/h)$$

Where: -

k : Boltzmann constant = $1.38 * 10^{-23}$ J.deg^{-1}

h: Plank's constant = $0.662 * 10^{-33}$ J.S^{-1}

The change in entropy of the transition state (ΔS*) was calculated from the following equation:

$$\Delta S^* = (\Delta H^* - \Delta G^*)/T$$

solation of (^{125}I-Anti hPRL Antibody /hPRL) Complex In Benign and Malignant Serous Ovarian Tumors Homogenate.

Gel filtration chromatography technique was used for the isolation of (^{125}I-anti hPRL antibody/hPRL) complex from the unbound ^{125}I-anti hPRL antibody in benign and malignant serous ovarian tumors.

- **Preparation of the Gel:-** The gel (Sephadex G-150) was allowed to swell in excess of buffer (1gm of the gel in approximately 50ml of the buffer) and left to stand for three days at room temperature without stirring to equilibrate with the buffer. The buffer was decanted and the gel was resuspended in excess volume of eluent buffer three times before bed packing.

- **Bed Packing:-** The de-gassed slurry was carefully mixed before pouring into the vertical column which contains 5ml of eluent buffer using a glass rod attached to the inner surface of the column. After the gel has settled, the column outlet was opened. Packing was continued until the gel reached a stable bed height 30cm. The column was equilibrated with Tris buffer for 24 hr with dimensions (1*30cm) and a bed volume 24ml.

- ***Void Volume (V_o) determination:*** The volume of the gel column was determined by using blue dexstran 2000 at concentration of (2mg/ml) in deionized water, 1ml of blue dexstran solution, was carried out with the same buffer, using a flow rate of (10ml/hour), fractions of 1ml then collected, and their absorbance were measured at 600nm to determine the void volume(V_o).

- ***Sample Addition:*** One milliliter of the (^{125}I-anti hPRL antibody/hPRL) complex of benign and malignant serous ovarian tumors, were applied to the column equilibrated with Tris buffer. The fractions were eluted with the same flow rate (10ml/hour). The radioactivity was measured by gamma counted and the absorbance for the eluted fractions was recorded at 280nm.

Solutions

1- A stock solution of Tris buffer were prepared by dissolving (24.2gm) of Tris (hydroxy methyl) aminomethane in (1000ml) of distilled water, the required pH (pH 7.4 and 7.8 for benign and malignant tumor) was adjusted by adding HCl solution (0.1N).

2- Sodium azid (0.02 %) (weight: volume) had been added to certain components as antibacterial agent.

Calculations

1- The radioactivity (c.p.m) and the absorbance were plotted against the number of fraction.

2- The fractions under each peak (complex and Free) were pooled and absorption spectrum was measured in the area (200-350nm) using a 0.5cm cuvette against Tris buffer pH 7.4 and 7.8 for benign and malignant tumor in reference beam.

Spectroscopic Studies on (^{125}I-Anti hPRL Antibody/hPRL) complex and The Unbound ^{125}I-Anti hPRL Antibody.

Using UV- visible spectrophotometer carried out absorption measurements

The U.V Spectra of hPRL, ^{125}I-Anti hPRL Antibody and (^{125}I- Anti hPRL Antibody/hPRL) Complex.

The U.V Spectrum of hPRL

Fifty – two microliters of hPRL contains (170ng/ml) provided by (IRMA Kit from DiaSorin- Italy) was completed to 1ml with Tris buffer 7.4 . Then placed in a 0.5cm cuvette in sample beam and the absorption spectrum was immediately measured against the same buffer in reference beam in the area of (200 –350nm).

The U.V Spectra of (^{125}I-Anti hPRL Antibody/hPRL) Complex and The Unbound ^{125}I-Anti hPRL Antibody

The gel filtration experiments in section (2.7) gave two peaks for premenopausal benign ovarian tumor homogenate. The first peak represented the complex (^{125}I-anti hPRL antibody/hPRL), while the second peak represented unbound (^{125}I-anti hPRL antibody). The fractions under each peak were pooled. A volume 100µl (300µg protein) was taken from fractions were pooled and represented the (^{125}I-anti hPRL antibody/hPRL) complex, the same volume 100µl was taken from fractions were pooled and represent the unbound ^{125}I-anti hPRL antibody, each volume was completed to 500µl with Tris buffer pH 7.4 then placed in a 0.5cm cuvette in a sample beam and the absorption spectrum was immediately measured against the same buffer in reference beam in the area of (200- 350nm).

Note: The experiment above was repeated for other groups, premenopausal malignant ovarian tumor homogenate.

Solution

Tris/HCl buffer was prepared by dissolving (2.42gm) of Tris (hydroxymethyl) aminomethane in 100ml of distilled water, the required pH (7.4) was adjusted by adding HCl solution (0.1N).

Factors Affecting the Absorption Properties of (^{125}I-Anti hPRL Antibody/ hPRL) Complex and The Unbound (^{125}I-Anti

hPRL Antibody) in Malignant Ovarian Tumors.

pH Effect

One hundred microliters (300μg protein) of (^{125}I-anti hPRL antibody/hPRL) complex was completed to 500μl with different buffers at different pH values (4 –12). Then each of which was placed in a 0.5cm cuvette in the sample beam and the buffer in each case was placed in reference cell and the absorption spectrum was measured in the area (200 – 350nm).

The buffers used were the following:
- Tris/HCl buffer at pH (7.4).
- Acetate buffer at pH (4).
- Glycine/ NaOH buffer at pH (12).

Note: the experiment above was repeated for the unbound (^{125}I-anti hPRL antibody/hPRL)

Solutions

1- **Tris/HCl buffer at different pH values was prepared as follows:**

Solution A: Tris 0.2M (2.4228gm Tris (hydroxymethyl) aminomethane

in 100ml distilled water).

Solution B: 0.1N HCl.

Working buffer pH (7.4) was prepared by mixing 25ml of solution A with an appropriate amount of solution B to adjust the pH required, then the volume was made up to 100ml with distilled water.

2- **Glycine/NaOH buffer was prepared as follows:**

Solution A: Glycine 0.1M in NaCl 0.1N (0.7507gm Glycin + 0.5844gm

NaCl in 100ml distilled water).

Solution B : NaOH 0.1N.

Working buffer pH (12) was prepared by mixing appropriate a mounts of solutions A and B in a final volume of 100ml

3- **Acetate buffer: was prepared as follows:**

Solution A: Sodium acetate 0.1N (0.8204gm $C_2H_5O_2Na$) in 100ml distilled water.
Solution B: Acetic acid 0.1 N.

Working buffer pH(4) was prepared by mixing appropriate amounts of solutions A and B to reach the pH required in a final volume of 100ml.

The Effect of Solvent Polarity:

- ### The Effects of 20 % Methanol
  One hundred microliters (300µg protein) of (^{125}I-anti hPRL antibody/hPRL) complex was completed to 500µl with Tris buffer contains 20 % methanol at pH 7.4, then placed in the sample beam. The absorption spectrum was measured in the area of (200 –350nm).

  Note: The experiment above was repeated for the fractions were pooled and represented the unbound (^{125}I- anti hPRL antibody).

- ### The Effect of 20 % Glycerol
  One hundred microliters (300µg protein) of (^{125}I-anti hPRL antibody/hPRL) complex was completed to 500µl with Tris buffer contains 20 % glycerol at pH 7.4, then placed in the sample beam by using 0.5cm cuvette against 20 % glycerol prepared in the same buffer in the reference beam. The absorption spectrum was measured in the area of (200 – 350nm).

  Note: The experiment above was repeated for the unbound (^{125}I- anti hPRL antibody).

- ### The Effect of 20 % Polyethylene glycol-6000
  One hundred microliters (300µg protein) of (^{125}I-anti hPRL antibody/hPRL) complex was completed to 500µl with Tris buffer contains 20 % polyethylene glycol-6000 at pH 7.4, then placed in the sample beam by using 0.5cm cuvette against 20 % poly ethylene glycol in the same

buffer in the reference beam. The absorption spectrum was measured in the area of (200 –350nm).

Note: The experiment above was repeated for the unbound (^{125}I- anti hPRL antibody).

- **The Effect of 20 % Chloroform**

    One hundred microliters (300µg protein) of (^{125}I-anti hPRL antibody/hPRL) complex was completed to 500µl with Tris buffer contains 20 % chloroform at pH 7.4, then placed in the sample beam using 0.5cm cuvette against 20 % chloroform prepared in the same buffer in the reference beam. The absorption spectrum was measured in the area of (200 – 350nm).

Note: The experiment above was repeated for the unbound (^{125}I- anti hPRL antibody).

- **The Effect o f 20 % Urea**

    One hundred microliters (300µg protein) of (^{125}I-anti hPRL antibody/hPRL) complex was completed to 500µl with Tris buffer contains 20 % urea at pH 7.4, then placed in the sample beam by using 0.5cm cuvette against 20 % urea prepared in the same buffer in the reference beam. The absorption spectrum was measured in the area of (200 – 350nm).

Note: The experiment above was repeated for the unbound (^{125}I- anti hPRL antibody).

- The Effect of 20 % KCl

    One hundred microliters (300µg protein) of (^{125}I-anti hPRL antibody/hPRL) complex was completed to 500µl with Tris buffer contains 20 % KCl at pH 7.4, then placed in the sample beam using 0.5cm cuvette against 20 % KCl prepared in the same buffer in the reference beam. The absorption spectrum was measured in the area of (200 – 350nm).

Note: the experiment above was repeated for the unbound (^{125}I- anti hPRL antibody).

Spectrophotometric Titration of (^{125}I- Anti hPRL Antibody/hPRL) Complex and The Unbound (^{125}I- Anti hPRL Antibody) In Malignant Ovarian Tumor Homogenate.

A series of (^{125}I- anti hPRL antibody/hPRL) sample (300µg protein in 100µl) were completed to 500µl with deionized water at pH range from 2 to 12. The maximum absorbance of each sample was measured at a wavelength of 295nm, the absorbance of λmax at each pH value was plotted versus the corresponding pH.

Another series of (^{125}I- anti hPRL antibody/hPRL) samples were completed to 500µl with deionized water at the same pH range form 2 to 12. The maximum absorbance of each sample was measured at a wavelength of 211nm. The absorbance of λmax at each pH value was plotted against the corresponding pH.

Note: The experiment above was repeated for the unbound (^{125}I- anti hPRL antibody).

Chapter Three

Tissue Collection and Preparation of Ovarian Tumors Tissues Homogenate.

Three groups of patients were included in this study. Group one consisted of (10) premenopausal patients with benign ovarian tumor (serous cystadenoma), group two contained (4) premenopausal patients with malignant ovarian tumor (serous cystadenocarcinoma), and group three contained (6) postmenopausal patients with benign ovarian tumor (serous cystadenoma) as confirmed by histopathological examination. The mean age of premenopausal patients with benign ovarian tumor (27) years and the age ranged from (17 – 38), while the mean age of premenopausal patients with malignant ovarian tumor was (31) years and the ranged from (29 – 33) years. The mean age of postmenopausal patients with benign ovarian tumor was (55) years and the age ranged from (51 – 60) years.

The weights of resected tissue samples ranged between (0.4 –6.2) grams. Tissue homogenization was carried out in 0.25M sucrose. Sucrose is a hypotonic solution that enhances the rupture of plasma cell membrane and preserves other cell organelle [116].

The homogenization was carried out in a cold medium (4 °C) in order to decrease the probability of the protein denaturation and the proteolytic enzyme activity [117]. The tissue homogenate was filtered through several layers of nylon gauze in order to remove any suspended pieces of unhomogenized tissue, fibers of connective tissues, and blood vessels, while homogenate centrifugation at 1500xg precipitates the unraptured cells and intact nuclei of the ruptured cells, leaving mitochondrial fraction and cell microsomes in the supernatant which was used as a source of hPRL in our study [118]. The amount of protein was (1300µg/ml) for premenopausal benign ovarian tumor, (1400µg/ml) for postmenopausal benign ovarian tumor, and (5000µg/ml) for premenopausal malignant ovarian tumor, as determined by **Lowry's** method [114].

Determination of hPRL Levels in Sera of Benign and Malignant Serous Ovarian Tumors Patients and Controls

Serum hPRL levels were measured with an Immunoradiometric assay (IRMA) in two groups of premenopausal patients with serous ovarian tumor, matched with one group of control subject. Group I contained (10) premenopausal patients with benign serous ovarian tumor, group II contained (4) premenopausal patients with malignant serous ovarian tumor. Table (3 –1) shows the results obtained form this study. The level of serum hPRL in premenopausal patient with benign ovarian tumor was founded to be (3.703ng/ml), whereas that of premenopausal patients with malignant ovarian tumor was founded to be (11.183ng/ml). But in controls, the level was found (12.99ng/ml). Student's T-test analysis revealed that there is a significant decrease of serum hPRL levels in benign tumor ($p > 0.001$) while there is no significant decrease of serum hPRL levels in malignant tumor ($p < 0.1$).

The measurement of hPRL showed a correlation of hPRL level with ovarian tumor. It may be concluded that serum prolactin level may be used as a tumor marker to monitor the therapeutic response in cases of ovarian tumor [119].

Table (3 –1): Serum Prolactin Levels (ng/ml) in patients with benign and malignant serous ovarian tumors. Details are described in section (2.3).

Group	No. of cases	Age (year)	Serum hPRL (ng/ml)

Premenopausal of benign serous ovarian tumor	10	17-38	3.703 ± 0.18
Premenopausal of serous ovarian cancer.	4	29-33	11.183 ± 0.23
Control	10	26-35	12.99 ± 0.75

Determination of hPRL Concentration in Benign and Malignant Serous Ovarian Tumors Tissue by IRMA

PRL was measured in benign and malignant ovarian tissues by Immunoradiometric assay (IRMA). The concentration in premenopausal patients with benign ovarian tumor tissue was found to be (2.8ng/ml) while in postmenopausal patients with benign ovarian tumor tissue the concentration was found to be (2.5ng/ml) and in premenopausal patients with malignant ovarian tumor tissue the concentration was found to be (3.2ng/ml). These results indicated that there was decrease in hPRL concentration in benign ovarian tumors tissues compared with that of malignant ovarian tumor tissue.

Binding Studies of hPRL in Benign and Malignant Serous Ovarian Tumors Homogenate with ^{125}I-Anti hPRL Antibody

Preliminary Test of the binding of hPRL in Benign and Malignant Serous Ovarian Tumors Homogenate with ^{125}I-Anti hPRL Antibody.

Benign and malignant ovarian tumor homogenate were used as the source of hPRL in this study. The homogenate was incubated with ^{125}I-anti hPRL antibody (mouse monoclonal IgG) for one hour. The ^{125}I-anti hPRL antibody/hPRL complex formed was separated form the unbound particular by centrifugation at 1500xg for 20min. This centrifugal speed was sufficient to precipitate the complex. After centrifugation the tubes were decanted in order to get rid of the unbound antibody or antigen present in the supernatant fraction. While the ^{125}I-anti hPRL antibody/hPRL complex remained as a pellet in the bottom of the tube. The preliminary conditions used in this experiment resulted in 29 % binding in the premenopausal patients with benign serous ovarian tumor, 26 % binding in the postmenopausal patients with benign serous ovarian tumor and 33% binding in the premenopausal patients with serous ovarian cancer patients, this result shown in table (3-2).

Table (3-2): Preliminary conditions of ^{125}I-anti hPRL antibody binding to hPRL in benign and malignant serous ovarian tumor. Details are described in section (2.5.1)

Group	No. of cases	B/T %	hPRL ng/ml
Postmenopausal patients of benign ovarian tumor	6	26%	2.5
Premenopausal patients of benign ovarian tumor	10	29%	2.8
Premenopausal patients of malignant ovarian tumor	4	33 %	3.2

The B/T % represents the binding percent of ^{125}I-anti hPRL antibody with hPRL in benign and malignant ovarian tumors, and then the concentration of prolactin. Accordingly, in premenopausal patients with malignant ovarian tumors, the binding percent (33 %) shows that hPRL concentration in tissue is higher than those of benign groups. In the premenopausal patients with benign tumors, the binding percent (29 %) also shows that hPRL concentration in tissue is higher than those of postmenopausal patients (26 %).

Most Appropriate Conditions of the Binding of hPRL in Benign and Malignant Serous Ovarian Tumors Homogenate with ^{125}I-Anti hPRL Antibody.

The Effect of Different Protein Concentration of Benign and Malignant Serous Ovarian Tumors Homogenate on the Binding of hPRL with ^{125}I-Anti hPRL Antibody.

To determine whether the different protein concentration of benign and malignant ovarian tumor effect the binding, increasing amounts of homogenate were incubated with ^{125}I-anti hPRL antibody.

Figure (3–1) shows the increasing values of (B/T %) with increasing amounts of protein concentration, until a point of maximum binding was reached, then a resultant decreases in the binding percent. One hundred (100µg/ml) of premenopausal patients with benign ovarian tumor, fifty (50µg/ml) of postmenopausal patients with benign ovarian tumor, and one hundred (100µg/ml) of premenopausal patients with malignant ovarian tumor, this result was shown to give maximum value of binding.

These results indicate that binding of hPRL is principally depended on the different amount of protein in the reaction mixture [120]. Accordingly, in all subsequent experiments, (50µg/ml and 100µg/ml) where used in the binding studies for benign and malignant ovarian tumor.

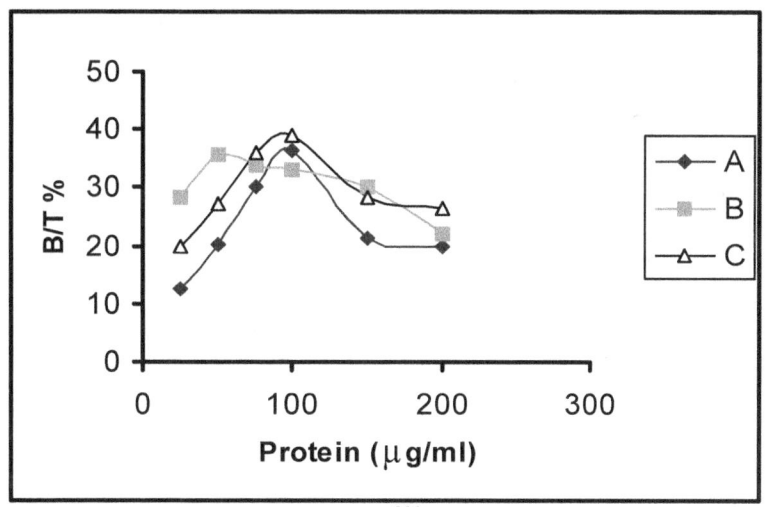

Figure (3-1): The effect of different protein concentration in:
   A: Benign premenopausal ovarian tissue homogenate
   B: Benign postmenopausal ovarian tissue homogenate
   C: Premenopausal ovarian cancer tissue homogenate
   Details are described in section (2.5.2.1)

The Effect of Different Concentrations of ^{125}I-Anti hPRL Antibody on the Binding with hPRL in Benign and Malignant Serous Ovarian Tumors Homogenate

One of the factors that effect the binding of hPRL with ^{125}I-anti hPRL antibody reaction is the concentration of the antibody. To fulfit this criterion and to estimate the suitable concentration of ^{125}I-anti hPRL antibody, the experiment was carried out in the presence of fixed amounts of (100µg/ml protein) for premenopausal patients with benign ovarian tumor, (50µg/ml protein) for postmenopausal patients with benign ovarian tumor, and (100µg/ml protein) for premenopausal patients with malignant ovarian tumor, and increasing concentration of ^{125}I-anti hPRL antibody.

Figure (3-2) is a representative of ^{125}I-anti hPRL antibody binding curve with hPRL in benign and malignant ovarian tissue homogenate. The results reveal that the percent of binding (B/T %) increased by increasing the amount of ^{125}I-anti hPRL antibody, until a point of maximum binding that was equivalent to (45.8µg/ml, 25µl) in premenopausal and postmenopausal patients with benign and malignant serous ovarian tumor homogenate. It is shown that the binding of ^{125}I-anti hPRL antibody with hPRL in benign and malignant ovarian tissue homogenate is a saturable process but complete saturation however is theoretically never reached unless the amount of hPRL used reached infinity [121]. According to the results of this experiment (45.8µg/ml protein) of ^{125}I-anti hPRL antibody were used in the binding studies in the subsequent experiments.

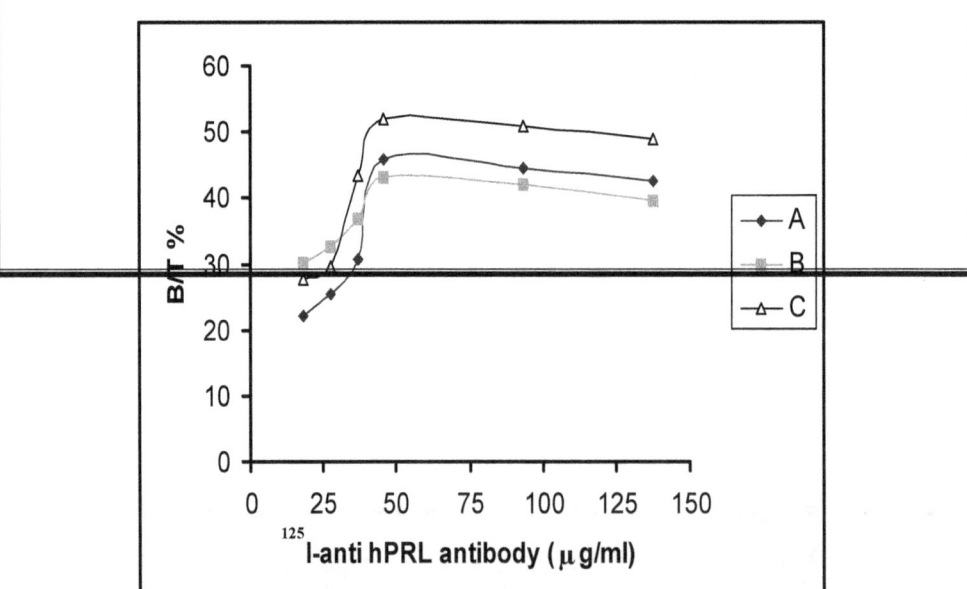

Figure (3-2): Effect of different concentrations of ^{125}I-anti hPRL antibody on the binding with hPRL in:
A: Premenopausal patients with benign ovarian tumor
B: Postmenopausal patients with benign ovarian tumor
C: Premenopausal patients with malignant ovarian tumor
Details are described in section (2.5.2.2)

The Effect of Different pH on the Binding of hPRL in Benign and Malignant Serous Ovarian Tumors Homogenate with ^{125}I-Anti hPRL Antibody

The analysis of the influence of pH on binding of hPRL in benign and malignant ovarian tumor homogenate to ^{125}I-anti hPRL antibody is stated in Figure (3-3). The optimum pH was found to be (7.4) for benign and malignant premenopausal ovarian tumor, while (pH 7.8) is the optimum pH for the binding of ^{125}I-anti hPRL antibody to the benign postmenopausal ovarian tumor.

The same Figure (3-3) shows a decreasing in the binding percent (B/T %) at the pH higher or lower than the optimum pH. These results indicate that the shift in the pH of the environment may affect the properties of the macromolecules involved in the binding. This effect includes the induction of protonation- deprotonation process occurring within the ionizable groups of the amino acids present in the binding domain of these macromolecules[122].

According to the results obtained in this experiment, the pH of incubation buffer in all subsequent experiments was adjusted at (7.4 and 7.8) as optimum pH for the three different groups used in this study.

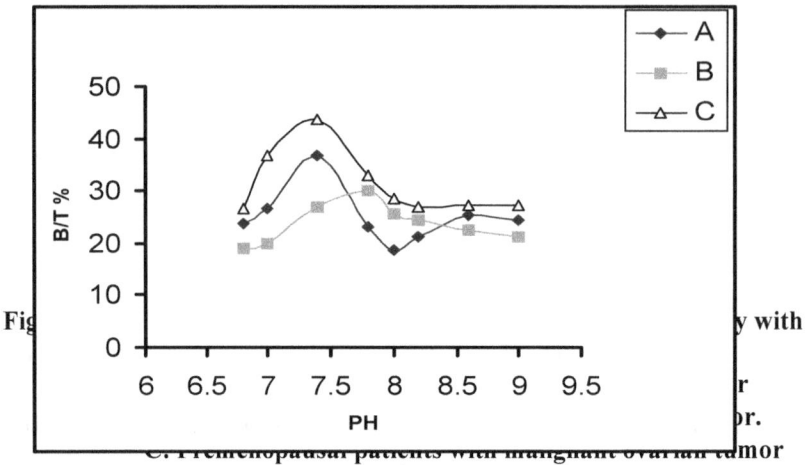

Fig ... with ... r. C. Premenopausal patients with malignant ovarian tumor

Effect of Temperature on The Binding of hPRL in Benign and Malignant serous Ovarian Tumors Homogenate with ^{125}I-Anti hPRL Antibody

The temperature dependency of the binding of ^{125}I-anti hPRL antibody to benign and malignant ovarian tissue was investigated. Figure (3-4) reveals that the binding of ^{125}I-anti hPRL antibody to hPRL in benign and malignant ovarian tissue was maximum at 10°C for premenopausal patients with benign ovarian tumor, while it was maximum binding at 4°C for postmenopausal patients with benign ovarian tumor, and a maximum binding obtained at 45°C for premenopausal patients with malignant ovarian tumor. It seemed that binding percent (B/T%) was increasing when the temperature was raised to a point of maximum binding and the binding was decreased as temperature increase after maximal value of binding. The loss of binding activity may be due to degradation of the hPRL [123], or may be due to the irreversible dissociation of the (^{125}I-anti hPRL antibody/hPRL) complex [124].

According to these results, (4°C, 10°C and 45°C) were used in all the subsequent experiments for benign and malignant serous ovarian tumor homogenate.

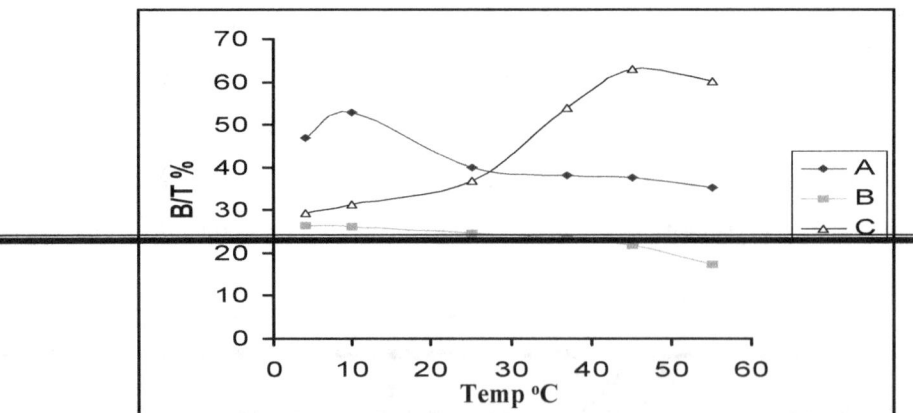

Figure (3-4): Effect of the temperature on the binding of ^{125}I-anti hPRL antibody with hPRL in:

A: Premenopausal patients with benign ovarian tumor
B: Postmenopausal patients with benign ovarian tumor
C: Premenopausal patients with malignant ovarian tumor
Details are described in section (2.5.2.4)

The Choice of the Most Appropriate Incubation Time for the Binding of hPRL in Benign and Malignant Serous Ovarian Tumors Homogenate with ^{125}I-Anti hPRL Antibody.

To choose the most appropriate incubation time at (10°C, 4°C, and 45°C) the experiment was carried out at different time intervals (30-180min).

Figure (3-5) shows that the optimum binding of ^{125}I-anti hPRL antibody to hPRL in premenopausal patients with benign ovarian tumor homogenate was occurred in 60min, while the optimum binding in postmenopausal patients with benign ovarian tumor was occurred in 30min, and the optimum binding obtained at 180min for premenopausal patients with malignant ovarian tumor. In view of these results, the incubation time (30min, 60min, and 180min) were used in all subsequent experiments for benign and malignant tumor.

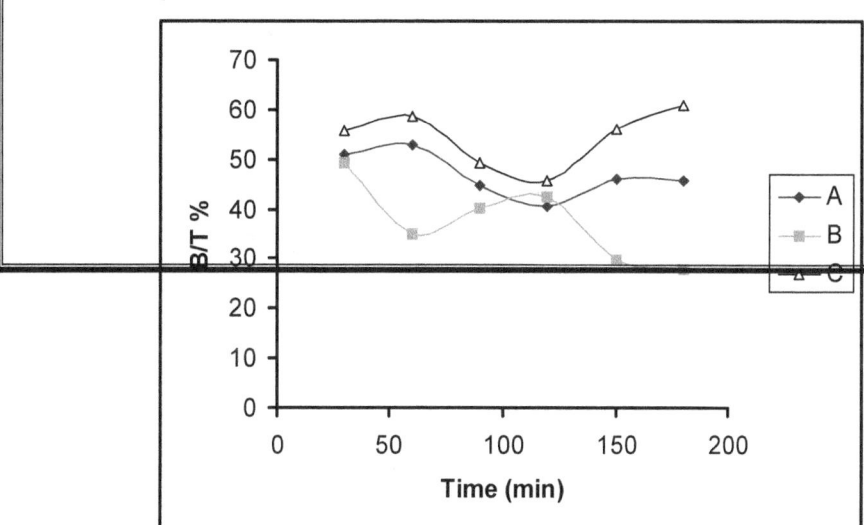

Figure (3-5): Time-course of ^{125}I-anti hPRL antibody binding with hPRL

in:

A: Premenopausal patients with benign ovarian tumor
B: Postmenopausal patients with benign ovarian tumor
C: Premenopausal patients with malignant ovarian tumor.
Details are described in section (2.5.2.5).

The Effect of Different Halides on the Binding of hPRL in Benign and Malignant Serous Ovarian Tumors Homogenate with ^{125}I-Anti hPRL Antibody.

Different sodium halides in a concentration of (0.1M) were investigated for their action on the binding of ^{125}I-anti hPRL antibody to benign and malignant ovarian tissue Homogenate. The results were illustrated in Figure (3-6 A, B&C).

The presence of sodium halides in the incubation medium tends to promote the binding of ^{125}I-anti hPRL antibody to benign and malignant ovarian tissue in the three groups according to the following sequence.

- Premenopausal benign ovarian tissue homogenate
    NaCl> NaF>NaI>NaBr
- Postmenopausal benign ovarian tissue homogenate
    NaI > NaBr>NaF>NaCl
- Premenopausal ovarian cancer tissue homogenate

    NaCl> NaI> NaBr>NaF

The maximal binding in the two groups of premenopausal benign and malignant ovarian tumor was in the presence of NaCl in the incubation medium, this could be due to that NaCl in Low concentration or in physiological concentration (0.15M) increase the binding of ^{125}I-anti hPRL antibody with hPRL in ovarian tumor tissue homogenate, while high salt concentrations lowers the affinity [125].

In the postmenopausal benign ovarian tissue homogenate the maximal binding was observed in the presence of NaI, this could be due to the large size of iodide ion, which could inhibit, the interaction of ^{125}I-anti hPRL antibody with benign ovarian tissue homogenate in lower extent than do other halides. In premenopausal ovarian cancer, NaF causes lower binding percent (B/T %), this could be due to the high interaction of fluoride with the positive residue in the active site of the ^{125}I-anti hPRL antibody which lead to decrease the interaction between ^{125}I-anti hPRL antibody and hPRL in ovarian tumor homogenate [126].

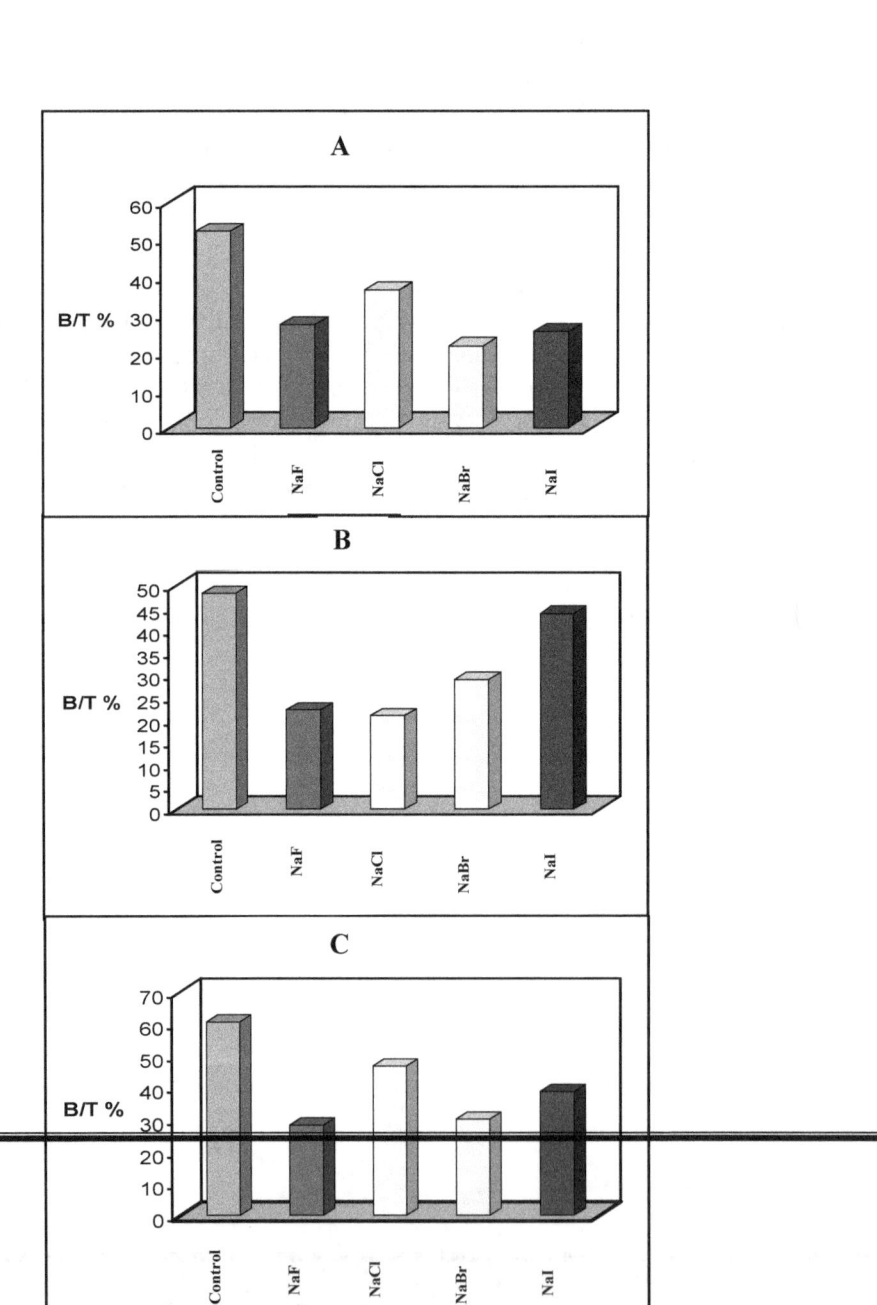

Figure (3-6): Effect of different halides on the binding of ^{125}I-anti hPRL antibody with hPRL in:

A: Premenopausal patients with benign ovarian tumor

B: Postmenopausal patients with malignant ovarian tumor

C: Premenopausal patients with malignant ovarian tumor

Details are described in section (2.5.2.6)

The Effect of Divalent Cations on the Binding of hPRL in Benign and Malignant Serous Ovarian Tumors Homogenate with ^{125}I-Anti hPRL Antibody.

Figure (3-7 A, B&C) shows the effect of divalent cations on the binding of ^{125}I-anti hPRL antibody to benign and malignant ovarian tissue homogenate. Some of divalent cations appeared to enhance the binding reaction, while others inhibit the reaction. Several cations have been used to study their action on the binding, these cations are Ca^{+2}, Mg^{+2}, Mn^{+2}, Cu^{+2} and Zn^{+2} in a (25mM) concentration.

The presence of divalent cations in the incubation medium tend to stimulate the binding of ^{125}I-anti hPRL antibody to benign and malignant ovarian tissue homogenate in the three groups according to the following:

- Premenopausal benign ovarian tissue homogenate.
  $Cu^{+2} > Ca^{+2} > Zn^{+2} > Mn^{+2} > Mg^{+2}$
- Postmenopausal benign ovarian tissue homogenate.
  $Zn^{+2} > Mn^{+2} > Mg^{+2} > Cu^{+2} > Ca^{+2}$
- Premenopausal ovarian cancer tissue homogenate

$$Ca^{+2} > Mg^{+2} > Mn^{+2} > Cu^{+2} > Zn^{+2}$$

As shown, the maximal binding in premenopausal benign tumor was occurred in the presence of copper (II) in the incubation mixture while, the maximal binding in postmenopausal benign tumor was observed in the presence of zinc (II) in the incubation mixture, and the maximal binding in premenopausal ovarian cancer was observed in the presence of calcium (II) in the incubation mixture.

One hypothesis assumes that, the effects of those metal ions may alter the nature of the hydrophobic forces necessary for the stabilization of biological membranes and affect the hydrophobic forces controlling the stabilization of the complex formed [127]. Several studies demonstrated the effect of different cations on the binding of ^{125}I-anti hPRL antibody with hPRL in ovarian tumor. It was reported that calcium (II) in a concentration ranging for (10-20mM) increases the association between ^{125}I-anti hPRL antibody and hPRL in ovarian tumor tissue [128]. Also the presence of zinc (II) at 20mM concentration seemed to increase the binding of ^{125}I-anti hPRL antibody with hPRL in ovarian tumor.

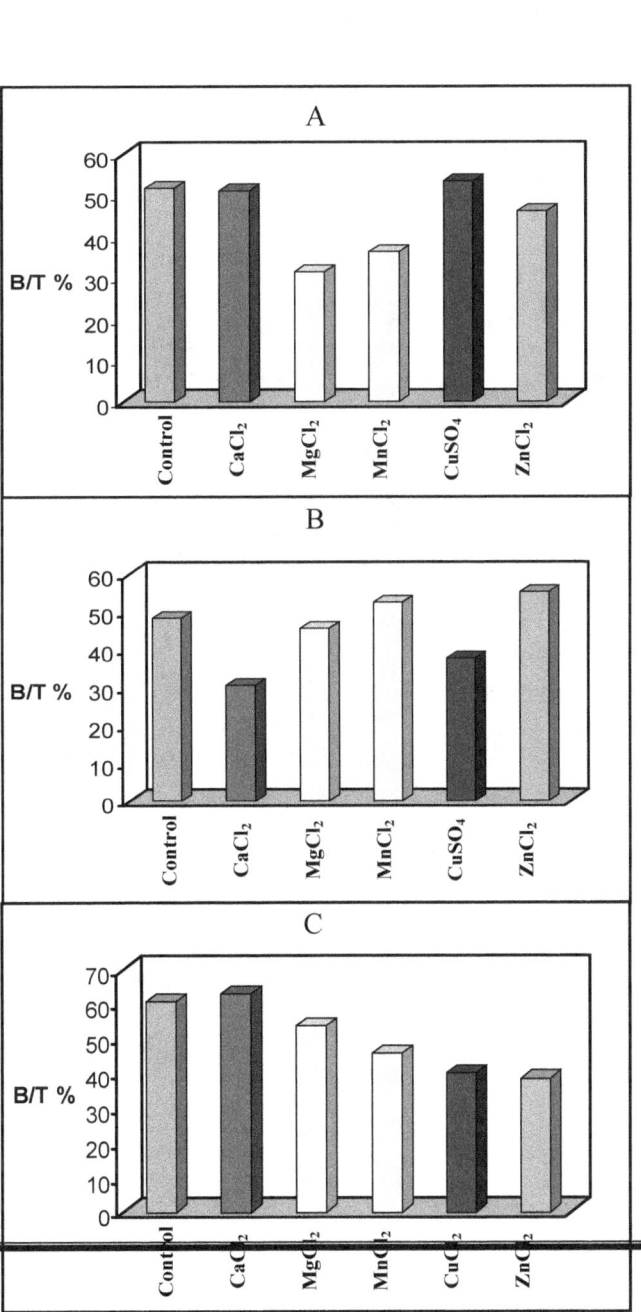

Figure (3-7): Effect of divalent cations on the binding of ^{125}I-anti hPRL antibody with hPRL in:
  A: Premenopausal patients with benign ovarian tumor.
  B: Postmenopausal patients with benign ovarian tumor.
  C: Premenopausal patients with malignant ovarian tumor.
Details are described in section (2.5.2.7).

The Kinetic and Thermodynamic Studies of hPRL Binding in Benign and Malignant Serous Ovarian Tumors Homogenate with ^{125}I-Anti hPRL Antibody.

The Kinetics of Interaction of ^{125}I-Anti hPRL Antibody with Benign and Malignant Serous Ovarian Tumors.

To examine the characteristics of the binding of ^{125}I-anti hPRL antibody with hPRL in benign and malignant ovarian tissue homogenate, the experiment was carried out at five temperatures and for different incubation time.

Figure (3-8 A, B and C) shows the time course of the formation of (^{125}I-anti hPRL antibody/hPRL) complex at five different temperatures (4, 10, 25, 37, and 45°C). The concentration of the ^{125}I-anti hPRL anti body /hPRL complex that formed after time (t) was calculated from the following equation:

$$B(mg/ml) = [B(c.p.m)/T(c.p.m)] * \text{Concentration of } ^{125}\text{I- anti hPRL antibody in the incubation medium in (mg/ml)}$$

The results of the time-course patterns at different temperatures revealed that the binding of ^{125}I-anti hPRL antibody to hPRL in benign and malignant ovarian tissue homogenate is a temperature and time dependent process with a maximum binding occurs at 10°C and the incubation time 60min for the premenopausal patients with benign ovarian tumor, and 4°C with 30min incubation for the postmenopausal patients with benign ovarian tumor, and 45°C with 180min incubation for the premenopausal patients with malignant ovarian tumors.

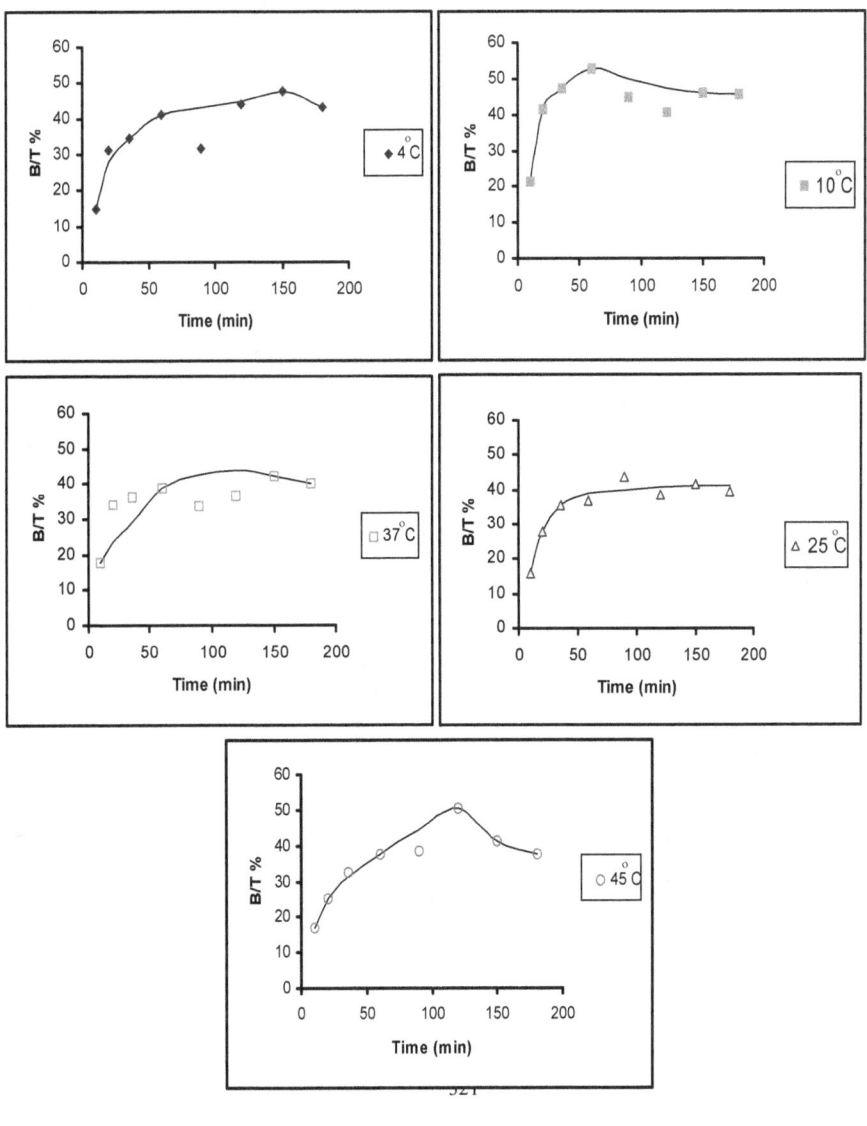

Figure (3-8): Time-course of ^{125}I-anti hPRL antibody binding with hPRL in:
  A: Premenopausal patients with benign ovarian tumor
  Details are described in section (2.6.1)

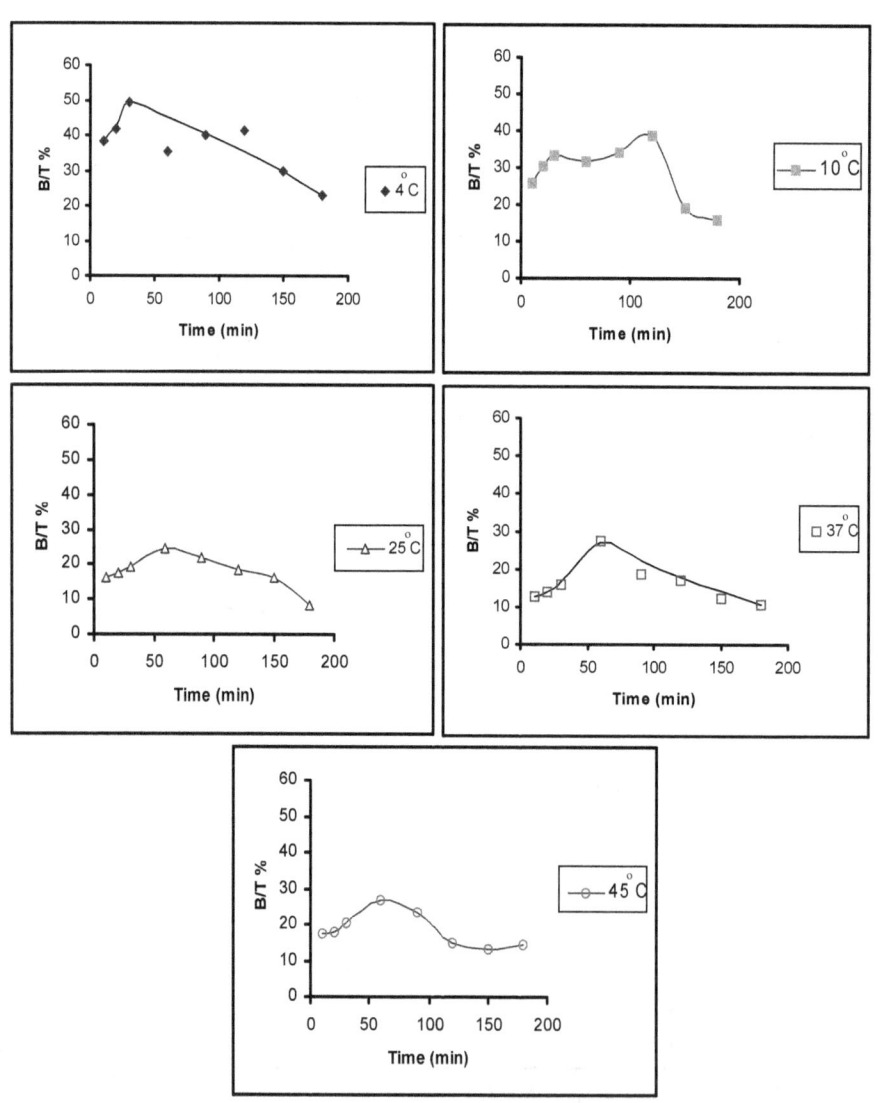

Figure (3-8): Time-course of ^{125}I-anti hPRL antibody binding with hPRL in:
  B: Postmenopausal patients with benign ovarian tumor
  Details are described in section (2.6.1)

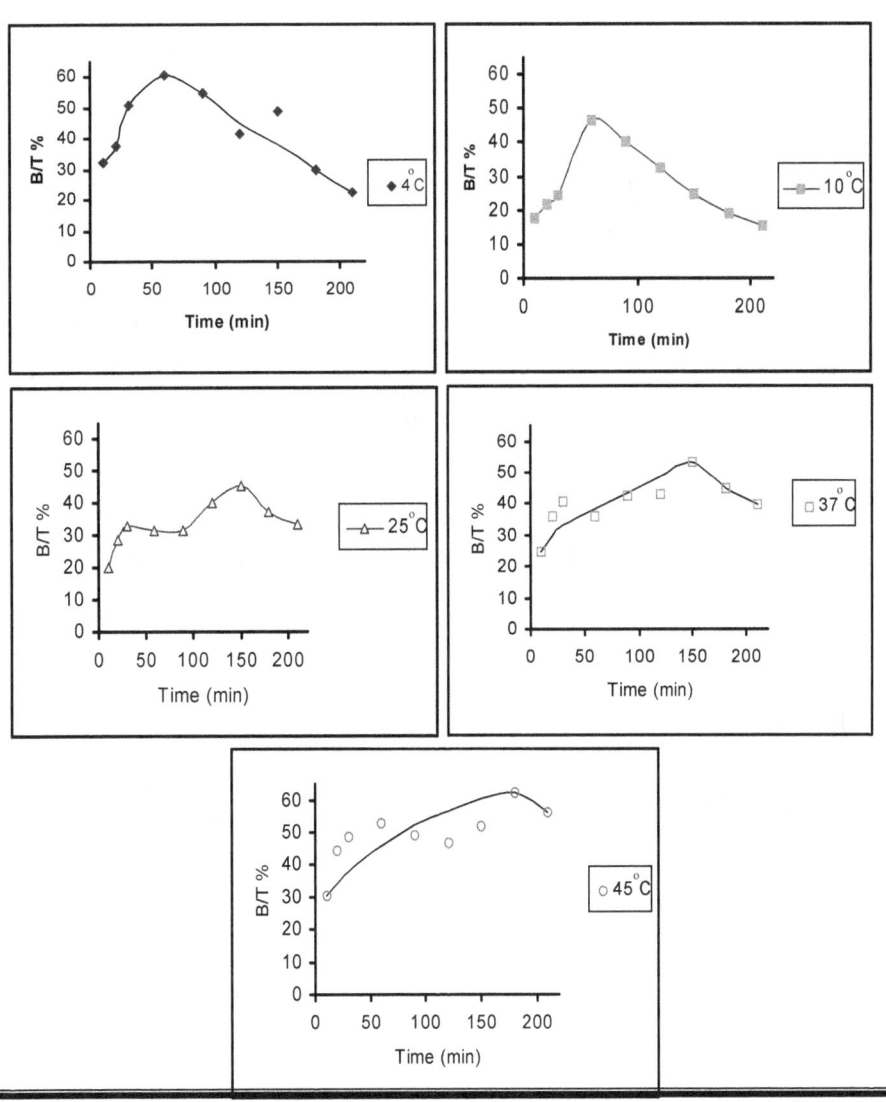

Figure (3-8): Time-course of ^{125}I-anti hPRL antibody binding with hPRL in:
    C: Premenopausal patients with malignant ovarian tumor
Details are described in section (2.6.1)

Determination of the Affinity Constant (Ka) and the Maximal Binding Capacity (Bmax) of hPRL in Benign and Malignant Serous Ovarian Tumors Homogenate Associated with ^{125}I-Anti hPRL Antibody.

The concentration of hPRL in benign and malignant ovarian tissue homogenate (Bmax) and the affinity constant (Ka) of the binding to ^{125}I-anti hPRL antibody has been measured in premenopausal and postmenopausal patients with benign and malignant ovarian tumors. The experiment was carried out at the optimal conditions. That was obtained in previous experiments. Scatchard plot analysis gave a straight line as shown in Figure (3-9). The results are summarized in table (3-3). The binding capacities of premenopausal patients with benign ovarian tumors in the optimal conditions were 0.021mg/ml while of postmenopausal with benign tumor were 0.0273mg/ml and of premenopausal ovarian cancer patients were 0.029mg/ml.

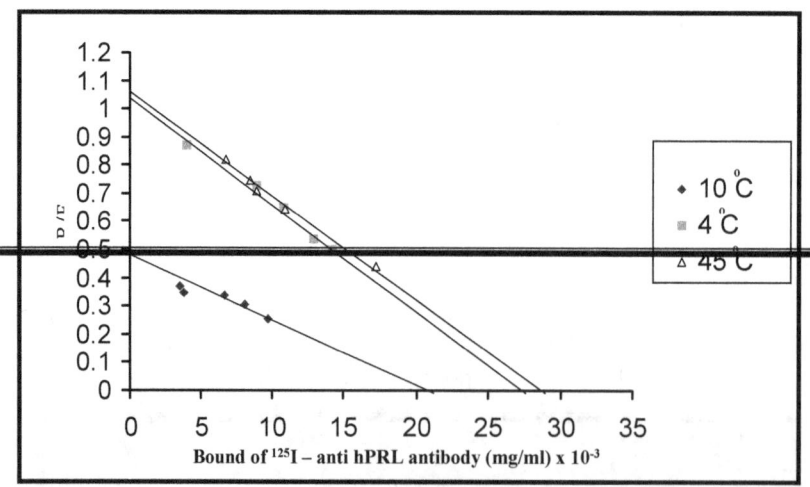

Figure (3-9): Scatchard plot of ^{125}I-anti hPRL antibody binding with hPRL in:

◆ Premenopausal patients with benign ovarian tumor.
▪ Postmenopausal patients with benign ovarian tumor.
△ Premenopausal patients with malignant ovarian tumor.

Table (3-3): Concentration and affinity constants of hPRL in three groups of serous ovarian tumor patients. Details are described in section (2.6.2)

Groups	o. of cases	Age (year)	Binding capacity $B_{max} *10^{-3}$ (mg/ml)	Ka (mg^{-1}.ml)
Premenopausal patients of benign ovarian tumor	10	17-38	21.0	22.857
Postmenopausal patients of benign ovarian tumor	6	51-60	27.3	35.897
Premenopausal patients of ovarian cancer	4	29-33	29.0	36.207

Determination of Kinetic Parameters of ^{125}I-Anti hPRL Antibody Binding with hPRL in Benign and Malignant Ovarian Tumors Homogenate

The time course of ^{125}I-anti hPRL antibody binding to hPRL in benign and malignant ovarian tumor was carried out to describe the kinetic parameters of the binding.

The simplest proposed model representing the interaction of ^{125}I-anti hPRL antibody with hPRL could be expressed by the following equation:

$$^{125}\text{I-anti hPRL antibody} + \text{hPRL} \underset{K_{-1}}{\overset{K_{+1}}{\rightleftharpoons}} {}^{125}\text{I-anti hPRL antibody/hPRL}$$

$$(^{125}\text{I-Ab}) \qquad (\text{Ag}) \qquad\qquad (^{125}\text{I-AbAg})$$

Where:-

K_{+1}: is the rate of the association of ^{125}I-anti hPRL antibody with hPRL.

K_{-1}: is the rate of the reverse reaction of the dissociation of the complex formed under the same condition.

At equilibrium: -

$$Ka = \frac{[^{125}\text{I- AbAg}]}{[^{125}\text{I- Ab}][\text{Ag}]} \quad \dots\dots\dots\dots(1)$$

$$Kd = \frac{[^{125}\text{I-Ab}][\text{Ag}]}{[^{125}\text{I-AbAg}]} \quad \dots\dots\dots\dots(2)$$

Thus,

$$Ka = \frac{1}{Kd} = \frac{K_{+1}}{K_{-1}} \quad \dots\dots\dots\dots(3)$$

Where:-

Ka: is the equilibrium constant of the association (affinity constant).

Kd: is the equilibrium constant of the dissociation of (^{125}I-AbAg) complex.

The values of Ka and maximal binding capacity (Bmax) were calculated form scatchard plot at five temperatures, as shown in Figure (3-10 A, B&C) and Table (3-4).

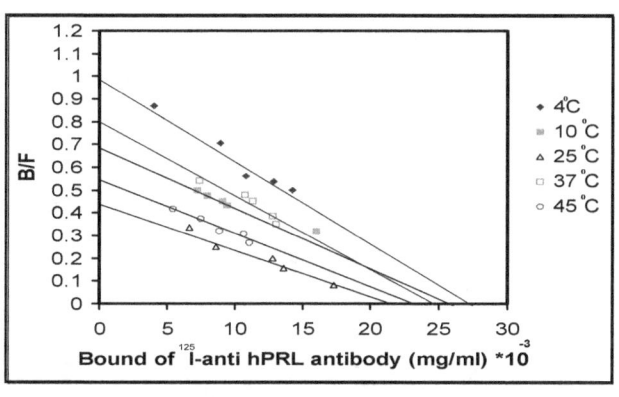

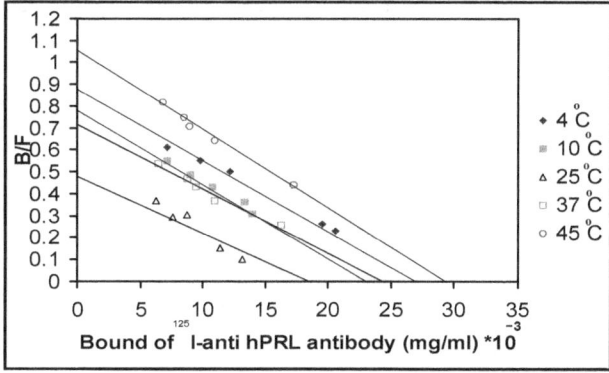

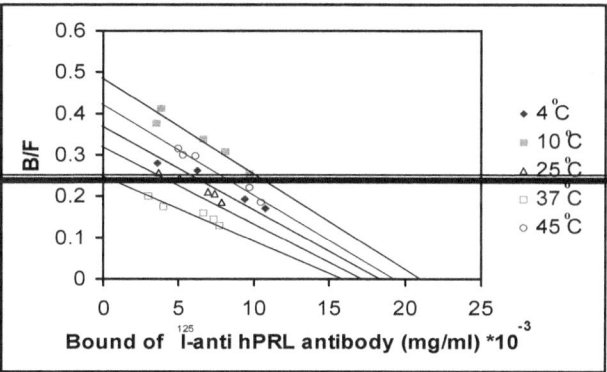

Figure (3-10): Scatchard plot of the ^{125}I-anti hPRL antibody binding with hPRL in:

A: Premenopausal patients with benign ovarian tumor.

B: Postmenopausal patients with benign ovarian tumor.

C: Premenopausal patients with malignant ovarian tumor.

Details are described in section (2.6.2).

Table (3-4): The Kinetic parameters of ^{125}I-anti hPRL antibody binding to hPRL in benign and malignant ovarian tumors.

Groups	Kinetic Parameters	Temperature (°C)				
		4	10	25	37	45
Premenopausal patients with benign ovarian tumors.	Binding Capacity $*10^{-3}$ (mg/ml)	18	21	17	16	19
	$Ka = K_{+1}/K_{-1}$ (mg^{-1}.ml)	20.0	22.857	18.824	15.625	22.105
	$Kd = K_{-1}/K_{+1} *10^{-3}$ (mg/ml)	50.0	43.8	53.1	64.0	45.2
Postmenopausal patients with benign ovarian tumors.	Binding Capacity $*10^{-3}$ (mg/ml)	27.3	26.0	21.3	24.5	23.0
	$Ka = K_{+1}/K_{-1}$ (mg^{-1}.ml)	35.897	26.154	20.657	32.653	23.478
	$Kd = K_{-1}/K_{+1} *10^{-3}$ (mg/ml)	27.8	83.2	48.4	30.6	42.6
Premenopausal patients malignant ovarian tumors.	Binding capacity $*10^{-3}$ (mg/ml)	27	23	18	24	29
	$Ka = K_{+1}/K_{-1}$ (mg^{-1}.ml)	32.593	33.913	26.667	30.0	36.207
	$Kd = K_{-1}/K_{+1} *10^{-3}$ (mg/ml)	30.7	29.5	37.5	33.3	27.6

Results in Table (3-4) show that Ka value at 10°C of premenopausal patients with benign ovarian tumors is higher than (4, 25, 37&45°C) and the Ka value at 4°C of postmenopausal patients with benign tumors is higher than (10, 25, 37&45°C) and the Ka value at 45°C of premenopausal patients with malignant tumors is higher than (4, 10, 25 &37). These results indicate that when the Ka value is high, then the binding affinity between hPRL and ^{125}I-anti hPRL antibody in benign and malignant serous ovarian tumors is increased.

The value of Kd calculated by using equation (3) shows that the lowest Kd values of (^{125}I-anti hPRL antibody/hPRL) complex occurs at (10 & 4 °C) in benign premenopausal and postmenopausal ovarian tumor homogenate and 45 °C for malignant premenopausal ovarian tumor homogenate.

Different equations are used for the determination of the association rate constant (K_{+1}) of ^{125}I-anti hPRL antibody with hPRL at five temperatures. These include the following:

$$Ln(AbAg)_e \left[\frac{(Ab)_T - (AbAg)_t (AbAg)_e / (Ag)_T}{(Ab)_T[(AbAg)_e - (AbAg)_t]} \right] = K_{+1} t \left[\frac{(Ab)_T(Ag)_T - (AbAg)_e}{(AbAg)_e} \right] \quad\quad (4)$$

This equation could be simplified to equation (5) in order to fit the data of the first order kinetics [129].

$$Ln \frac{(AbAg)_e}{(AbAg)_e - (AbAg)_t} = K_{+1} t[(Ab)_T(Ag)_T /(AbAg)_e] \quad\quad (5)$$

Where: -
  K_{+1}: is the kinetic association constant.
  $(Ab)_T$: is the total concentration of ^{125}I-anti hPRL antibody.
  $(Ag)_T$: is the total concentration of hPRL in ovarian tissue homogenate.
  $(AbAg)_e$: is the concentration of (^{125}I-anti hPRL antibody /hPRL)

complex formed at equilibrium.

$(AbAg)_t$: is the concentration of (^{125}I-anti hPRL antibody /hPRL) complex formed after time (t).

Since in some cases of our work the percent of binding was small. And most of the ^{125}I-anti hPRL antibody remained free and only a small fraction of ^{125}I-anti hPRL antibody is bounded even at equilibrium (pseudo-first order conditions). So that the following equation could be used in order to fit the data of first order kinetic:

$$Ln \frac{(AbAg)_e}{(AbAg)_e - (AbAg)_t} = t\, K_{obs} \quad \text{------(6)}$$

Figure (3-11 A, B&C) shows that the plotting of $Ln \dfrac{(AbAg)_e}{(AbAg)_e - (AbAg)_t}$ against time (t) gives a straight line with a slope equal to the observed value of first order rate constant (K_{obs}) in min^{-1}. The association rate constant (K_{+1}) was calculated from the following formula:

$$K_{obs} = K_{+1} \frac{(Ab)_T (Ag)_T}{(AbAg)_e} \quad \text{------(7)}$$

The half-life time of association (t ½)ass., which represents the time needed for the formation of half amounts of the complex at equilibrium, was determined from the concentration of the complex at equilibrium and the time course curve, while the half-life time of dissociation (t ½)diss. was determined from:

$$(t\, \tfrac{1}{2})diss = \frac{Ln\, 2}{K_{-1}} = \frac{0.693}{K_{-1}} \quad \text{------(8)}$$

The values of K_{obs}, K_{+1}, K_{-1}, (t ½)ass. and (t ½)diss. at different temperatures are summarized in Tables (3-5) and (3-6).

Table (3-5): The effect of different temperatures on the kinetic parameters of ^{125}I-anti hPRL antibody binding with premenopausal benign and malignant ovarian tumors (All details are described in section 2.6.2)

Groups	Kinetic Parameters	Temperatures (°C)				
		4	10	25	37	45
Premenopausal patients with benign ovarian tumors	Kobs (min^{-1})	0.0429	0.0781	0.0417	0.0565	0.0242
	K_{+1}(mg^{1}.ml.min^{-1})	113.542	196.661	107.192	149.51	63.937
	K_{-1} (min^{-1})	5.677	8.604	5.694	9.569	2.892
	(t½)diss.*10^{-2}(min)	12.209	8.056	12.173	7.244	23.968
	(t ½)ass. (min)	14	12	15	11	19
Premenopausal patients with malignant ovarian tumors	Kobs (min^{-1})	0.0521	0.0323	0.0277	0.0278	0.043
	K_{+1}(mg^{-1}.ml.min^{-1})	111.386	65.120	26.212	61.747	91.931
	K_{-1} (min^{-1})	3.417	1.923	0.989	2.058	2.539
	(t½)diss.*10^{-2}(min)	20.282	36.058	70.101	33.674	0.273
	(t½)ass. (min)	180	24	13	11	11

Table (3-6): The effect of different temperatures on the kinetic parameters of ^{125}I-antibody binding with postmenopausal benign ovarian tumors. (All details are described in section 2.6.2).

Groups	Kinetic Parameters	Temperatures (°C)			
		10	25	37	45
Postmenopausal patients with benign ovarian tumors	Kobs (min^{-1})	0.042	0.0692	0.0357	0.0581
	K_{+1} (mg^{-1}.ml.min^{-1})	62.761	79.888	40.086	66.193
	K_{-1} (min^{-1})	2.399	3.867	1.228	2.819
	(t ½)diss.* 10^{-2} (min)	28.885	17.923	56.462	24.585
	(t ½)ass. (min)	146	168	11	139

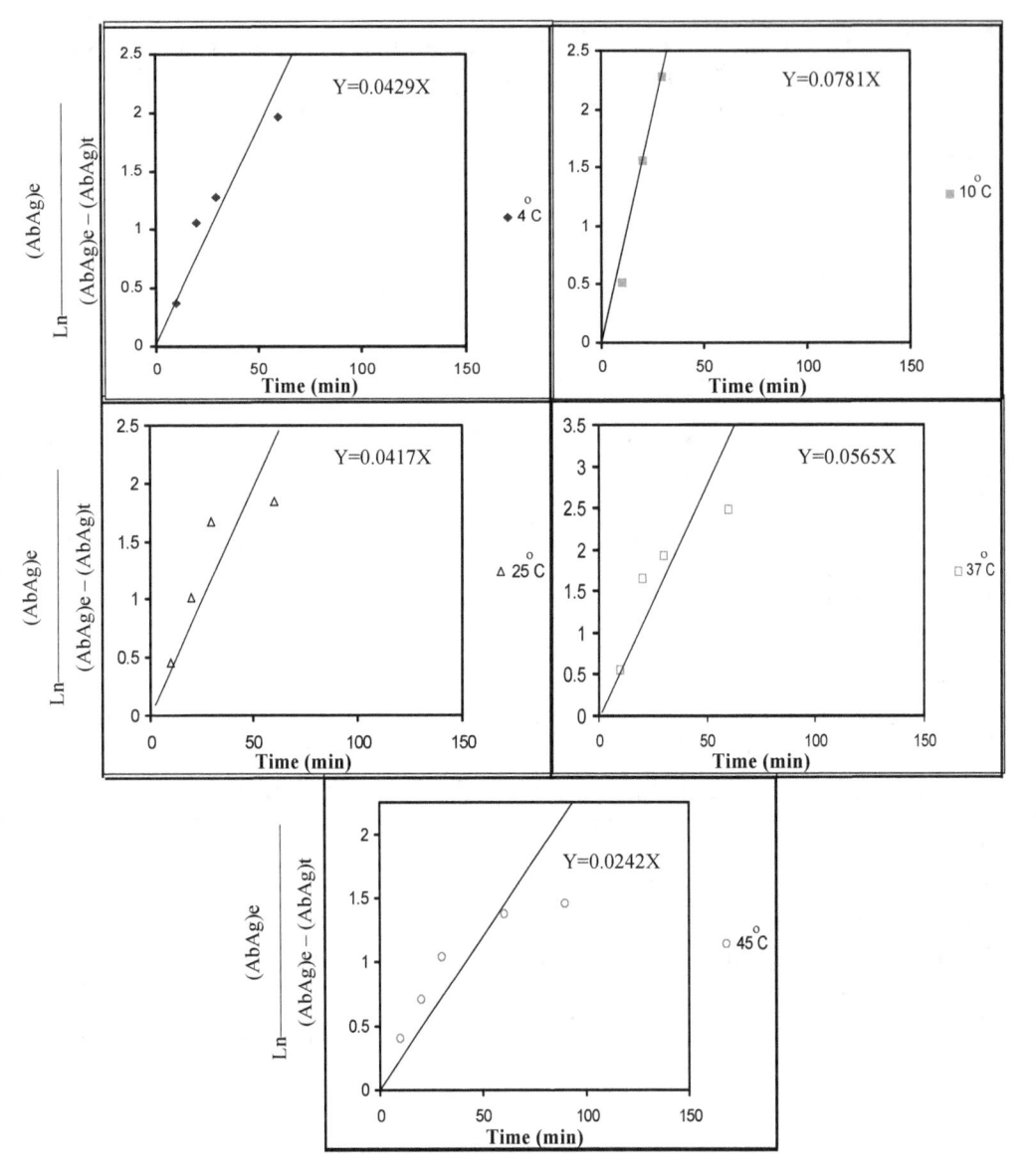

Figure (3-11): Kinetics of ^{125}I-anti hPRL antibody binding with hPRL in:
A: Premenopausal patients with benign ovarian tumor.

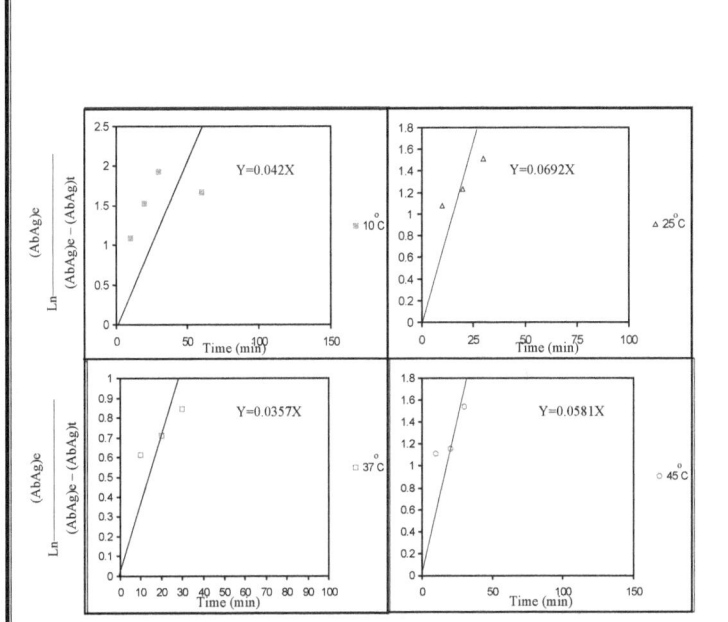

Figure (3-11): Kinetics of ^{125}I-anti hPRL antibody binding with hPRL in:
B: Postmenopausal patients with benign ovarian tumor.

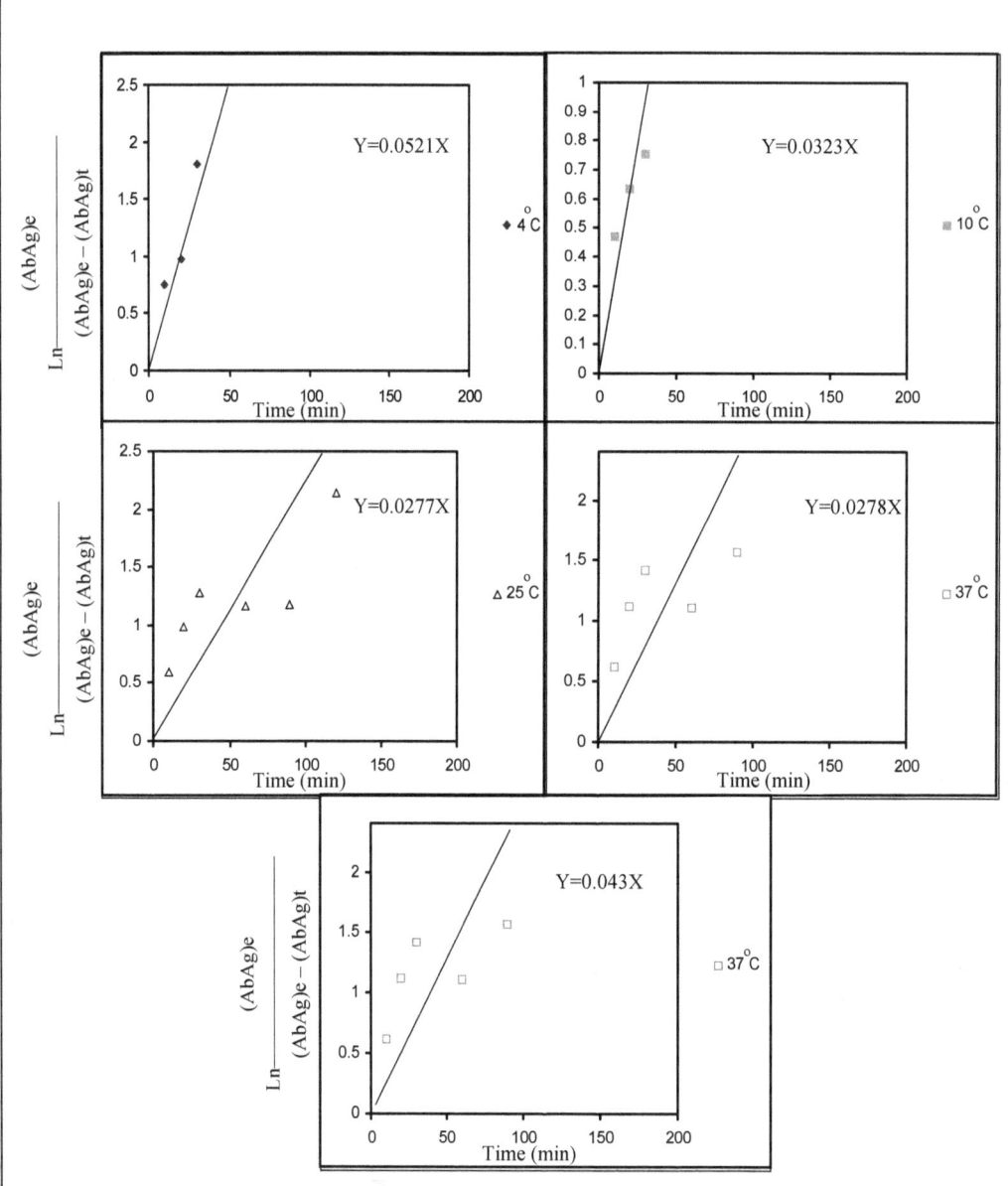

Figure (3-11): Kinetics of ^{125}I-anti hPRL antibody binding with hPRL in:
C: Premenopausal patients with malignant ovarian tumor.

The Thermodynamic Studies of hPRL Binding in Benign and Malignant Serous Ovarian Tumors Homogenate with ^{125}I-Anti hPRL Antibody

3.6.1 Thermodynamic Parameters of Standard State

Figure (3-12 A, B, &C) represents the dependence of the equilibrium binding constant (affinity constant) for the binding of ^{125}I-anti hPRL antibody with hPRL in benign and malignant serous ovarian tumors on the temperature (**Van't Hoff Plot**). The results obtained from Van't Hoff Plot revealed that ΔH° in general had small values and their positive sign ascertain that the reaction was nearly endothermic.

Table (3-7) shows the value of thermodynamic parameters of standard state of ^{125}I- anti hPRL anatibody with hPRL in benign and malignant ovarian tumor. The negative values of ΔG° reflect the stability of the complex hence, the high affinity of the reactants. So our system is characterized by the sole contribution of ΔS° to the stability of the complex formed, while ΔH° has little or no effect [130].

A high values of positive ΔS° suggest that the reaction spontaneity was entropically driven. Entropy was the driven force for the occurrence of the binding reaction. This indicates that the hydrophobic interactions played an important role in stabilizing the complex [131].

The small positive ΔH° may indicate a favorable interaction between ^{125}I- anti hPRL antibody with hPRL in benign and malignant ovarian tumor tissue. These include the non-covalent interactions which are fundamentally electrostatic in nature, such as charge-charge, charge-dipole, dipole-dipole, charge-induced dipole, dipole-induced dipole interactions and hydrogen bonds. The sum of these types of interactions can yield some stabilization to the folded structure of the complex [91].

Table (3-7): Thermodynamic parameters at standard state of ^{125}I-anti hPRL antibody binding with hPRL in benign and malignant ovarian tumors.
All details are described in section (2.6.3)

Group	Thermodynamic parameters	Temperatures (°C)				
		4	10	25	37	45
Premenopausal patients with benign ovarian tumors	ΔH° (KJ.mole^{-1})	11.083	11.083	11.083	11.083	11.083
	ΔG° (KJ.mole^{-1})	-6.899	-7.363	-7.272	-7.085	-8.185
	ΔS° (J.mole^{-1}.K^{-1})	64.916	65.178	61.593	58.604	60.589
Postmenopausal patients with benign ovarian tumors	ΔH° (KJ.mole^{-1})	13.851	13.851	13.851	13.851	13.851
	ΔG° (KJ.mole^{-1})	-8.246	-7.679	-7.502	-8.984	-8.344
	ΔS° (J.mole^{-1}.K^{-1})	79.773	76.081	71.656	73.663	69.797
Premenopausal patients with malignant ovarian tumors	ΔH° (KJ.mole^{-1})	20.785	20.785	20.785	20.785	20.785
	ΔG° (KJ.mole^{-1})	-8.024	-8.291	-8.135	-8.766	-9.489
	ΔS° (J.mole^{-1}.K^{-1})	104.003	102.74	97.047	95.326	95.203

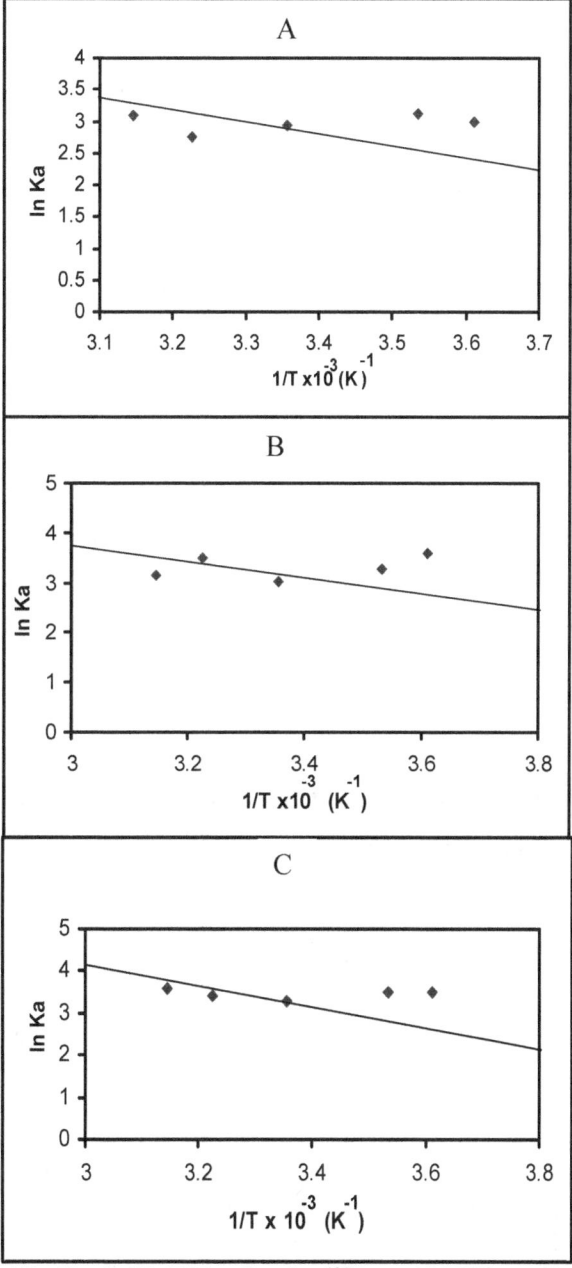

Figure (3-12): Van't Hoff Plot for the ^{125}I- anti hPRL antibody binding to hPRL in:

    A: Premenopausal patients with benign ovarian tumor.
    B: Postmenopausal patients with benign ovarian tumor.

C: Premenopausal patients with malignant ovarian tumor.
Details are described in section (2.6.3).

Thermodynamic Parameters of Transition State

The transition state theory proposes that the association of two substances to form the final product proceed through the formation of an activated complex (Transition State). Consequently, the interaction of ^{125}I-anti hPRL antibody with hPRL in benign and malignant ovarian tissue can be represented as follows: -

^{125}I-anti hPRL antibody + hPRL ⟶ [^{125}I-anti hPRL antibody/hPRL] ⟶
an activated complex
(Transition State)

^{125}I-anti hPRL antibody/hPRL
(Product)

The thermodynamic parameters of the transition state (ΔH^*, ΔG^* & ΔS^*) could be determined from **Arrhenius equation** and the Kinetic constant. Figure (3-13 A, B&C) shows the Arrhenius plots of $\ln K_{+1}$ against $1/T$ values. The slope of the straight line represents the activation energy (Ea).

Tables (3-8) and (3-9) show the values of thermodynamic parameters of the transition state(Ea*, ΔH^*, ΔG^* and ΔS^*). The high positive value of ΔG^* indicate that the formation of an activated complex was a non-spontaneous process and required a lot of energy (equal to Ea.) to overcome the transition state energy barrier and giving the final product, whereas the high negative ΔS^* revealed that the activated complex had a more order structure than the reactant species, ($\Delta S^* < 0$). The positive values of ΔG^* is mainly attributed to decrease in entropy of the transition state ($\Delta S^* < 0$). In addition, the positive value of ΔH^* shows that the heat content of the activated complex is more than that of isolated species [132].

The thermodynamic data indicate that the binding of ^{125}I-anti hPRL antibody to hPRL in benign and malignant ovarian tissue are entropy driven and in agreement with the concept that hydrophobic play an important role in (^{125}I-anti hPRL antibody/hPRL) interactions.

Table (3-8): Thermodynamic parameters at transition state of ^{125}I- anti hPRL antibody binding with hPRL in premenopausal benign and malignant serous ovarian tumors. All details are in section (2.6.3)

Group	Thermodynamic parameters	Temperatures (°C)				
		4	10	25	37	45
Premenopausal patients with benign ovarian tumors	Ea (KJ.mole^{-1})	20.785	20.785	20.785	20.785	20.785
	ΔH*(KJ.mole^{-1})	18.482	18.432	18.307	18.208	18.141
	ΔG*(KJ.mole^{-1})	56.774	56.761	61.401	63.118	67.060
	ΔS*(J.mole^{-1}.K^{-1})	-138.237	-135.439	-144.611	-144.872	-153.833
Premenopausal patients with benign ovarian tumors	Ea (KJ.mole^{-1})	27.711	27.711	27.711	27.711	27.711
	ΔH* (KJ.mole^{-1})	25.408	25.358	25.233	25.133	25.067
	ΔG* (KJ.mole^{-1})	56.818	59.359	64.891	65.397	66.1
	ΔS* (J.mole^{-1}.K^{-1})	-113.394	-120.146	-133.08	-129.884	-129.036

Table (3-9): Thermodynamic parameters at transition state of ^{125}I-anti hPRL antibody binding with hPRL in Postmenopausal benign ovarian tumors.
All details are described in section (2.6.3)

Group	Thermodynamic Parameters	Temperatures (°C)			
		10	25	37	45

Postmenopausal patients with benign ovarian tumors	Ea (KJ.mole^{-1})	24.942	24.942	24.942	24.942
	ΔH* (KJ.mole^{-1})	22.589	22.464	22.365	22.298
	ΔG* (KJ.mole^{-1})	59.448	62.129	66.511	66.969
	ΔS* (J.mole^{-1}.K^{-1})	-130.246	-133.105	-142.407	-140.473

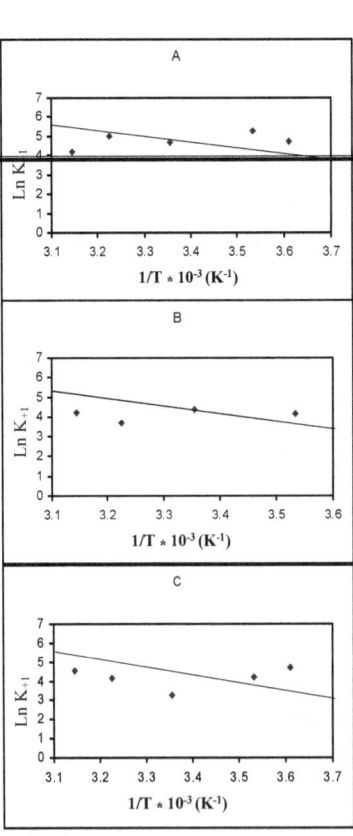

Figure (3-13): Arrhenius plots for the ^{125}I-anti hPRL antibody with PRL in:
A: Premenopausal patients with benign ovarian tumor.
B: Postmenopausal patients with benign ovarian tumor.

Isolation of (^{125}I-Anti hPRL Antibody/ hPRL) Complex of Benign and Malignant Serous Ovarian Tumors Homogenate.

Figure (3-14 A, B&C) shows the results of gel filtration technique used to separate (^{125}I-anti hPRL antibody/hPRL) complex from unbound (^{125}I-anti hPRL antibody) for benign and malignant serous ovarian tumors, respectively. In this experiment the amount of protein and radioactivity was measured for every fraction.

For premenopausal groups with benign ovarian tumors all trials of this experiment revealed two peaks of radioactivity profile, the first peak represents the complex with maximum radioactivity in fraction number (10), and the second peak represents the unbound (^{125}I-anti hPRL antibody) with maximum radioactivity in fraction number (27), while three absorbency peaks for protein content were obtained with maximum absorbency in fraction number (10, &25), for the complex, the unbound (^{125}I-anti hPRL antibody) and in fraction number (30) for a medium proteins because the homogenate was crude.

For postmenopausal groups with benign ovarian tumors all trials of this experiment revealed two peaks of radioactivity profile, the first peak represents the complex with maximum radioactivity in fraction number (10), and the second peak represents the unbound (^{125}I-anti hPRL antibody) with maximum radioactivity in fraction number (27), while two absorbency peaks for protein content were obtained with maximum absorbency in fraction number (11) for the complex and in fraction number (27) for the unbound (^{125}I-anti hPRL antibody).

For premenopausal groups with malignant ovarian tumors all trials of this experiment revealed two peaks of radioactivity profile, the first peak represents the complex with maximum radioactivity in fraction number (10) and the second peak represents the unbound (^{125}I-anti hPRL antibody) with maximum radioactivity in fraction number(25), while two absorbency peaks for protein content were obtained with maximum absorbency in fraction number (10) for the complex and in fraction number (28) for the unbound (^{125}I-anti hPRL antibody).

The isolation by gel filtration depends upon the difference of molecular weight of the compounds and because that the molecular weight of the complex is greater than of the unbound ^{125}I-anti hPRL antibody, so the results indicate that the first peak was assigned for the complex and the second was assigned for unbound (^{125}I-anti hPRL antibody). The studies demonstrate the molecular weight of the complex (182,000 Dalton).

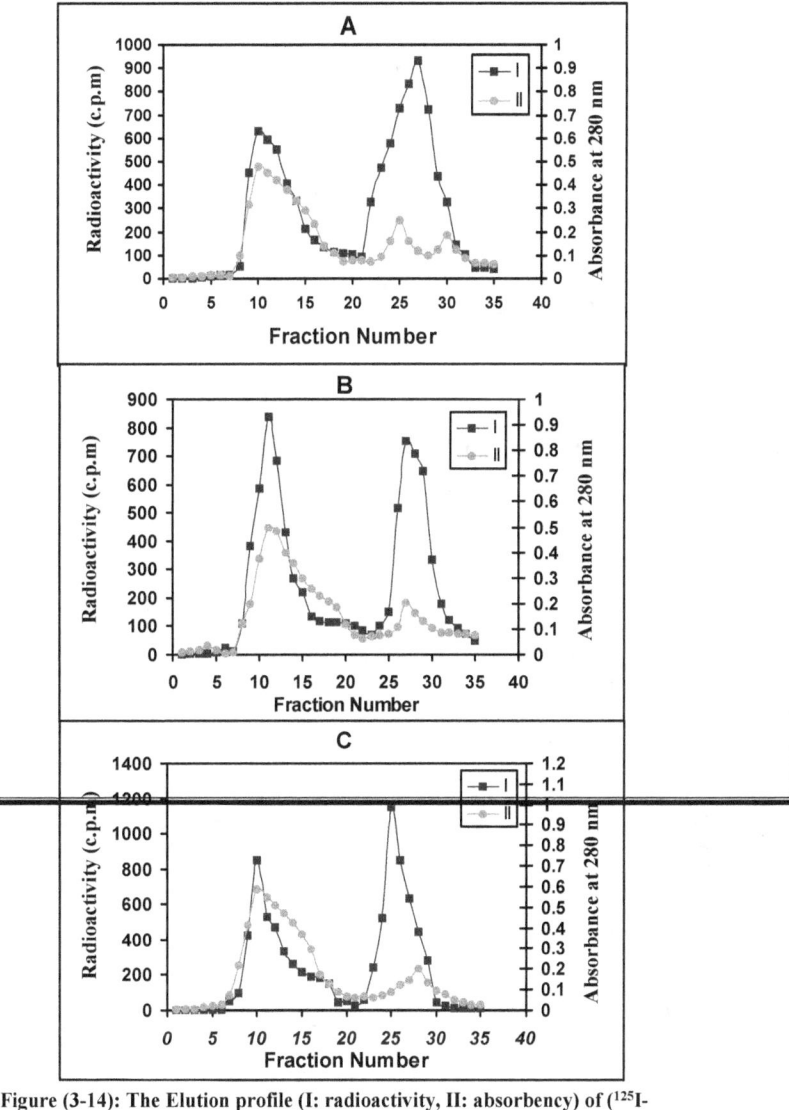

Figure (3-14): The Elution profile (I: radioactivity, II: absorbency) of (^{125}I-anti hPRL antibody) binding with PRL in:
A: Premenopausal patients with benign ovarian tumor.
B: Postmenopausal patients with benign ovarian tumor.
C: Premenopausal patients with malignant ovarian tumor.

Spectroscopic Studies On (*125I-Anti hPRL Antibody/hPRL*) Complex and the Unbound *125I-Anti hPRL antibody*.

The U.V Spectra of hPRL, 125I-Anti hPRL Antibody and 125I-Anti hPRL Antibody /hPRL) complex.

The U.V Spectrum of hPRL

Figure (3-15) illustrates the U.V spectrum of hPRL (provided by hPRL IRMA kit, DiaSorin-Italy) at pH 7.4 . The spectrum shows that the λmax for hPRL is consists of two peaks at 224.2 nm and 273.4 nm. As a result, hPRL has a characteristic spectrum and can be identified by its peaks, which are assigned to the peptide bond and tyrosine residues, respectively [133]. It seems that tyrosine residues in hPRL molecule is located in a way, that part of it is on the surface of the protein molecule while the other part is buried [134].

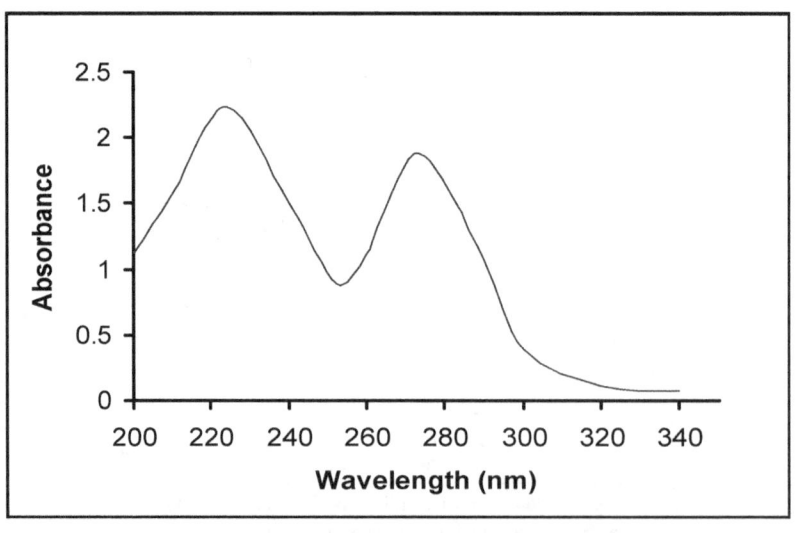

Figure (3-15): The U.V spectrum of hPRL at neutral pH.
Details are described in section (2.8.1.1)

The U.V Spectra of (^{125}I-anti hPRL antibody/hPRL) Complex and the unbound ^{125}I-Anti hPRL Antibody in Benign and Malignant Serous Ovarian Tumors.

Figure (3-16 A, B&C) illustrates U.V spectrum of (^{125}I-anti hPRL antibody/hPRL) complex and the unbound (^{125}I-anti hPRL antibody) for premenopausal patients with benign and malignant serous ovarian tumors. For benign tumors the spectrum shows that the λmax for the complex consists of two peaks at 227.2 nm and at 278.1 nm. The absorption at 227.2 nm is due to the amide group in the poly peptide bond of the protein molecule with contribution of histidyl residues, while the absorption at 278.1 nm is due to the tyrosine residues. It seems that each of tyrosyl and histidyl residues in hPRL molecule is located in way, that part of it is on the surface of the protein molecule while the other part is buried [135].

The spectrum for malignant ovarian tumors shows that the λmax for the complex consists of two peaks at 220.1 nm and at 278.5 nm and the spectrum shows that λmax for the unbound ^{125}I-anti hPRL antibody consists of one peak at 206.4 nm. As a result, the complex has a characteristic spectrum and can be identified by its peaks which are assigned to the tyrosine residues, while the unbound (^{125}I-anti hPRL antibody) can be identified by its peak which is assigned to the phenylalanine residues [134].

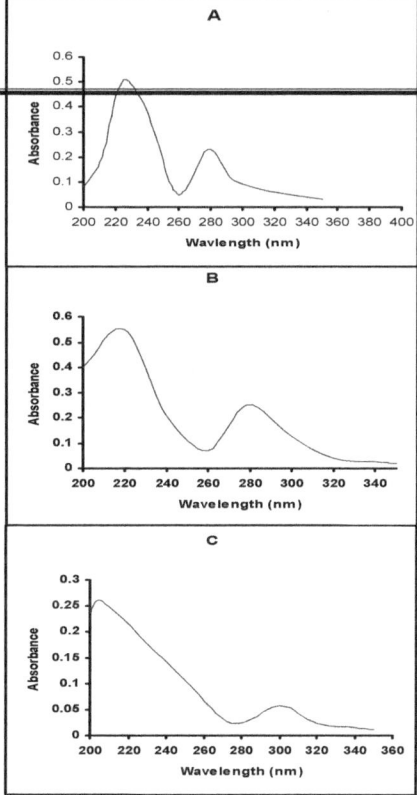

Figure (3-16): The U.V spectrum of:
A: (^{125}I-anti hPRL antibody/ hPRL) complex for premenopausal patients with benign ovarian tumor.
B: (^{125}I-anti hPRL antibody /hPRL) complex for premenopausal patients with malignant ovarian tumor.
C: Unbound (^{125}I-anti hPRL antibody)Details are described in section (2.8.1.2).

Factors Affecting the Absorption Properties of (^{125}I-Anti hPRL Antibody/hPRL) Complex and the Unbound (^{125}I-Anti hPRL Antibody) in Malignant Ovarian Tumors.

The absorption spectrum of a chromophore is primarily determined by the chemical structure of the molecule. However, a large number of environmental factors produce detectable changes in λmax and absorbance. Environment factors such as pH and polarity of the solvent provide the basis for the use of absorption spectroscopy in characterizing macromolecule [134].

pH Effects

The pH of the solvent determines the ionization state of ionizable chromophore in the protein molecule [134]. Table (3-10) shows the λmax values of (^{125}I-anti hPRL antibody/hPRL) and unbound ^{125}I-anti hPRL antibody, respectivily, at different pH (4, 7.4 & 12).

When the pH value of (^{125}I-anti hPRl antibody/hPRL) complex and the unbound (^{125}I-anti hPRL antibody) were increased from (4- 7.4) the $λmax_1$, was increased from (210.2 nm to 220.1 nm) for the complex and from (203.6 nm to 206.4 nm) for the unbound (^{125}I-anti hPRL antibody), so that $λmax_2$ was increased from (276.0 nm to 278.5 nm) for the complex (^{125}I-anti hPRL antibody/hPRL) while there is no another λmax for the unbound (^{125}I-anti hPRL antibody). Further increase in pH to 12.0 has shown an increase in both $λmax_1$, $λmax_2$ and the absorency for the complex and the unbound (^{125}I-anti hPRL antibody), the change in $λmax_1$ of the polypeptide bond could be due to a conformation change in the protein while the increase in $λmax_2$ is due to the dissociation of the phenolic OH of the tyrosine (pKa 10.07).

The spectral shifts of proteins produced by pH cannot be simply attributed to the inductive effects of vicinal charges, such spectral changes must therefore be attributed mainly to rearrangement of secondary and tertiary structure, although the possibility of field effects due to unusually close conjunction of charges to aromatic groups is not excluded [136].

Table (3-10): The pH effect on λmax of (^{125}I-anti hPRL antibody /hPRL)complex and the unbound (^{125}I-anti hPRL antibody). Details are described in section (2.8.2.1).

pH	(^{125}I-anti hPRL antibody /hPRL) complex		(^{125}I-anti hPRL antibody)	
	λmax_1 (nm)	λmax_2 (nm)	λmax_1 (nm)	λmax_2 (nm)
4.0	210.2	276.0	203.6	-----
7.4	220.1	278.5	206.4	-----
12.0	227.8	281.6	216.0	-----

The Effect of Solvent Polarity

The importance of this study comes from studying of the internal configuration of protein [137].

- **The Effect of 20 % Methanol**

Table (3-11) shows the effect of 20 % methanol at pH 7.4 on the (^{125}I-anti hPRL antibody /hPRL) complex and the unbound (^{125}I-anti hPRL antibody) U.V spectrum. The data obtained show that λmax for the complex at PH 7.4 (λmax_1= 220.1 nm and λmax_2 = 278.5 nm) while λmax for the unbound ^{125}I-anti hPRL antibody at the same pH (λmax_1= 206.4 nm shown in previous experiments). The presence of 20 % methanol showed a decrease in λmax_1 from 220.1 nm to 218.8 nm while λmax_2 increased from 278.5 nm to 280.0 nm for the (^{125}I-anti hPRL antibody /hPRL) complex, and the λmax for the unbound (^{125}I-anti hPRL antibody) increased from 206.4 nm to 210 nm . The values of λmax 218.8 nm and 280.0 nm are assigned to tryptophane residues, while 210 nm is referred to histidine residues.

The appearance of new λmax values indicates that the protein was folded to change in the secondary and tertiary structure of the protein that bring the histidine and tryptophane to expose to absorbence [134].

- **The Effect of 20% Glycerol**

    Table (3-11) shows the λmax values of (^{125}I-anti hPRL antibody /hPRL) complex and the unbound (^{125}I-anti hPRL antibody) at PH 7.4 . The presence of 20 % glycerol shows a decrease in λmax_1 from 220.1 nm to 218.2 nm while λmax_2 remained constant (278.5 nm) for the (^{125}I-anti hPRL antibody /hPRL)complex , and the λmax for the unbound (^{125}I-anti hPRL antibody) increased from 206.4 nm to 217.6 nm . The values of λmax (218.2 and 217.6 nm) are assigned to tryptophane and tyrosine risdues. According to these results the λmax is rather shifted toward longer wavelength (red shift), 206.4 nm 217.6 nm . This shift is due to the $\pi \longrightarrow \pi^*$ transition of the benzene ring . On the other hand, the shift toward shorter wavelength (blue shift), 220.1 to 218.2 nm is due to the $n \longrightarrow \pi^*$ transitions [137].

-
- **The Effect of 20 % Polyethylene glycol-6000**

    Table (3-11) shows the effect of 20 % polyethylene glycol (PEG) at pH 7.4 on the (^{125}I-anti hPRL antibody /hPRL)complex and the unbound (^{125}I-anti hPRL antibody) spectra. The presence of 20 % polyethylene glycol has shown decrease in λmax_1 from 220.1 nm to 216.2 nm while λmax_2 remained constant (278.5 nm)for the (^{125}I-anti hPRL antibody /hPRL)complex, and the λmax for the unbound (^{125}I-anti hPRL antibody) increased from 206.4 nm to 219 nm . These values of λmax 216.2 nm and 219 nm are assigned to tyrosine and tryptophane respectively. According to these results , the λmax is rather shifted toward longer wavelength (red shift), 206.4 nm to 219 nm . This shift is due to the π   π* transition of the aromatic ring of tyrosine , on the other hand , the shift toward shorter wavelength (blue shift) , 220.1 nm to 216.2 nm is due to the n   π* transitions[138].

- ### The Effect of 20 % chloroform
  Table (3-11) shows the effect of 20 %chloroform at pH 7.4 on the (^{125}I-anti hPRL antibody /hPRL) complex and the unbound (^{125}I-anti hPRL antibody) spectra. The presence of 20 % chloroform shows an increase in λmax_1 from 220.1 nm to 222.2 nm while λmax_2 decreased from 278.5 nm to 274 nm for the complex, and the λmax for the unbound (^{125}I-anti hPRL antibody) increased from 206.4 nm to 224.8 nm . The vlues of λmax 222.2 nm, 274 nm and 224.8 are assigned to tyrosine residues. According to these results, the λmax is rather shifted toward longer wavelength (red shift), (220.1 to 222.2 nm) and (206.4nm to 224.8 nm). This shift is due to the π   π* transition of the aromatic ring of tyrosyl residue. On the other hand, the shift toward shorter wavelength (blue shift), 278.5 nm to 274.0 nm is due to the the n   π* transitions[138].

- ### The Effect of 20 % Urea
  Table (3-11) shows the λmax values of (^{125}I-anti hPRL antibody /hPRL) complex and the unbound (^{125}I-anti hPRL antibody) at PH 7.4 . The presence of 20 % urea shows an increase in λmax_1 from 220.1 nm to 221.9 nm while λmax_2 decrease from 278.5 nm to 273.6 nm for the (^{125}I-anti hPRL antibody

/hPRL) complex and the λmax for the unbound (^{125}I-anti hPRL antibody) remained constant (206.4 nm). The value of λmax 221.9 nm and 273.6 nm are assigned to tyrosine residues. This shift (red shift) is due to the $\pi \longrightarrow \pi^*$ transition of the aromatic ring of tyrosine, while the blue shift is due to n $\longrightarrow \pi^*$ transitions.

- **The Effect of 20 % KCl**

Table (3-11) shows the effect of 20 % KCl at pH 7.4 on the (^{125}I-anti hPRL antibody/hPRL) complex and the unbound (^{125}I-anti hPRL antibody) U.V spectrum. The presence of 20% KCl shows a decrease in λ max$_1$ from 220.1 nm to 209.6 nm while λmax$_2$ increased from 278.5 nm to 291.6 nm, for the complex(^{125}I-anti hPRL antibody/hPRL), and the λmax$_1$ for the unbound (^{125}I-anti hPRL antibody) increased from 206.4 nm to 214.6 nm. Also a new λmax at 294.8 nm was obtained in 20 % KCl. The values of λmax 209.6 nm is refereed to phenylalanine residues, and 214.6 nm, 294.8 nm are assigned to tyrosine residues while 291.6 nm is referred to tryptophane residues.

The appearance of new chromophore indicates that the protein was folded due to the presence of KCl at this concentration. When 20 % KCl was used, there was significant red shift (206.4 nm to 214.6 nm) and (278.5 to 291.6 nm) this shift is due to the $\pi \longrightarrow \pi^*$ transition of the aromatic ring of tyrosyl residue. Also the blue shift 220.1 nm to 209.6 nm is due to the n π^* transitions. Such a blue or a red shift can a rise by introducing positive(K^+) or negative (Cl^-) charges near the chromophore (the amide group) which might interact directly with the π electron system of the amide group [137].

Table (3-11):The effect of polarity on the λ max of (^{125}I-anti hPRLantibody/ hPRL) complex and the unbound (^{125}I-anti hPRLantibody) . Details are described in section 2.8.2.2

Solvent	(^{125}I-anti hPRL antibody / hPRL) Complex λ max (nm)	(^{125}I-anti hPRL antibody) λ max (nm)
20% Methanol	218.8 , 280.0	210.0
20% Glycerol	218.2 , 278.5	217.6
20% Polyethylene glycol	216.2 , 278.5	219.0
20% Chloroform	222.2 , 274.0	224.8
20% Urea	221.9 , 273.6	206.4
20% KCl	209.6 , 291.6	214.6 , 294.8

Spectrophotometric Titration of (^{125}I-Anti hPRL Antibody /hPRL) complex and the Unbound (^{125}I-Anti hPRL Antibody) in Malignant Ovarian Tumor Homogenate

Spectrophotometric titration is the following of the change in absorbency of the chromophore with increasing pH [134]. Many studies of protein structure require the determination of pKa values for proton dissociation from ionizable amino acid side chains, because these values give an indication of the location of the amino acid in the protein. This can often be done spectrophotometrically because dissociation often changes the spectrum of one of the chromophore, the observation of tyrosine dissociation was performed by measuring the absorption at 295 nm (λmax for the ionized form of tyrosine), and the observation of histidine dissociation was carried out by measuring the absorption at 211 nm.

Figure (3-17 A&B) shows the titration curve of (^{125}I-anti hPRL antibody /hPRL) complex and the unbound (^{125}I-anti hPRL antibody). Curve (A) shows that the pKa for tyrosine is (10.2) for the complex (^{125}I-anti hPRL antibody / hPRL) and (9.1) for the unbound (^{125}I-anti hPRL antibody), while the pKa for histidine is (6.2) for the complex (^{125}I-anti hPRL antibody /hPRL) and (5.1) for the unbound (^{125}I-anti hPRL antibody), these results are shown in curve (B).

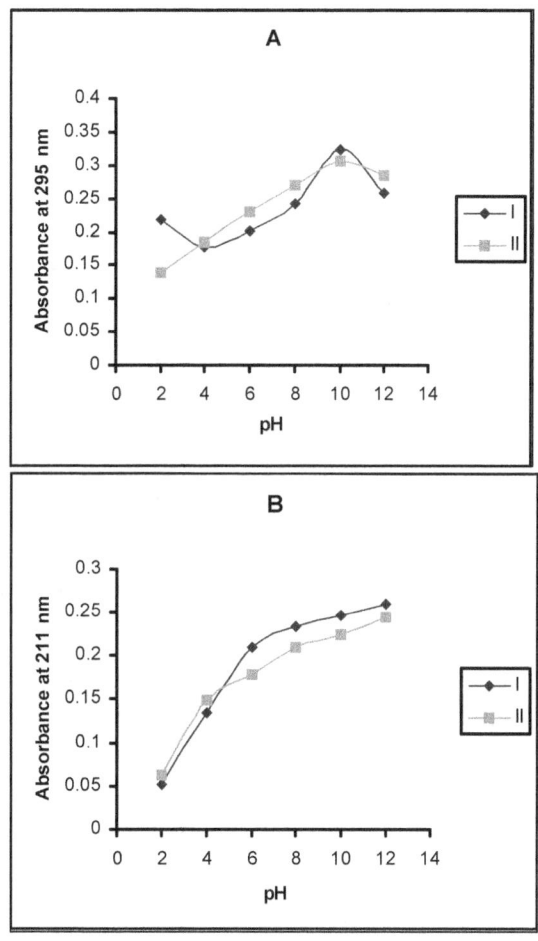

Figure (3-17): Spectrophotometric titration of I:[^{125}I-anti hPRL antibody/hPRL]complex, II:[^{125}I-anti hPRL antibody] at two wavelengths.
A: 295 nm for tyrosine residues.
B: 211 nm for histidine.

Details are described in section (2.8.3).

References

1- L.Carlos Junqueiva, Jose Carneiro, Robert O. Kelley. ***Basic Histology***. 8 th. ed. Lange medical book. 1995, PP. 423-425.

2- Balint Kacsoh. ***Endocrine Physiology***. The McGraw-Hill companies. 2000 , P.503.

3- Jean D.Wilson, Daniel W.Foster, Henry M. Kronenbry , P.Reed Larsen. ***Williams Text Book of Endocrinology***. 9th.ed.W.B. Saunders Company. 1998, PP.193, 210,211,288-289, 757-771.

4- K.S.Clifford Chao, Carlos A. Pere Z, luther W.Brady. ***Radiation Oncology Management Decisions***. Lippincott-Raven Publishers. 1999, P.515.

5- Ivan Damjanov, James Linder. ***Anderson's Pathology***. 10th.ed. Mosby-Year book. 1996, P.2278.

6- Zhang S.X. ***An Atlas of Histology***. Springer-Verlag, Inc.1998, P.298.

7- Francis S. Greenspan, David G.Gardner. ***Basic and Clinical Endocrinology***. 6th.ed. The McGraw-Hill. 2001, PP.453,460-461.

8- Robert G. Edwards, Fiona Bennett. ***Reproductive BioMedicine Online***.2001; 2:194.

9- Geoff Barnard, and fortune Kohen. ***Clinical Chemistry***.1998;44:1520.

10- William Jubiz. ***Endocrinology: A Logical Approach for Clinicians***. 2nd.ed. McGraw-Hill book company. 1987, P.436.

11- Arthur C. Guyton, John E.Hall. ***Text book of Medical Physiology***. 9th.ed. W.B.Saunders company. 1996 ,PP.1017-1022.

12- William F. Ganong. ***Review of Medical Physiology***. 17th.ed. Appleton and Lange. 1995,pp.389-390, 399.

13- Treloar AE , Boynton BE , Behn BG. ***Int. J. Fertil***. 1967; 12:77-126.

14- Rod R. Seeley, Trent D. Stephens, Philip Tate. ***Essentials of Anatomy And Physiology***. 4th.ed.McGraw-Hill book company. 1998,PP.528, 935-942.

15- Murray R. K., Granner D. K., Mayes P. A., Rodwell V. W., ***Harper's Biochemistry***. 25th.ed. Appleton and Lange.2000, pp.552, 603-604.

16- Groon MP, ***J.Clin. Endocrinol.Metab***.1996;81:1401-1405

17- Gore-Langton RE, Armstrong DT. ***The Physiology of Reproduction***. 2th.ed. NewYork .1994,pp.516-628.

18- Michael L.Bishop, Janet L., Edward P. Fody. ***Clinical Chemistry***. 4th.ed.Lippincott Williams and Wilkins.2000,pp.375-392.

19- Lipsett M., Jaffe RB. ***Pathophysiology and Clinical Management***. 2nd.ed.WB Saunders company.1986, pp.140-153.

20- Margaret A. Shupnik. ***Gene Engineering in Endocrinology***. Human Press Inc. 2000, p.239.

21- Richard C. Tilton, Albert Balows, David C. Hohnadel, Robert F. Reiss. ***Clinical Laboratory Medicine***. Mosby-year book. 1992, p.285.

22- Lawrence M. Tierney, Stephen J. Mcphee, Maxine A. Papadakis. ***Current Medical Diagnosis and Treatment***. McGraw-Hill Companies. 2001, p.746.

23- Vincent T. Devita, Samuel Hellman ,Steven A. ***Cancer Principles and Practice of Oncology***. 5th.ed. Lippincott-Raven. 1997, pp. 1502-1507, 1514.

24- Parker SL, Tong T, Bolden S, Wingo PA. ***Cancer Statistics***. 1996;46:5.

25- James Homer. ***The Lancet***. 2000; 355:1028.

26- Leonard L. Gunderson, Joel E. Tepper. ***Clinical Radiation Oncology***. Churchill Livingstone. 2000, pp.940-944.

27- Scully RE. *Int. J. Gynecol. Obstet*. 1995;49:9-15.

28- Powell DE, Puls L,Van Nagell J. *Hum Path*.1992;23:46-47.

29- Poels LE. Powell De, De Priest PD. *Gynecol. Oncol*. 1992;47:53-57.

30- Walter H. Gotlieb, Ben Davidson, Yaacov Korach. *Int.J.Cancer*. 1998;82:141.

31- Smita Jain, Chien Sheng Tsai. *J. Reprod.Med*.2001;46:267.

32- Michael Peckham, Herbert Pinedo, Umberto Veronesi. *Oxford Text Book of Oncology*. Oxford University Press Inc. 1995,pp.1294,1298.

33- Kirby I. Bland, John M. Daly, Constantine P. Karakousis. *Surgical Oncology*. McGraw-Hill companies. 2001,pp.911-915, 920, 926-928.

34- Nelson Fausto, Steven L. Kunkel, Henry Carter, Tamara Carlson. *Am.J.Pathol*.1999; 154:119.

35- Jan P. Neijt. *N. Engl.J.Med*.1996; 334:50.

36- Hal W. Hirte, Jutta S. Kaiser, Silvia Bacchetti. *Int.J.Cancer*. 1994;74:900.

37- Raghavan, M.L Brecher, D.H.Johnson, N.J.Meropol, P.L.Moots, J.T. Thigpen. *Text Book of Uncommon Cancer*. 2th.ed. John Wiley and Son Inc.1999,p.653.

38- Yancik R, Ries LG, Yates JW.*Am.J.Obstet. Gynecol*. 1998;154:639.

39- Greene MH, Clark JW, Blayney DW. *Semin.Oncol*. 1984; 11:209.

40- Casagrande JT. *Lancet*. 1979; 2:170.

41- Roberta. B. Ness, Jeane Ann Grisso, Jennifer Klapper, Ron Vergona,Mark Morgan, James E. Wheeler. *Am.J.Epidemiol*. 2000; 152:233.

42- Bewtra Cetal. *Int. J. Gynecol. Pathol*. 1992; 11:180.

43- Tbomas S. Frank. *Cancer Control*.1999; 6:327.

44- JJ Nieto, KJ Rolfe, AB Maclean, P Hardiman. *Lancet*.1999;354:649.

45- Joellen M. SchildKraut, N.Keith Collins, J. Allen Tucker, J. Carl Barrett, *Am. J. Obstet. Gynecol*.1995; 172:912.

46- J.E. Roulston, R.F.Leonard, K.D.Bagshawe. ***Serological Tumor Markers***. Langman singapora. 1993,pp.60-61.

47- Jane Bradbury.*Lancet*.2000; 356:1826.

48- James F. Holland, Robert C. Bast, Donald L.,Emill Frei, Donald W. Kufe, Ralph R. Weichselbaum. ***Cancer Medicine***. 4th.ed.Williams and Wilkins a waverly company. 1997,p.284.

49- Daniel L. Clark-Pearson, M. Yousif Dawood. ***Green's Gynecology: Essentials of Clinical Practice***. 4th.ed. Little, Brown and company .1990,pp.531-541.

50- Gerardo Zanetta, Cristina Bonazzi, Maria Grazia, Sergio Bini, Anna Locatelli, Giorgio Bratino, Costantino Mangioni. *J. Clin. Oncol*. 2001; 19:1015.

51- Pollock R.E. ***Manual of Clinical Oncology***. 7th.ed.Wiley-liss, Inc.1999, p.542.

52- Yanick R.*Cancer*.1993; 71:517.

53- Young RC. *N.Engl.J.Med*. 1990; 332:1021.

54- Mskoto Emoto, Hiroshi Lwasaki, Kumi Mimura, Tatsuhiko Kawara bayashi, Masahiro Kikuchi. *Int. J. Cancer*.1997; 80:899.

55- Fritshe A.A., Bast R.C. *Clinical Chemistry*. 1998; 44:1379.

56- Rubin S., Hoskins W., Halces T. *Am.J.Obstet.Gynecol*. 1989; 160:667.

57- Franco Causio, Rita Fischetto, Teresa Leonetti, Luca Marea Schonauer. *J. Repred.Med*. 2000; 45:236.

58- L. Kovacs, E. Toldy, M. Wenczl. *Clinical Chemistry*. 2001; 47:124.

59- Burtis C.A., Ahwood. ***Tietz Text book of Clinical Chemistry***. 3th.ed. Philadelphia W.B. Saunders company. 1999,pp.722-747.

60- Jacobs, Bast R. C., ***Hum Reprod*** .1989; 4:1-12.

61- Gordon J.S. Rustin, Ann E. Nelstrop, Soren M. Bentzen, Simon J. Bond. *J. Clin.Oncol*. 2000; 18:1733.

62- Jonathan S Berek. *Lancer* .2000; 365:6.

63- Rosenoff SH, DeVita VT, Hubbard S. *Semin. Oncol*.1975; 61:1537-1560.

64- Trimbos JB. *Gynecol.Oncol*. 1990; 37:374.

65- Toshiki Lwasaka, Shinbu Umemura, Kochi Kakimoto, Harudo Kozumi. *Journal of Histochemistry and Cytochemistry*. 2000;48:389.

66- Charles C.J.Carpenter, Robert C. Griggs, Josehp Loscalzo, *Cecil Essentials of Medicine*. 5th.ed. W.B.Saunders Company .2001, pp.547-556.

67- C.R.Kannan. *Essential Endocrinology*. Plenum Publishing Corporation. 1998,pp.28-61.

68- Carl A. Burtis, Edward R. Ashwood. *Tietz Text book of Clinical Chemistry*. 2th.ed. W.B.Saunders Company. 1994,pp.1672-1674.

69- Neill JD, Martini L, Ganong WF. *Frontiers in Neuroendocrinology*. New York. 1980,pp.129-155.

70- Senogles SE. *J.Endocrinology*. 1994; 134:783-789.

71- M. Pawlikowski, J kunert-Radek. *J.Endocrin*. 1996; 148:193.

72- A Lafuente, J Marco, Esquifino. *J. Endocrin*.1994; 142:581.

73- Sinha YN. Gilligan TA. **J. Clin. Endocrinol. Metab**. 1984; 58:752-754.

74- Li C.H. *Chemistry of Ovine Prolactin In: Hand Book of Physiology*. Am. Physiological Soc. 1974,p.103.

75- Li C.H. *Hormonal Proteins and Peptides: Growth hormone and related proteins*. Academic Press. 1977,p.61.

76- David Horrobin. *Prolactin: Effects and Clinical Significance*. Eden Press Inc. 1978,pp.21,40,56.

77- Vermeulen A, Sug E, Rubens R. *J.Clin. Endocrinol. Metab*. 1977; 44:989-1222.

78- Posner BI. *J. Endocrinol*. 1976; 99:1168.

79- Sasakai N., Tanaka Y., Mai Y., Tushima T., Matsuzaki F. *J.Biochem.* 1982; 203:653.

80- Herrington, veith. *J.Endocrinol.* 1977; 101:984.

81- Marja T.Nevalainen, Eeva M.Valve, Patricia M. Ingleton, Paula M. Martikainen. *J.Clin.Invest.* 1997; 99:618.

82- Sinha, Y.N. *Endocrinol. Rev.*1995; 16:354-369.

83- Wilson, J.D. *Am. J. Med.* 1980; 68:745-756.

84- Sissom, J.F., M.L.Eigenbrodt, J.C. Porter. *Am.J. Pathol.* 1988; 133:589-595.

85- Nakamura, T. Shirai, K. Ogawa, S. Wada, N.A. Fujimoto. *Cancer.* 1990; 53:151-157.

86- Costello, R.B. Franklin. *The Prostate.* 1994; 24:162-166.

87- Perez-Villamil. E. Bordiu, M. Puente Cueva. *J. Endocrinol.* 1991; 132:449-459.

88- Prins. *Endocrinology.* 1987; 120:1457-1464.

89- Thomas, M. Manadhar. *J. Endocrinol.* 1975; 65:149-150.

90- Mc Nelly A.S. *J. Reprod. Fert.* 1980; 58:537.

91- Al-Khayat T.H.A., *"Molecullar Characterization of Prolactin Receptors in Human Prostate"*. Ph.D. thesis suspervised by Al-Mudhaffar, S.A., Collage of Science, Baghdad University. (1991), pp.13, 23-24.

92- Franchimont P, Dourcy C, Legros JJ, Reuter A, Van Cauwenberge. *Clin.Endocrinol.* 1976; 5:673.

93- Hiroshi Nagasawa, *Prolactin and Lesions in Breast, Uterus and Prostate*. Todyo, CRC Press, Inc. 1989,p.109.

94- Patrick Schmit, Jean Thix, Jean-Paul Hoffman, and Rene-Louis Humbel. *J. Clin. Chem.* 2001; 47:331.

95- Michael Fahie-Wilson, Penelope Brunsden, John Surrey, Anthony Everitt. *J.Clin.Chem.*2000; 46:1993.

96- Cavaco B, LeiteV, Santos MA, Arranhado E. *J. Clin.Endocrinol. Metab*. 1995; 80:2342.

97- Singh, R.J., O kane. *J.Clin.Chem*. 1999; 45:95.

98- Heaney, I. Laing, Lwalton, MW Seif, Beard Well, Davis. *Lancet*. 1999; 353:720.

99- Philip Rubin, Jacqueline P. Williams. *Clinical Oncology*. 8th.ed.W.B.Saunders company.2001,p.661.

100- Christopher Haslett. Edwin R. Chilvers, John A. A. Hunter, Nicholos A. Boon. *Davidson's:Principles and Practice of Medicine*. 18th.ed.Harcourt Brace and company. 1999,p.551.

101- Alby J.D., Fernandez H., Gervaise A., frydman R. *Hum.Reprod*. 2000; 15:14.

102- Frands replies, *N. Engl. J. Med*.1996; 334:668.

103- Sonya Kashyap, Paul Claman. *J.Reprod. Med*.2000; 45:991.

104- RI-Cheng Chian, Wiliam M. Buckett, Seang-Lin Tan. *N. Engl. J. Med*. 1999; 341:1624.

105- Lakhani K., Tai N., Seifalian A., Hardiman P. *Hum. Reprod*. 2001; 16:213.

106- Bahn R.C., Bates R.W. *J.Clin.Endocrinol. Metab*. 1956; 16:1337.

107- Mary C. Martin, Jon E.Block, Sarah D. Sanchez, Claude D.Arnaud. *Am. J. Obstet. Gynecol*. 1993; 168:1840.

108- Rosalyn S. Yalow. *Methods in Radioimmunoassay of Peptide Hormones*. North-Holland Publishing company. 1976,p.126.

109- M.Wallis, S.L.Howell, K.W.Taylor. *The Biochemistry of the Polypeptide Hormones*. John Wiley and Sons Inc.1985, pp.29-36.

110- Abraham G.E. *Handbook of Radioimmunoassay*. 2th.ed.Marcel Dekker. Inc. New Yourk. 1977, pp. 179-208.

111- Rillema J. A. *Fed. Proc*. 1980; 29:2893.

112- Lutz Bernbaumer, Bert W.O' Malley. *Methods In Enzymology: Hormone Action*. Academic Press, Inc. 1985,pp.156-164.

113- Al-Said H., "*Molecullar Characterization of ^{125}I-FSH Receptors in Prostatic Tumors*" M.Sc. Thesis Collage of Science University of Baghdad. 1995,p.41.

114- Lowry O.H., Rosebrough N.J, Farr A.L., *J.Biol.Chem*. 1951; 93:265.

115- Scatchard G., *Ann NY Acad. Sci*. 1949; 51:660.

116- Chamberlain J., Jargarinec N. and Ofner P., *J.Biochem*. 1966; 99:610.

117- Thompson S.A., Johnson M.P., Brook S.C., *The Prostate*. 1982;3:45

118- keenan E.J., Kem E.D., Ramsy E.F., et al. *J.Urol*. 1966;99:610.

119- Jha. P, Faroog. A, Agarwal. N, Buckshee.K. *Int. J. Gynecol. Obstet*. 1991; 36:8-33.

120- Brinkinshaw M. and Falconer I.R., *J. Endocrinol*. 1977; 55:323.

121- Shiu P.R.C and Friesen H.G., *J.Biochem*. 1974;140:310

122- Haro L.S. and Talaments F. G., **Mol. Cell. Endocrinol**. 1985; 43:199.

123- Daxembichler G., Grill H.J., Wittliff J.L., Dapunt O., *Multiple Molecular Forms of Steroid Hormone Receptors*. A garwal M.K. editor, Elsevier, North Holland Biomedical Press. 1977,p. 163.

124- Sairam, M.R. and Li, C.H. *Hormonal Proteins And Peptides*, Vol.6. Academic Press, New York. 1978,pp.1-56.

125- Williams, E.P. *Fundemental Immunology*. 4th.ed. Philpadelphia, Lippincott. Raven. 1998,pp.75-110.

126- Leach, S.J. *physical Principles and Techniques of Protein Chemistry*. New York, Academic Press. Part B, 1970,pp.365-427.

127- Sakai S., J.Diary. *Science*. 1994 ; 77:433-438

128- Cumningham, Bass. S, Wells. J.A. *Science*. 1990; 250:1709-1712.

129- Weiland G.A. and Molinoff P.B. *Life Science*; 1981; 29:314.

130- Nemethy G and Scheraga H.A. *J.Phys.Chem*.1962; 66:1773.

131- Walebroeck M., Van Obberghen E. DeMeyts P. *J. Biol. Chem.* 1979; 254:7736.

132- Ross P.D. and Subramanian S. *Biochemistry*. 1981; 20:3096.

133- Devlin T.M. ***Textbook of Biochemistry with Clinical Correlation***. 2th.ed. John Wiley and Sons, Inc. 1986,p.66.

134- Freifelder, D. ***Physical Biochemistry: Application to Biochemistry and Molecular Biology***. 2th.ed. Freeman and Company.1982, pp.500-512.

135- Leach, S.J. ***Physical Principles and Techniques of Protein Chemistry***. New York, Academic press. Part A,1969, pp.102-170.

136- Yanari S. and Bovey. F.A. *J. Biol. Chem.* 1960; 235:2818-2825.

137- Leach S.J. and Scheraga H.A. *J. Biol. Chem.*1960; 235:2827.

138- Silvestien, R.M., Bassler, G.C., Morril, T.C. ***Spectrophotometric Identification of Organic Compounds***. New York, John Wiley and Sons. 1981,pp.25-331.

www.ingramcontent.com/pod-product-compliance
Lightning Source LLC
Chambersburg PA
CBHW062211220526
45471CB00009B/3163